Thirst and Sodium Appetite

Thirst and Sodium Appetite
Physiological Basis

Sebastian P. Grossman

Department of Psychology
University of Chicago
Chicago, Illinois

ACADEMIC PRESS, INC.
Harcourt Brace Jovanovich, Publishers
San Diego   New York   Boston
London   Sydney   Tokyo   Toronto

Academic Press, Inc.
San Diego, California 92101

United Kingdom Edition published by
Academic Press Limited
24–28 Oval Road, London NW1 7DX

Library of Congress Cataloging-in-Publication Data

Grossman, Sebastian Peter.
    Thirst and sodium appetite : physiological basis / Sebastian P.
Grossman.
        p.   cm.
    Includes bibliographical references.
    ISBN   0-12-304300-X   (alk. paper)
    1. Thirst--Physiological aspects. 2. Water-electrolyte balance
(Physiology) 3. Sodium--Metabolism. I. Title.
    [DNLM: 1. Thirst--physiology. 2. Sodium--physiology.   WI 102
G878t]
    QP139.G76   1990
    612.3'91--dc20
    DNLM/DLC
    for Library of Congress   89-18107
                                                                   CIP

Printed in the United States of America
90 91 92 93   9 8 7 6 5 4 3 2 1

Contents

10 Sodium Appetite

11 Retrospect and Prospect

Preface

Research on the physiological basis of thirst and sodium appetite has been the subject of explosive growth in the last decade. When Fitzsimons (1979) reviewed the field in the late 1970s he commented on the arduous task of keeping the manuscript for his monograph up-to-date and suggested that it might be no more than an interim account. The extraordinarily rapid progress in this field during the past decade has supported Fitzsimons' prophetic vision and required another review after little more than a decade. The information explosion in the past ten to fifteen years unfortunately also made it necessary to depart from the style of Fitzsimons' monograph, which presented extensive detail on a large number of experiments. Instead, I have provided extensive bibliographic documentation to give the reader access to the primary literature.

Not only has there been a general explosion of information about the physiological, endocrinological, and pharmacological mechanisms that influence water intake, but the emphasis of contemporary concerns has shifted significantly. Where Fitzsimons did not find it necessary to include a chapter on brain mechanisms in his extensive monograph, the 1980s have produced such a plethora of information on the subject that I found it necessary to devote a significant portion (three chapters) of the present work to it.

The general organization of this book is designed to take the reader from a basic description of the phenomenon of thirst to an analysis of the basic physiological mechanisms that determine the need for water (the distribution and exchange of water between cellular and extracellular compartments and the depletion that occurs during periods of water deprivation). Much of this is classic physiology, although significant developments have occurred in recent years. Next, there is a discussion of the various experimental paradigms that have led to the dual-depletion theory of thirst which states, in essence, that water deprivation results in the loss of fluid from both cellular and extracellular compartments. Both result in the sensations we identify as "thirst" but quite different neural and hormonal mechanisms are involved in transmitting cellular and extracellular thirst signals to the brain. The distinction between cellular and extracellular thirst also applies when one considers satiety signals that terminate drinking. The former requires only the ingestion of water, the latter is slaked only when both salt and water are available.

The next three chapters deal with the neuroanatomical, neuroendocrinological, and neuropharmacological brain mechanisms that respond to various peripheral signals to give rise to the sensation of thirst. As I have already suggested, this is the area that has experienced the most extensive and fundamental developments in the last decade. Last, but not least, there is a chapter which attempts to do for sodium appetite what the preceding chapters have done for thirst. Although the relevant literature is far less extensive, there have been major recent advances in our understanding of the role of sodium appetite in extracellular thirst and the neural and hormonal mechanisms which mediate it. The final chapter presents a brief retrospective review of the principal questions that have occupied investigators in this field and the direction future research may take.

Sebastian P. Grossman

Chapter 1

The Nature of Thirst

Introduction

Life evolved in the sea, and the basic component of all living organisms, the cell, still contains a mixture of water and salts that is, in many respects, similar to seawater. In many marine animals, there is a continuous and automatic exchange between the environment and the intracellular fluids. In others, seawater is reflexly ingested and excess salt automatically excreted.

In the course of evolution, some ocean dwellers began to enter into rivers and lakes that contained water but not sufficient concentrations of the salts found in the oceans. To live in these environments marine organisms developed mechanisms that promote the retention of electrolytes, reduce the influx of water, and facilitate its excretion.

Eventually, life ventured onto dry land where water is often a scarce commodity. In such an environment, water and salts are continually lost because of evaporation and the need to excrete products of essential metabolic processes. In complex terrestrial vertebrates such as humans, this involves evaporation from the skin and lungs, secretion by sweat glands, and excretion of urine and feces (Fig. 1.1).

This water loss is obligatory because it is essential for temperature regulation and the removal of potentially toxic metabolic waste products. In an average adult human, who consists of 40–60% water, the daily obligatory water loss amounts to about 2.5 l. Along with the water, several electrolytes (mainly sodium, potassium, and magnesium) that are an essential part of the internal environment are lost.

To survive on dry land, organisms had to evolve mechanisms that conserve salt and water and assure their prompt resupply. Different species achieve this goal in different ways. Some, such as various small desert mammals, have evolved extremely efficient kidneys that excrete very small quantities of highly concentrated urine. They also have developed temperature control mechanisms that do not rely on sweating. These conservation techniques reduce the water

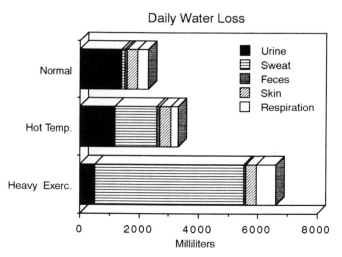

Fig. 1.1. Obligatory daily water loss. Data from: Guyton, A. C. (1987). "Human Physiology and Mechanisms of Disease." 4th Ed., W. B. Saunders, Philadelphia.

needs of these animals to the point where they can be met, under normal circumstances, by foraging vegetation that contains water. Drinking occurs rarely.

Most mammals do not obtain sufficient water from their diet but rely on thirst for the initiation of water ingestion. The intake must be sufficient to match the obligatory water loss within a fairly short time frame because water cannot be stored in significant quantities (Fig. 1.2).

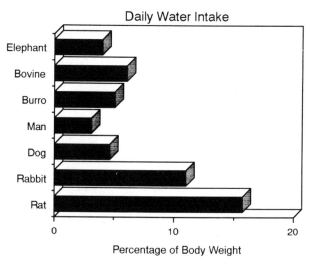

Fig. 1.2. Daily water intake in several mammalian species. Data from: Adolph, E. F. (1943). "Physiological Regulations." Jacques Cattell Press, Lancaster, Pennsylvania.

Carnivores obtain a sufficient supply of sodium and other electrolytes from their diet to permit "passive" (as opposed to "behavioral") regulation of the organism's salt balance by the kidney, which controls the rate of their excretion. Herbivores, on the other hand, often survive on sodium-deficient diets and rely on an innate salt appetite to insure an adequate intake (potassium and magnesium are abundant in all diets, and there is no known appetite for these electrolytes and only inefficient renal mechanisms for their conservation).

Because the water and electrolyte concentrations of body fluids are essential for metabolic functions, they are closely regulated by the interplay of several neural and hormonal mechanisms. In recent years, many of these have been investigated in detail and their action is, as we shall see, becoming increasingly elucidated. We still struggle, however, to understand the nature of the essential integrative action of the brain that results in our perception of the need for action that culminates in the ingestion of salt or water. The resolution of this important problem is complicated by the fact that there is still little agreement on the nature of the sensations that we call "thirst" or "sodium appetite."

The Sensation of Thirst

Historical Perspectives

Prescientific attempts to account for the urge to drink were based on the assumption that thirst was a sensation arising as a result of stimulation of receptors in peripheral organs. Aristotle, for instance, suggested that thirst sensations might arise directly from the stomach. Galen, the medical authority of the pre-Christian era, thought it might originate in the heart and lungs. Hippocrates first suggested an interpretation that has played an important role in more recent scientific investigations. Thirst, according to his views, refers to the sensations that arise from the mouth and throat when they become dry and parched because of a loss of body fluids.

This *dry-mouth theory* of thirst was revived by the German physiologist Haller in 1764. It continued to be popular well into the early decades of the twentieth century, at least in part because the eminent physiologist Walter B. Cannon strongly supported it. According to Cannon's version of the theory, thirst sensations are due to the activation of receptors in the mouth and throat that are sensitive to the moisture content of the surrounding mucosa. As the body loses water, the viscosity of the blood is maintained by the withdrawal of fluid from tissues, much of it coming from the salivary glands, which are known to contain a good deal of water. As a consequence, the rate of salivation drops and this reduces the moisture of the mouth and throat. The resulting dryness irritates the postulated thirst receptor and gives rise to the "burning" sensations we recognize as thirst.

Scientific interest in thirst dates back to the physiological research centers that began to flourish at French and German universities during the eighteenth and nineteenth centuries. An extensive summary of research and theory related to the "urge to drink" was published in France as early as 1821 (Rullier, 1821). It contained such a bewildering variety of observations and contradictory theoretical interpretations that Magendie (1822), one of the great pioneers of French physiology, suggested that thirst should be considered an "instinctive sentiment which does not admit of any explanation."

Much of the early research in this field was concerned with the dry-mouth theory of thirst. The most famous of these pioneering experiments is Claude Bernard's (1856) demonstration that wetting the mouth and throat does not alleviate thirst. Bernard cut the esophagus of a horse and brought both ends to the surface of the throat. When the animal became thirsty and began to drink, the water wetted the mouth and throat but gushed out of the cut esophagus before reaching the stomach. The animal drank for a very long time and consumed large quantities of water before stopping, it seemed to Bernard, only when exhausted. When the cut ends of the esophagus were reconnected so that water could reach the stomach, drinking stopped after the animal had consumed a normal quantity of water. Bernard repeated the experiment in a dog and concluded that the dry-mouth theory could not account for thirst or satiety.

Other physiologists of the nineteenth century reached similar conclusions after demonstrating that rinsing the mouth with water produced little effect on thirst in humans (Schiff, 1867) and that cutting the principal nerves that carry sensory information from the mouth and throat did not reduce the water intake of dogs (Longet, 1868).

As early as 1867, the German physiologist Schiff proposed an alternative theory, which stated, in essence, that thirst is a general sensation that cannot be referred to any particular part of the body. Schiff also made the important suggestion that this general sensation might be related to a lack of water in the blood.

Schiff's proposal was put to experimental test at the turn of the century when A. Mayer obtained a measure of the concentration of the blood by recording the osmotic pressure of blood plasma taken from water-deprived dogs. Mayer (1900, 1901) reported that prolonged water deprivation increased the osmotic pressure of the blood (see The Exchange of Body Fluids, p. 13), whereas intravenous infusions of hypotonic saline that returned the osmotic pressure to normal levels abolished drinking. He proposed, therefore, that thirst was a result of an increase in the concentration of solutes in the body fluids, which stimulated receptors located in the walls of blood vessels.

Wettendorf (1901) published similar results within a few months of Mayer's first report but noted that the osmotic pressure increased significantly only after 24 h of deprivation. Wettendorf believed that the concentration of solutes in blood might be maintained at nearly normal levels during the initial stages of water deprivation, by a movement of water from tissue into the vascular bed. He did not accept Mayer's view that osmotic pressure changes of the blood could be directly responsible for thirst because he observed significant changes only after far longer periods of deprivation than those known to give rise to the sensations we associate with thirst. Wettendorf's hypothesis that water deprivation results in a movement of water between different fluid compartments in the body continues to play a major role in contemporary theories of thirst.

Contemporary Views

Perusal of modern treatises on the subject of thirst (e.g., Fitzsimons, 1979; Rolls and Rolls, 1982) reveals that definitional problems have remained with us. Everyone agrees that thirst is a "general sensation" that cannot be referred to a particular sense organ, but most investigators proceed to point out that "associated" sensations from the mouth do seem to play a role under normal circumstances.

Contemporary investigators also agree that thirst arises as a direct consequence of a loss of water from the cellular and/or extracellular stores of the body. In the laboratory, it can be shown that water deprivation depletes both of these stores and results in water intake that is proportional to the total deficit. We shall discuss the mechanisms that appear to be responsible for the tight control of such "homeostatic" or *primary drinking* in some detail.

It is also generally agreed, however, that many species, including humans, drink far more than the body requires when water or other fluids such as tea, coffee, soft drinks, etc. are freely available. Such *secondary drinking* (Fitzsimons, 1979) does not appear to be based on a physiological "need" (although it can be argued that it anticipates need) and thus does not, by commonly accepted definition, represent a response to true thirst. Just how important a role secondary drinking plays in the regulation of body water has been the subject of considerable debate, as we shall see. We are, in any case, forced to consider the implications of the fact that the behavior used to measure thirst may, in many situations, not be motivated by it. The alternative—to include the many causes of secondary drinking in an "operational" definition of thirst—is not acceptable to most investigators in the field.

Oral Influences

Salivation

Cannon's (1919, 1934) version of the dry-mouth theory of thirst is compatible with more recent experimental findings, which indicate that water deprivation causes cellular dehydration (which in turn reduces the ability of cells in the salivary glands to secrete saliva).

In humans, the rate of salivation is an essentially linear function of body water over a considerable range. Salivation decreases promptly during water deprivation and ceases entirely when a fluid deficit of about 8% of body weight is incurred (Adolph 1947a,b,c). The correlation between water loss and rate of salivation is good enough (-0.74 in one study) to suggest to some that salivary flow could serve as a useful, albeit not always practical, objective measure of thirst (Adolph, 1947a,b,c).

Much experimental evidence indicates, however, that this strong correlation does not reflect the causal relationships envisioned by Cannon and other proponents of a dry-mouth explanation of thirst.

Drugs such as pilocarpine that elicit profuse salivation do not alleviate thirst or reduce water intake (Adolph, 1947a,b,c). Similarly, drugs such as atropine that suppress salivation do not increase drinking when water is available ad libitum (Montgomery, 1931) and may even depress it (Adolph, 1948).

Reduced salivation due to congenital dysfunctions of salivary glands in human patients (Steggerda, 1941) or experimental removal (Montgomery, 1931) of salivary glands in dogs also has been reported to have little or no effect on water intake under normal circumstances, although the pattern of drinking may shift toward more frequent smaller drinks. Salivarectomized (Epstein et al., 1964; Epstein, 1967; Kissileff and Epstein, 1969) as well as atropine-treated (Chapman and Epstein, 1970) rats maintained on a dry diet do develop a pattern of prandial drinking that alternates each mouthful of food with a small draught of water. Total water intake is increased in both paradigms, apparently because the rat requires water to chew and swallow dry food, not because thirst itself is increased. This conclusion is supported by the observation that intragastric infusions of quantities of water that suppress drinking in control rats did not reduce the excessive prandial drinking in these experiments. Intraoral injections of very small quantities of water, timed to coincide with the ingestion of dry pellets, on the other hand, did so effectively (Kissileff, 1969b).

Further evidence against a dry-mouth theory comes from modern replications of some of the pioneering research of the French physiologists of the nineteenth century. Extensive denervation of the mouth and throat (including transection of the trigeminal, glossopharyngeal, and chorda tympani nerves), for instance, has been shown to have no significant effect on total water intake in dogs (Bellows and Van Wagenen, 1939).

Drinking Associated with Eating

The very tight coupling of food and water intake observed in salivarectomized or atropine-treated animals (Epstein et al., 1964; Epstein, 1967; Kissileff and Epstein, 1969; Chapman and Epstein, 1970) is not typical of the ingestive behavior of rats under normal circumstances. However, drinking is clearly "meal-associated" in the rat as well as many other species (Siegel and Stuckey, 1947; Cizek and Nocenti, 1965), occurring mainly immediately before, during, and after each discrete meal (Kissileff, 1969a; Fitzsimons and LeMagnen, 1969) (Fig. 1.3). In the rat, the total amount of water drunk each day is highly correlated with the total amount of food consumed (Fitzsimons and LeMagnen, 1969).

The association of food and water ingestion is most striking when animals are maintained on a dry diet such as the pellet chow typically fed to laboratory rats. This suggests that drinking may be controlled, at least in part, by oral and esophageal stimuli related to the ingestion of food.

Postingestional factors such as osmotic effects of the ingested food and the attendant urinary requirements for solute excretion may also contribute to meal-associated drinking. The influence of these variables has been demonstrated in experiments showing that the amount of water ingested is closely related to the nature of the diet [a high-protein diet being associated with larger water/food ratios than diets high in carbohydrates and fats (LeMagnen and Tallon, 1967)].

A change from a high-protein to a high-carbohydrate or high-fat diets resulted in a gradual decrease in meal-associated drinking in these experiments. A change in the opposite direction increased daily water intake without delay but the normal pattern of meal-associated drinking was temporarily replaced by a nearly random pattern of intake. Because of these transient errors in correlation or synchrony, Fitzsimons (1979) suggested that diet-related changes in water intake may reflect secondary, learned adaptations rather than only primary reactions to the differential water requirements of the ingested food.

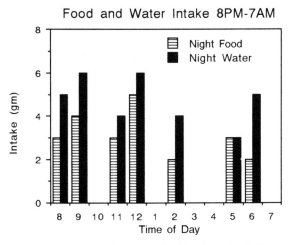

Fig. 1.3. Correlation between food and water intake. Data from: S. P. Grossman, unpublished observations.

Interactions between Oral Sensations and Thirst

The experimental evidence leaves little doubt that a dry-mouth theory of thirst cannot be correct. Yet all of us associate thirst with dryness of the mouth and throat and would agree that intense stimulation of oral sensory receptors as a result of the ingestion of highly spicy or "hot" foods results in thirst.

Wolf (1958) has suggested that the apparently fortuitous association between oral sensations and thirst may be a result of classical conditioning. According to this view, oral receptors lose water and may therefore become irritated whenever cellular dehydration (which is the primary result of water deprivation, as we shall see) occurs elsewhere in the body. Cellular dehydration is believed to stimulate special osmoreceptors in the brain that give rise to the sensation of thirst (the unconditioned stimulus in Wolf's schema). The concurrent sensations from the mouth and throat would presumably become conditioned stimuli for thirst because of their ubiquitous close temporal association. Although Wolf's hypothesis is plausible, it is essentially untestable and we cannot reject the possibility of a purely fortuitous association between oral sensations and thirst.

There is some evidence suggesting that human subjects can distinguish the sensation of thirst from the sensation of dryness of the mouth and throat that normally accompanies it. Wolf (1950), for instance, reported that intravenous injections of fairly concentrated salt solutions produced a dry throat long before a desire to drink was reported. The sensation of dryness disappeared immediately after the intravenous injection of glucose, whereas the desire for water persisted for some time afterward.

More recent attempts to investigate the sensations arising after 24 h of water deprivation quantitatively (Rolls *et al.*, 1980b) resulted in subjective ratings indicating that human subjects can distinguish not only dryness of the mouth but also an accompanying, unpleasant or "putrid" sensation from thirst itself.

The available evidence thus indicates that a dry mouth may well accompany thirst under normal conditions and can initiate drinking under some circumstances (i.e., during a meal consisting of dry or spicy food) even when the body's fluids do not require replenishing.

Ad Libitum Drinking

Patterns of Ingestion

When water is readily available, many animals as well as humans drink frequently and in excess of physiological need. In one study, laboratory rats maintained normal food intake and growth when their daily water ration was reduced to only 62% of their average ad libitum intake. The adjustment was made mainly by a reduction in urine excretion (Dicker and Nunn, 1957).

Animals display patterns of drinking that remain remarkably constant under controlled laboratory conditions. Most species are subject to diurnal cycles of sleep and waking, which are reflected in the pattern of their ingestive behavior. Rats, for instance, are nocturnal animals that consume about 80% of their daily water ration at night (Fitzsimons and LeMagnen, 1969). Rats modify their drinking pattern when the light–dark cycle is reversed, but the change occurs only gradually, suggesting an underlying circadian rhythm. This conclusion is supported by the fact that the 24-h periodicity persists for several days in the absence of external cues (Fitzsimons, 1971c).

The close association between food and water intake has been the subject of much experimental investigation (e.g., Fitzsimons and LeMagnen, 1969; Kissileff, 1969a). The ingestion of food (particularly the dry pellets fed to rats in most laboratories) generates a need for water in several independent ways: (a) water is needed to chew and swallow many diets, (b) the ingestion of food promotes the secretion of digestive juices, which removes water from the extracellular fluids, and (c) many foods represent an osmotic load that eventually depletes intracellular fluids.

Environmental Variables Affecting Water Intake

The total amount of water ingested varies as a function of a number of factors that may or may not influence the fluid economy of the body, including the following.

1. Ambient temperature. Sweating and evaporation from the mouth and skin surfaces are major components of temperature regulation in many species. Their water loss and thus water need increase dramatically in hot climates (Adolf, 1947a). The laboratory rat does not sweat or pant but has developed its own way of keeping cool. When it gets hot, the animal spreads saliva over its body and achieves relief by its evaporation. It too must increase water intake in the heat to replace the water lost in this unusual manner (Hainsworth, 1967; Epstein and Milestone, 1968).

2. Diet. Variations in the diet have significant effects on thirst because the metabolism of protein-rich foods requires more water for the excretion of metabolic breakdown products and excess sodium than foods rich in fats or carbohydrates (LeMagnen and Tallon, 1967).

3. Availability of food. The pattern of eating also has significant effects on water intake, not only because the digestion and metabolism of nutrients require water but also because drinking in many species occurs mainly in association

with eating. The rat, for instance, consumes about 70% of its total daily water ration in association with meals (Fitzsimons and LeMagnen, 1969; Kissileff, 1969a) and often drinks little when food-deprived (Strominger, 1947; Siegel and Stuckey, 1947).

4. Taste. Human subjects report that water itself has a "pleasant" taste after 24 h of deprivation (Rolls et al., 1980b). When the hedonic properties of water are improved by the addition of artificial sweeteners or various artificial flavors, rats as well as human subjects increase their water intake, particularly when a choice of several odors or flavors is available (Ernits and Corbit, 1973; Rolls et al., 1978; Rolls et al., 1980a). Conversely, when the water supply is adulterated with bitter-tasting quinine, rats curtail their daily intake (Nicolaidis and Rowland, 1975a) and drink far less than normal in response to various experimental procedures that elicit drinking in intact animals (Rolls et al., 1972; Rowland, 1977). It is interesting to note that quinine adulteration all but abolishes drinking responses to experimentally induced cellular dehydration, whereas most extracellular thirst stimuli continue to be effective (Burke et al., 1972; Nicolaidis and Rowland, 1975a; Rowland and Flamm, 1977).

5. Water temperature. Following deprivation, rats drink significantly more water at body temperature than of cold (12°C) water (Kapatos and Gold, 1972a). They also display a lasting preference for warm water (after an initial selection of cold water) when both are offered simultaneously (Kapatos and Gold, 1972b).

Review and Conclusions

Terrestrial mammals incur a steady obligatory water and electrolyte loss due to evaporation from skin surfaces and lungs, digestive processes, and urinary losses required to excrete waste products of cellular metabolism. The water content of the diet is not sufficient, for most mammals, and the often sizable residual needs must be met by ingestion of fluids and salts (mainly NaCl).

The impetuses for this are complex sensations that we call *thirst* (or *salt appetite*). Although they have been the subject of extensive investigation, we cannot, as yet, precisely define the nature or origin of these essential sensations, although they are readily identifiable introspectively and seem to be ubiquitous in many species other than humans.

We do know that oral sensations accompany and may, under normal circumstances, represent a significant component of the sensory input associated with "thirst." In many species, including humans, drinking is associated with eating; "dry mouth" and other unpleasant oral sensations arise during water deprivation; and stimuli that irritate oral receptors, such as very salty or spicy ("hot") foods, initiate thirst. Yet numerous experiments have shown that water intake can be regulated when oral influences are excluded. A possible explanation of this apparent paradox is Wolf's notion that oral sensations may become conditioned stimuli for thirst.

True thirst arises as a consequence of cellular or extracellular dehydration, as we shall see shortly. When water or other palatable fluids are readily available, many species including the laboratory rat as well as humans drink far in excess of actual need and rarely experience primary thirst. This "secondary drinking" occurs mainly in association with a meal and is influenced by the nature of the diet.

Chapter 2

The Body's Water Stores

Cellular and Extracellular Compartments

The body stores water and electrolytes in two "compartments" that are separated by a semipermeable membrane. In humans, about 60% of total body weight (more in infants, less in older people) consists of water. Two-thirds of the body's water is contained inside cells. The semipermeable cell membrane separates this cellular water from the fluid that forms a thin film on the outside of each cell and fills the spaces between adjacent cells. This interstitial fluid represents about 80% of the total extracellular water. The remaining 20% consists of blood plasma that is confined to the heart, arteries, and veins. Water enters and leaves this system only via the vasculature (Fig. 2.1).

The composition of cellular fluids differs in essential ways from that of extracelullar fluids. Cells contain large amounts of protein and phosphate. Because the the protein and phosphate ($HPO_4{}^{2-}$) molecules are relatively large, they constitute approximately 97% of the mass of a cell. The cellular compartment is also rich in potassium (K^+) and magnesium (Mg^{2+}), which are found only in low concentrations in the extracellular fluid. The extracellular fluid is rich in sodium (Na^+) and chloride (Cl^-), which are found only in low concentrations inside the cell. Plasma contains approximately 25% as much protein as cells do and there is very little protein (only about one-fourth as much as in plasma) in the interstitial fluid. Water, as well as ions and smaller lipid-insoluble molecules, diffuses constantly across the single-layer capillary walls at slit-like openings between adjacent endothelial cells. Because of their size, proteins cannot cross most of these "pores." Their concentration in the interstitial fluid is further reduced because they are taken up into vessels of the lymphatic system (Fig. 2.2).

The Exchange of Body Fluids

All molecules and ions, including water molecules, are in constant motion. This is called *diffusion*. Enough water diffuses through cell membranes per second to

13

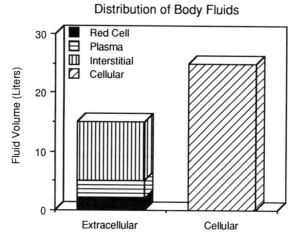

Fig. 2.1. Distribution of body fluids. Data from: Guyton, A. C. (1987). "Human Physiology and Mechanisms of Disease." 4th Ed., W. B. Saunders, Philadelphia.

equal as much as 100 times the volume of the entire cell. Because the direction of diffusion is random, there is no *net* movement of water into or out of the cell. Only when the concentration of solutes that cannot cross the cell membrance differs between the intra- and extracellular environment does a net movement of water occur, which is the result of osmotic forces.

When solutions containing unequal concentrations of solutes are separated by

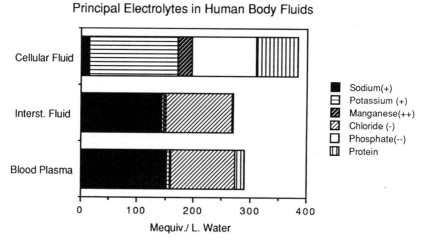

Fig. 2.2. Distribution of principal electrolytes. Data from: Guyton, A. C. (1987). "Human Physiology and Mechanisms of Disease." 4th Ed., W. B. Saunders, Philadelphia.

a membrane that is impermeable to the solutes but permeable to the solvent, the latter will move into the region of higher concentration until the concentration differences are eliminated. The process is called *osmosis*. The movement of the solvent can be reduced or prevented by increasing the mechanical pressure on the more concentrated solution. The amount of pressure that prevents pure water from moving into a solution represents *absolute osmotic pressure*. The pressure required to prevent the movement of water between two solutions of unequal concentration is called *relative* or *effective osmotic pressure*.

The osmotic pressure of molecules or ions in a solution is determined by the number of particles, not their mass. For nondissociated molecules this is equal to the *molar concentration*. The term *osmole* is used to express the concentration of a solution in terms of the number of particles it contains. One osmole equals the number of particles in 1 gram molecular weight of undissociated solute. If the solute dissociates into two (or more) ions, each is osmotically active (e.g., 1 gram molecular weight of sodium chloride equals 2 osmoles). The term *osmolality* is used to refer to the number of osmoles per kilogram of water. (Osmolarity is used to refer to the number of osmoles per liter.) The relationship is approximated by the following: osmotic pressure (mm Hg) $= 19.3 \times$ osmolality (mOsm/kg). Because osmotically effective solutes increase the freezing point of water, their concentration (i.e., the absolute osmotic pressure of a solution) can be measured by recording the freezing point of a solution.

Human plasma has an osmolality of 290 mOsm/kg water. Solutions of identical osmolality (such as a 0.9% or 0.15 M solution of sodium chloride in water) exert no osmotic pressures against plasma or other body fluids in osmotic equilibrium—they are *isotonic*. Solutions of higher or lower osmolality promote the movement of water across cellular membranes. They are called *hypertonic* and *hypotonic*, respectively.

The exchange of water (and various solutes) between plasma and interstitial fluid is subject to several forces. Water and solutes (except proteins) diffuse freely and constantly between the two compartments, but the net flow of water from plasma into the interstitial spaces is quite small. The excess water (as well as the few proteins that escape from capillaries through some large pores) is returned to the vascular system by the lymphatic system.

The pumping action of the heart creates *capillary pressure*, which is greater at the arterial end of the capillary bed than at the venous end. This provides the principal force that moves fluid from plasma into interstitial spaces. The movement of water into the interstitial spaces is aided by two factors, (a) negative pressure of the interstitial fluid (the pressure is slightly less than atmospheric pressure) and (b) interstitial fluid oncotic (or colloid osmotic) pressure of proteins in the insterstitial fluid. These forces are opposed by plasma oncotic (or colloid osmotic) pressure, generated by the high concentration of negatively charged proteins in plasma that cannot pass through most capillary pores. For the average human, the following values (data from Guyton, 1987) have been estimated:

Forces moving fluid out of capillaries	
Capillary pressure	30.0 mm Hg
Negative pressure of interstitial fluid	5.3 mm Hg
Oncotic pressure of interstitial fluid	6.0 mm Hg
Total outward force	41.3 mm Hg
Forces opposing outward flow	
Oncotic pressure of plasma	28.0 mm Hg
Net outward force	13.3 mm Hg

The principal force that returns water to the capillaries is the high oncotic pressure of plasma proteins and the positive ions captured by them. The movement of fluid into capillaries is opposed by capillary pressure (relatively low at the venous end), the negative interstitial fluid pressure, and the oncotic pressure of proteins in the interstitial fluid. The values (data from Guyton, 1987) estimated for an average human are as follows:

Forces moving fluid into capillaries	
Oncotic pressure of plasma	28.0 mm Hg
Forces opposing inward flow	
Capillary pressure	10.0 mm Hg
Negative pressure of interstitial fluid	5.3 mm Hg
Oncotic pressure of interstitial fluid	6.0 mm Hg
Total forces opposing inward flow	21.3 mm Hg
Net inward force	6.7 mm Hg

As Starling pointed out nearly 100 years ago, the end result of this interplay of forces is a near equilibrium so that the amount of water filtered into the interstitial fluid compartment at the arterial capillary bed is almost matched by the return of fluid into plasma and the venous capillaries. This is true in spite of the sizable difference between the total outward force at the arterial end of capillaries and the reabsorption pressure at the venous end because venous capillaries are more numerous and more permeable. There is a very small *net filtration* into interstitial spaces, which is balanced by a movement of water into the *lymphatic* system, which returns the excess to the vascular bed.

Water enters this system via the gastrointestinal tract, which permits the absorption of water (as well as nutrients and electrolytes) into blood plasma. From here, water and solutes diffuse into the interstitial spaces so that the entire extracellular fluid becomes diluted. This sets up an osmotic pressure gradient, which results in the movement of water into the more concentrated cellular fluid compartment.

During water deprivation, this process is reversed. Water continues to be lost from plasma because of salivation, urination, digestive needs, and evaporation from skin and lungs. This produces an increase in the concentration of solutes in plasma. As a result, water is drawn into venous capillaries from interstitial fluid, which, in turn, becomes increasingly concentrated and encourages cellular water to exit into the extracellular environment. In the short term, the movement of water from the cells into the extracellular compartment is sufficient to postpone a severe depletion of blood plasma. The resulting cellular dehydration becomes a signal for thirst as well as renal conservation of water.

As deprivation continues, the intracellular fluid also becomes increasingly concentrated and this reduces the osmotic gradient across the cell membrane and the resulting movement of water. The volume of extracellular fluid then decreases, and this hypovolemia activates pressure-sensitive neural and endocrine mechanisms, which contribute additional signals for thirst and renal conservation.

The Role of the Kidney

Cellular metabolism produces toxic waste products, which must be removed from the body. The kidney does so by continually filtering blood and forming urine. In performing this essential function, the kidney also controls the volume and composition of blood. When more water is ingested than is needed for the maintenance of homeostasis, the kidney secretes large quantities of dilute urine. Conversely, in times of water deprivation, or after excessive salt ingestion, the kidney conserves water and rids the body of unwanted salt by excreting highly concentrated urine.

The rate of urine formation and its concentration are controlled by the interplay of several hormones. When water or sodium needs to be conserved, the kidney releases renin, which acts on its substrate in plasma to form angiotensin I (A-I). A converting enzyme then changes angiotensin I into angiotensin II (A-II).

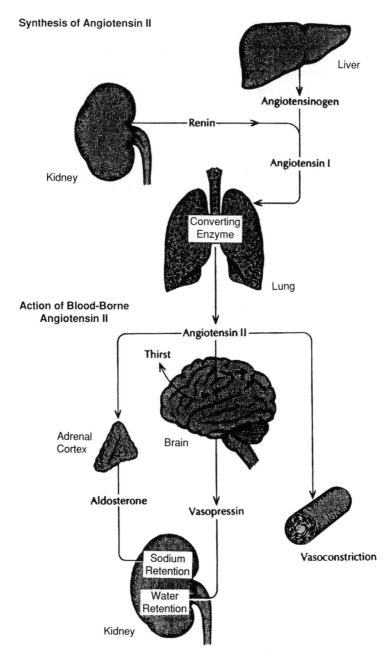

Synthesis of Angiotensin II

Liver

Angiotensinogen

Kidney —Renin—→

Angiotensin I

Converting Enzyme

Lung

Action of Blood-Borne Angiotensin II

Angiotensin II

Thirst

Adrenal Cortex

Brain

Aldosterone

Vasopressin

Vasoconstriction

Sodium Retention

Water Retention

Kidney

Fig. 2.3. The kidney plays a major role in the regulation of the organism's sodium and fluid balance. It exerts its influence in part by releasing renin in response to a decrease in the volume and pressure of its blood supply (upper left). Renin is converted to angiotensin, which promotes renal sodium and water retention, peripheral vasoconstriction, and thirst. The details of these events will be discussed in a later chapter. From: Ramsay, D. J., and Ganong, W. F. (1980). CNS regulation of salt intake. In: "Neuroendocrinology." (D. T. Krieger and J. C. Hughes, eds.), pp. 123–129. Sinaur, Sunderland, Massachusetts. Reproduced with permission of the authors, Hospital Practice, and the artist, N. L. Graham Marks.

Renin and A-I are physiologically inactive, but A-II has numerous central as well as peripheral effects that affect the body's fluid and sodium balance (Fig 2.3).

Renin is released in response to a decrease in the blood volume (and pressure) in the arteries that supply the kidney (note that a decrease in plasma sodium results in its dilution, a movement of water into cells, and, consequently, vascular hypovolemia). The resulting elevation of circulating A-II increases blood pressure because of a powerful direct vasoconstrictor action on arterial smooth muscle, aided by a facilitatory effect on noradrenergic nerve endings of sympathetic nerves and activation of central noradrenergic pressor mechanisms.

Angiotensin II also stimulates the synthesis and release of the adrenal hormone *aldosterone*, which promotes sodium reabsorption in the kidney. Aldosterone is also secreted in response to an increase in plasma potassium and promotes the renal secretion of potassium in urine. In addition, angiotensin-II stimulates the release of antidiuretic hormone (or vasopressin) from neurosecretory cells in the supraoptic and paraventricular nuclei of the hypothalamus, which store and release the hormone in the posterior pituitary. This hormone increases the permeability of the distal portion of the renal tubules and thus increases the reabsorption of water into interstitial fluid. It also promotes vasoconstriction and thus aids in maintaining blood pressure. The tubular reabsorption of sodium and water is also facilitated by a direct local action of angiotensin.

The release of antidiuretic hormone is also stimulated by cellular dehydration, which results in the activation of osmoreceptor mechanisms in the preoptic area.

Most interesting in the context of our discussion of thirst is the fact that angiotensin II is a powerful stimulus for drinking as well as for a delayed salt appetite. The dipsogenic effects of A-II may reflect peripheral effects of the hormone on baroreceptors in the great veins and heart as well as a direct action on brain mechanisms concerned with extracellular thirst and sodium appetite.

Effects of Water Deprivation

Terrestrial mammals continually lose water through the skin, lungs, kidneys, and intestines. When the body is in positive water balance, urine contains water and solutes in roughly the same proportions as they exist in body fluids. During the first few hours of water deprivation, fluid appears to be lost mainly from the extracellular compartment (Elkinton and Taffel, 1942; Blass and Hall, 1976). The resulting vascular hypovolemia promotes the efflux of interstitial fluid into plasma. As deprivation continues, the extracellular fluid becomes increasingly concentrated and begins to draw water from cells due to osmotic forces. The resulting cellular dehydration activates osmoreceptor mechanisms in the brain, which stimulate the release of antidiuretic hormone (ADH). ADH then acts on the kidney to conserve water.

The loss of water and electrolytes from extracellular fluid also stimulates the

adrenal secretion of aldosterone, which acts on the kidney to promote the retention of sodium. This further increases the osmolality of extracellular fluid relative
to cellular electrolyte concentrations and thus stimulates the movement of water
from cells into interstitial fluid and plasma by osmosis. Cellular water is also
released due to the continuing renal excretion of potassium. Increased urinary
potassium excretion (relative to sodium) is a sign that the body is using cellular
water to sustain extracellular (mainly vascular) volume. When water deprivation

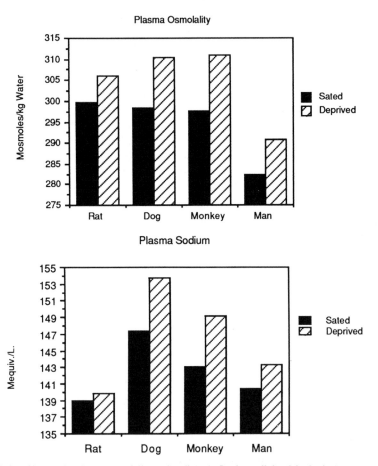

Fig. 2.4. Changes in plasma osmolality and sodium (reflecting cellular dehydration) as a result of
water deprivation (21 h for the rat; 24 h for dog, monkey, and human). Data from: Rolls, B. J.,
Wood, R. J., and Rolls, E. T. (1980a). Thirst: The initiation, maintenance, and termination of
drinking. *In*: "Progress in Psychobiology and Physiological Psychology." Vol. 9 (J. M. Sprague, and
A. N. Epstein, eds.), pp. 263–321. Academic Press, New York.

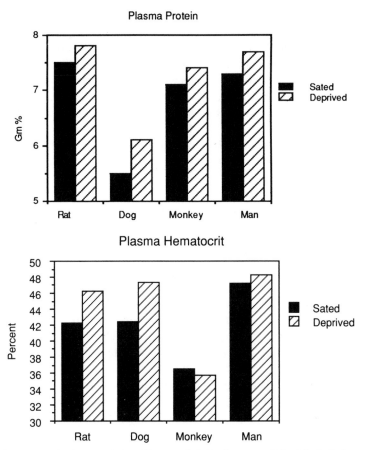

Fig. 2.5.   Changes in plasma protein and hematocrit (reflecting extracellular dehydration) as a result of water deprivation (21 h for the rat; 24 h for dog, monkey, and human). Data from: Rolls, B. J., Wood, R. J., and Rolls, E. T. (1980a). Thirst: The initiation, maintenance, and termination of drinking. *In*: "Progress in Psychobiology and Physiological Psychology." Vol. 9 (J. M. Sprague, and A. N. Epstein, eds.), pp. 263–321. Academic Press, New York.

is prolonged, cells may be forced to give up additional water by breaking down protein in order to defend plasma volume (Figs. 2.4 and 2.5).

The body's fluid stores can also be seriously compromised as a result of sodium deprivation, particularly when it is combined with sudden salt losses due to sweating, diarrhea, or medication that promotes diuresis. Initially, the body attempts to defend the osmolality of the extracellular fluids by excreting extremely dilute urine. If sodium deprivation continues, the volume and osmolality of plasma decrease. The resulting extracellular hypovolemia gives rise to thirst and a delayed and persisting sodium appetite in spite of cellular overhydration.

The Dual Depletion Theory of Thirst

During extended periods of water deprivation, extracellular hypovolemia coexists with cellular dehydration. Both provide inputs to brain mechanisms that give rise to the complex sensations associated with thirst, although the relative contribution of cellular dehydration and extracellular hypovolemia changes as a function of the length of the deprivation period. It is this combination of cellular and extracellular influences that explains the observation that had puzzled Adolph and other pioneers in this field, that water deprivation produces far more drinking than salt loads calculated to produce the same degree of cellular dehydration (Adolph, 1964; Kanter, 1953).

The relative contribution of cellular and extracellular influences on thirst have been estimated by administering water (which restores cellular hydration with little or no persisting effect on vascular volume) or isotonic saline (which restores extracellular volume without affecting its osmolality) after an overnight deprivation.

These experiments have shown that oral, intragastric (ig), or intravenous (iv) preloads of water, calculated to restore cellular hydration, reduced the water intake of rats allowed to drink to satiation during a 1-h test, by 64–68% (Ramsay et al., 1977a). This is an estimate of the contribution of cellular dehydration to the thirst produced by an overnight period of deprivation. (Some cellular dehydration may have persisted in these studies in spite of the water load because solute is lost during the deprivation period.)

Oral, ig, or iv preloads of isotonic saline that restored plasma volume without significant changes in osmolality reduced the 1-h water intake of the same rats by 20–26%, an indication of the magnitude of the contribution of extracellular thirst to the effects of overnight deprivation (Ramsay et al., 1977a).

The exact numbers apply, of course, only to the particular deprivation period, and the quantity of the water and salt loads, but the general conclusions that both water and saline appear to be required for complete satiety and that water is far more effective than isotonic saline are supported by the results of other investigations (e.g., Adolph, 1950; O'Kelly et al., 1954; Fregley et al., 1986). There are also considerable species differences although quite similar data have been reported for the dog in a somewhat different test situation.

In these experiments (Ramsay et al., 1977b), an attempt was made to specifically rehydrate putative central osmoreceptors by infusing water into the lateral carotid artery, which supplies much of the forebrain. This procedure left the osmolality of the general circulation largely unaffected but reduced the water intake of deprived dogs by 72%. Restoration of plasma volume without significant shifts in osmolality by iv infusions of isotonic saline resulted in a 27% decrease in deprivation-induced water intake in the same dogs. Doubling the size of the saline infusion did not further decrease water intake, indicating that expansion of the extracellular fluid volume beyond baseline levels had no inhibitory effect on drinking in this species (see Corbit, 1967 for similar results in the rat). When the water and saline infusions were combined, water intake was inhibited all-but-completely.

The results of similar studies in monkeys (Wood *et al.*, 1980, 1982) emphasize that the relative contribution of cellular and extracellular thirst signals may be quite different in other species. When enough water was infused intravenously to return the osmolality of plasma to predeprivation levels, monkeys reduced their oral intake by 85%. Larger amounts of iv water virtually abolished drinking. Similar infusions of isotonic saline, which restored plasma volume to predeprivation levels, reduced oral intake by only 5% on the average. Increases in the injection volume that raised plasma volume above baseline levels produced only minor further decreases in oral intake. It would appear that this species relies far more extensively on cellular deprivation cues than either the rat or the dog.

The additivity of cellular and extracellular thirst stimuli has also been demonstrated directly in experiments that consistently show that the amount of water drunk in response to hypertonic saline injections (which give rise to cellular dehydration thirst) sums, often quite precisely, with the amount of water consumed in response to experimental procedures that arouse extracellular thirst, such as hemorrhage (Fitzsimons and Oatley, 1968), ligation of the inferior vena cava (Fitzsimons, 1969b), polyethylene glycol (Corbit and Tuchkapsky, 1968; Stricker, 1969), and iv angiotensin (Fitzsimons and Simons, 1969). The combination of cellular and extracellular thirst stimuli has also been reported to mimic the temporal pattern of drinking (as well as the amount consumed) normally seen in the rat after 24 h of water deprivation (Almli *et al.*, 1975).

Review and Conclusions

All living cells contain water. In humans and other large mammals, about two-thirds of the body's water is stored in cells. The semipermeable cell membrane separates cellular water from interstitial fluid, which constitutes the immediate environment of cells. Interstitial fluid communicates with blood plasma via the capillary bed of the vascular system. Together, they form the extracellular pool of water.

The exchange of water between the extracellular and cellular compartments is due to the action of osmotic forces that arise as a consequence of changes in the concentration of various positively and negatively charged electrolytes in the extracellular or cellular compartment.

Ingested water first "dilutes" plasma and interstitial fluid. This, in turn, results in osmotic pressure gradients that cause the movement of water into cells. Conversely, during periods of water deprivation, plasma and the interstitial environment become more concentrated and osmotic pressure gradients result in the movement of water out of cells. The resulting "cellular dehydration" is a primary stimulus for thirst.

As the cellular compartment becomes increasingly dehydrated during water deprivation, osmotic pressure gradients across cell membranes decline and the outflow of cellular water no longer compensates for the water lost from plasma. The resulting vascular hypovolemia is the second major signal for thirst.

Decreased blood volume (and/or pressure) releases renin from the kidney. This, in turn, results in increased plasma levels of angiotensin II, which has several physiological effects relevant to the regulation of body water and salt. Angiotensin acts directly as well as indirectly (via sympathetic neurons) on blood vessels to alleviate low blood pressure by vasoconstriction. It also releases vasopressin from stores in the posterior pituitary and aldosterone from cells in the adrenal gland. Vasopressin (or antidiuretic hormone) promotes reabsorption of water in the kidney; aldosterone facilitates sodium reabsorption. Angiotensin is also an extremely potent stimulus for thirst when administered systemically or directly into the ventricles or some tissues of the brain.

Renin release and the resulting increase in blood levels of angiotensin II are probably not the only extracellular thirst signals relayed to the brain. Hypovolemia and the resulting decrease in blood pressure also affect baroreceptors in the great veins and atria of the heart. Neural signals from these receptors also appear to be an important input to thirst-related brain mechanisms. Angiotensin may exert its dipsogenic effects by modulating the sensitivity of this baroreceptor mechanism and/or by acting directly on brain pathways involved in the regulation of behavioral as well as hormonal reactions to vascular hypovolemia.

Chapter 3

Cellular Dehydration Thirst

Introduction

At the turn of the Century, Mayer (1900) demonstrated experimentally that prolonged water deprivation increased the absolute osmotic pressure of plasma. He suggested that the elevated tonicity of plasma might irritate receptors in the walls of blood vessels, which, in turn, give rise to the sensation of oral dryness that is commonly associated with thirst.

Wettendorff (1901) replicated Mayer's basic finding but reported that the osmotic pressure of blood did not increase significantly during the first 24 h of deprivation. He pointed out that the subjects of his experiments (dogs) lost a significant amount of water during that time and would have drunk large quantities of water (presumably because they were thirsty) had it been offered. He also noted that most other large mammals, including humans, replenish body fluids after much shorter periods of water deprivation, apparently long before the osmolality of plasma changes.

On the basis of these observations, Wettendorff proposed that the loss of water from the circulation results in osmotic pressure gradients that force water out of cells. This maintains the volume and concentration of the blood constant until the cellular supply becomes depleted. Thirst, according to his view, arises not because of an increase in the osmotic pressure of blood as Mayer had suggested but, instead, because of cellular dehydration.

Osmotic influences on thirst became readily apparent in many subsequent experiments, which demonstrated thirst and copious drinking in humans (Arden, 1934; Holmes and Gregersen, 1947) as well as experimental animals (Gilman, 1937; Holmes and Gregersen, 1950; Fitzsimons, 1969b) after the ingestion or injection of hypertonic solutions that increase the osmolality of the extracellular fluid and draw water out of cells.

25

Water Intake after Different Hypertonic Solutions

That cellular dehydration rather than an increase in the absolute osmotic pressure of plasma is responsible for the increased water intake seen in these classic experiments has been demonstrated in a series of investigations of the differential effectiveness of various solutes (Gilman, 1937; Bellows, 1939; Adolph et al., 1954; Fitzsimons, 1961b, 1963).

Drinking was found to be stimulated promptly and strongly by injections of sodium chloride or other solutes, such as sucrose, that are rigorously excluded from cells but not by injections of solutes such as glucose, methyl glucose, or fructose that readily enter cells and thus increase the osmotic pressure of cellular and extracellular fluids equally. Injections of solutions containing solutes such as mannitol, which penetrate cells more readily than sodium but not as readily as glucose, produced intermediate drinking responses, which were due, in part, to renal water loss since they are powerful osmotic diuretics that are subject to little renal reabsorption.

Urea, which enters most cells readily, has been shown to produce significant drinking in the rat and dog although the response is much smaller than that elicited by equiosmotic sodium chloride (Gilman, 1937; Bellows, 1939; Adolph et al., 1954). That urea should produce drinking puzzled early investigators until it was shown that urea crosses the blood–brain barrier only slowly and thus produces an osmotic pressure gradient between the brain and the rest of the body that results in cellular dehydration of the brain (Reed and Woodbury, 1962; Crone, 1965; Kleeman et al., 1962). It is interesting to note that urea does not appear to produce drinking in the goat (Erickson et al., 1971; Olsson, 1972), a fact that has led Andersson et al. (1982) to propose that the receptor mechanisms for cellular thirst must reside on the blood side of the blood–brain barrier (possibly in the lining of the anterior third ventricle) in this species.

The results of these pioneering experiments left no doubt that the injection or ingestion of sodium chloride as well as other hypertonic solutions that are excluded from cells elicit thirst in humans and drinking in many diverse species of animals. However, when one examines the relationship between osmotic stimuli and water intake over a range of stimulus intensities and across species, it rapidly becomes apparent that it is curiously variable and in many instances unpredictable.

The classic experiments of Gilman (1937) indicated that dogs injected with hypertonic saline drank just enough to correct the osmotic effects on plasma. Subsequent investigations have not agreed with this conclusion. Holmes and Gregersen (1950), for instance, report that some of their dogs consistently failed to drink enough water to achieve osmotic equilibrium after intravenous injections of hypertonic solutions. Others drank too much and became overhydrated (Fig. 3.1). Kanter (1953) similarly found that some dogs (which he called "minimal

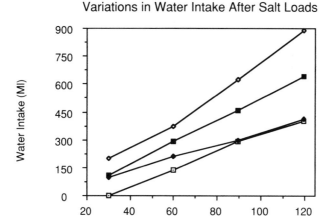

Fig. 3.1. Water intake in response to iv injections of 5, 10, 15, or 20% NaCl in four normal dogs. After: Holmes, J. H., and Gregersen, M. I. (1950). Observations on drinking induced by hypertonic solutions. *Am. J. Physiol.* **162**, 326–337. With permission of the authors and the American Physiological Society.

internal regulators") responded to stomach loads of hypertonic saline by drinking large amounts of water while others (called "maximal internal regulators") drank little water but excreted the salt load in highly concentrated urine.

Pronounced species differences have also been reported. While few animals drink more water than is needed to replace the fluid deficits incurred during deprivation [cellular overhydration prior to the cessation of drinking has been reported in the rat, by Blass and Hall (1976)], many, such as the donkey, camel, sheep, mule, and deer, drink enough to assure cellular rehydration. Others, such as the rabbit, hamster, guinea pig, human, and, in most studies, the rat, drink more slowly and tend to sustain some "voluntary dehydration" until the ingestion of food imposes prandial and digestive needs (see Adolph, 1964, for more detailed review).

Renal Effects of Hypertonicity of Body Fluids

The reason for these wide individual and species differences in the drinking response to increased plasma osmolality is the fact that it stimulates hormonal mechanisms that promote the renal retention of water and excretion of sodium and other solutes. Indeed, some solutes, such as potassium, seem to activate renal mechanisms exclusively. In this case, osmotic homeostasis is achieved through renal excretion and diuresis, not by drinking and dilution (Arden, 1934; Janssen, 1936). Sodium chloride elicits drinking as well as renal excretion in dogs as well as rats, but the relative contribution of the two regulatory mechanisms is curiously variable.

Verney's (1947) classic studies demonstrated nearly 50 years ago that an increase in the osmolality of plasma elicits a prompt release of antidiuretic hormone (ADH) (also called vasopressin), which acts on the collecting ducts of the kidney to retain water. More recent quantitative studies of this relationship (Robertson et al., 1976; Robertson and Athar, 1976) have demonstrated the exquisite sensitivity of this system. In these experiments, normal human subjects in water balance had plasma osmolality values averaging 286 mOsm/kg and ADH levels adequate to utilize approximately 50% of the renal capacity to retain water. A 2% decrease in body water resulted in a plasma osmolality of 294 mOsm/kg and ADH levels that were maximally effective for urine concentration. Conversely, ingestion of water sufficient to increase body water by 2% over baseline suppressed ADH secretion completely and thus induced maximal urine dilution.

Andersson et al. (1982) have commented on the sensitivity and precision of this system by suggesting that "osmo-regulatory thirst in man may be regarded as an emergency mechanism that intervenes only when the water in food and anticipatory or habitual drinking, in combination with fully utilized effect of ADH, are insufficient to maintain extracellular Na concentrations below a certain level."

Most contemporary investigators would agree that food- and feeding-related water ingestion provide an adequate resupply of body fluid, as long as both food and water are available ad libitum. This may well be the norm for segments of modern human civilization whose populations may rarely experience true thirst and seldom engage in regulatory drinking. However, cellular dehydration thirst probably does play a significant role for humans in many regions of the world and undoubtedly represents the principal stimulus for drinking for many animal species that do not have ready access to water and cannot obtain sufficient water from their diet.

The sensitivity of thirst-related osmotic mechanisms has been elegantly demonstrated in animals that cannot excrete solutes because their kidneys have been surgically removed.

Cellular Dehydration in Nephrectomized Animals

When nephrectomized rats are given intravenous infusions of sodium chloride or other solutes that are excluded from cells, and are then allowed to drink to satiety, a nearly perfect relationship can be demonstrated between the initial

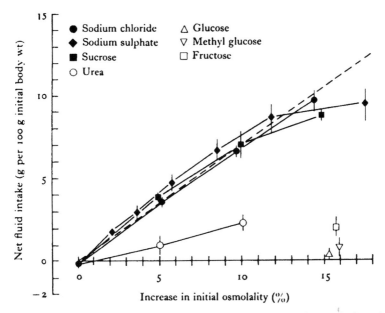

Fig. 3.2. Net water intake (expressed as an increase in body weight) of nephrectomized rats during 6 h after ip injections of various osmotically active solutions. Those rigidly and permanently excluded from cells (sodium chloride, sodium sulfate, and sucrose) resulted in drinking that precisely diluted the injected solute load to isotonicity (the dashed line indicates theoretical values calculated to represent the water required to achieve isotonicity and restore cell size). Solutes that penetrate cells relatively easily (urea, fructose, glucose, and methylglucose) produced little drinking in these experiments. After: Fitzsimons, J. T. (1979). "The Physiology of Thirst and Sodium Appetite." Cambridge University Press, Cambridge. With permission of the author and Cambridge University Press.

increase in osmolality of plasma and total water intake (Fitzsimons, 1961a, 1963, 1971c) (Fig. 3.2). Normal rats begin to drink when the osmotic pressure of plasma is increased by 1.6% regardless of the rate of increase. In nephrectomized rats, this value has been shown to rise slightly to 2.0%. Drinking continues until the osmotic pressure returns to ad libitum levels (Fitzsimons, 1963). When access to water is delayed by 12 or 24 h after the injection of hypertonic saline, nephrectomized rats drink as much as those allowed to drink immediately (Fitzsimons, 1971c).

Since water intake of salt-loaded, nephrectomized rats declines and stops as the ingested water rehydrates the cellular fluid compartment, satiety for pure cellular thirst may reflect simply the reversal of the conditions that were responsible for it (Fitzsimons, 1963).

Matters are complicated, however, by the fact that nephrectomy prevents the excretion of salts in these experiments. Because sodium cannot enter cells, the extracellular fluid absorbs a large quantity of water after an experimental salt load. This increase in extracellular fluid volume could itself account for the termination of drinking.

Such an interpretation appears unlikely, however, because drinking continues in spite of the hypervolemia until the extracellular fluid returns to isotonicity with cellular fluid. That an expansion of the extracellular fluid volume is, itself, not a significant satiety signal is further indicated by the results of experiments that have shown that infusions of isotonic saline (which increase extracellular fluid volume without changing cellular hydration) do not reduce the magnitude of the drinking response to hypertonic saline administered immediately afterward (Fitzsimons, 1961a,b).

Cellular Rehydration as a Satiety Signal

The precision of osmotic regulation seen in nephrectomized animals suggests that cellular rehydration is the satiety signal that stops drinking after cellular dehydration. There have been numerous clinical (Elkinton and Squires, 1951; Strauss, 1957) as well as experimental (Holmes and Cizek, 1951) reports of thirst or excessive water intake due to prolonged exposure to salt-deficient diets, which reduce the osmotic pressure of extracellular fluids and thus overhydrate cells. In the rat, drinking is also induced by acute sodium depletion (Falk, 1965a; Jalowiec and Stricker, 1970a,b), but in other species this produces no effects (Darrow and Yannet, 1935) or even long-lasting inhibition of drinking (Huang, 1955).

This "sodium depletion thirst" (see p. 46) would seem to contradict the conclusion that cellular rehydration represents a satiety signal, but it should be noted that sodium depletion produces cellular overhydration at the expense of extracellular fluid. Drinking thus may be sustained in spite of the cellular satiety signal by extracellular thirst signals arising as a consequence of vascular hypovolemia and renin release (Gross et al., 1965; Falk and Tang, 1973). This, rather than cellular overhydration, is probably responsible for the increased water intake (see the discussion of extracellular thirst, Chapter 4).

Adolph et al. (1954) reported that rats not allowed to drink until 8 h after ip injections of hypertonic saline drank large quantities of water even though most or all of the excess salt had been excreted. It has been suggested that only about 50% of the water intake seen 8 h after a salt load is due to obligatory water loss (Corbit, 1965). The nature of the stimulus for the additional water intake is not understood (see Fitzsimons, 1979, pp. 145–146).

Adolph et al. (1954) concluded from their observations that drinking was not related in any simple and straightforward way to either the osmotic pressure of a salt load or the severity of the resulting cellular dehydration. They proposed, instead, that thirst was determined by multiple factors. More recently, Blass and Hall (1976) similarly suggested that the cessation of drinking following deprivation appeared to be related more directly to the length of the deprivation period than to the degree of rehydration achieved.

Receptor Mechanisms for Cellular Thirst

Osmoreceptors

This brings us directly to the question of how cellular dehydration may be sensed or "metered" so that ADH secretion, water intake, and related physiological processes can be adjusted accordingly.

Verney (1947) postulated that the effects of IV infusions of hypertonic solutions on ADH secretion were mediated by osmoreceptors, which are excited by a decrease in their own volume (or by the efflux of water across their cell membrane). He suggested further that under conditions of *euhydration* these osmoreceptors maintained a certain baseline level of activity sufficient to release ADH in the quantities needed to stimulate 50% renal efficiency as seen in normohydrated subjects.

Verney's experiments have been replicated and extended (Erickson *et al.*, 1971; McKinley *et al.*, 1978), and similar experiments have shown (see Water Intake after Different Hypertonic Solutions, above) that solutes that are excluded from cells, including such nonelectrolytes as sucrose and sorbitol, elicit thirst as well as ADH release. Verney's hypothesis has accordingly been extended to cellular dehydration thirst.

It is generally believed that thirst-related (as well as ADH-related) osmoreceptors are located in the brain, although they have also been found in other organs. That brain osmoreceptors mediate cellular thirst is supported by many experimental observations (see Brain Osmoreceptors below), including the fact that intracarotid infusions of slightly hypertonic saline that increase the osmolality of the blood perfusing the forebrain within physiological limits but have no significant effect on the osmolality of the general circulation elicit drinking in dogs (Wood *et al.*, 1977) (Fig. 3.3).

Osmoreceptors have also been demonstrated in the stomach, liver (Hunt, 1956; Haberich, 1968), and duodenum (Hunt and Stubbs, 1975). There is some evidence that information from osmoreceptors in the hepatic-portal system reaches the hypothalamus (Schmitt, 1973) via the vagus nerve (Adachi *et al.*, 1976). Several investigators have suggested that this information may influence drinking under some conditions, in the rat (Kraly *et al.*, 1975) as well as dog (Kozlowski and Drzewiecki, 1973).

Sodium Receptors

Some investigators, notably Andersson and his colleagues (Andersson, 1978; Andersson *et al.*, 1967, 1969, 1982), have argued that the organism's principal

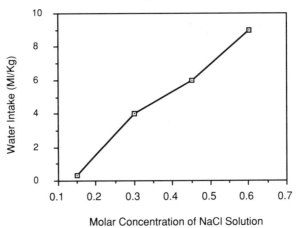

Fig. 3.3. Water intake of fluid-replete dogs during the last 5 min of a 10-min carotid infusion of hypertonic saline solutions. The 0.15 M control injection was administered iv. Data from: Wood, R. J., Rolls, B. J., and Ramsay, D. J. (1977). Drinking following intracarotid infusions of hypertonic solutions in dogs. *Am. J. Physiol.* **232**, 88–92.

goal must be the protection of sodium concentrations in plasma (because more than 90% of the osmolality of extracellular fluid is, in fact, due to sodium and its anions) and that this is most appropriately accomplished by receptors specifically sensitive to sodium.

According to this hypothesis, receptors that control ADH release, as well as similar ones that control cellular dehydration thirst, reside in circumventricular organs of the brain and are sensitive to the concentration of sodium in the cerebrospinal fluid (CSF).

The theory is supported by experiments showing that intracerebroventricular (icv) injections of hypertonic sucrose or electrolytes such as potassium do not elicit ADH release or drinking in the goat whereas equiosmolar sodium chloride solutions are effective (Olsson, 1969, Andersson *et al.*, 1969; Andersson, 1971). In the goat, icv injections of hypertonic fructose, sucrose, and mannitol, which increase the effective osmotic pressure of CSF but decrease its Na concentration, have been shown to inhibit ADH secretion (Olsson *et al.*, 1976) and reduce or abolish the normal dipsogenic and antidiuretic effects of intracarotid injections of hypertonic sodium chloride (Olsson, 1972, 1973, 1975).

A Combination of Sodium and Osmoreceptors

Denton and colleagues have presented evidence for both sodium-receptor and osmoreceptor mechanism in sheep (McKinley *et al.*, 1974, 1978, 1980). In this species, icv hypertonic sucrose (but not mannitol) elicits water drinking provided it is dissolved in artificial cerebrospinal fluid, which reduces the depletion of CSF sodium and other ions that occurs when water is used as the solvent. However, the response is significantly smaller than that elicited by equiosmolar solutions of sodium chloride (Fig. 3.4).

Sodium receptors are further implicated by the observation that icv infusions of mannitol in artificial CSF that lowered the sodium concentration of cerebrospinal fluid significantly reduced drinking in water-deprived sheep (Leksell *et al.*, 1981). Treatments that decrease the sodium content of cerebrospinal fluid also elicit sodium appetite in this species, and an existing sodium appetite can be suppressed in sodium-depleted sheep by increases in CSF sodium (Weisinger *et al.*, 1982, 1985). These observations suggest that sodium appetite as well as thirst may be affected by the concentration of sodium in CSF in this species.

Osmoreceptors are further implicated by the results of experiments that demonstrate that intracarotid infusions of 4.6 *M* urea caused a far greater increase in CSF sodium but less drinking than comparable infusions of 2 *M* sucrose (McKinley *et al.*, 1978). It has been suggested (McKinley *et al.*, 1978), that in sheep, thirst-related sodium sensors may be located inside the blood–brain barrier (BBB) whereas osmoreceptors are located at least in part outside the BBB.

In the rat, icv injections or infusions of hypertonic saline also have been reported to have a more potent dipsogenic effect than equiosmolar sucrose (Buggy, 1977a,b; Osborne *et al.*, 1987). The effects of microinjections of equiosmolar sucrose and sodium into the anteroventral third ventricle have been reported

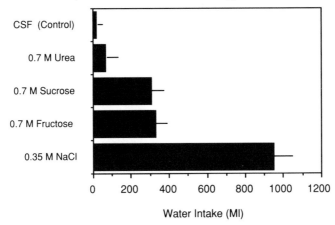

Fig. 3.4. Water intake during infusions of hypertonic solutions into the lateral ventricle of sheep. The substances were dissolved in artificial cerebrospinal fluid (CSF). Data from: McKinley, M. J., Denton, D. A., and Weisinger, R. S. (1978). Sensors for antidiuresis and thirst-osmoreceptors or CSF sodium detectors? *Brain Res.* **141**, 89–103.

to be essentially comparable (Buggy *et al.*, 1979). Microinjections of slightly hypertonic sucrose into the lateral preoptic region also appear to be as effective as injections of equiosmolar sodium chloride in eliciting water drinking in the rat (Blass, 1974; Peck and Blass, 1975). It has been suggested that in this species, water intake may be controlled, at least in part, by osmoreceptors in the preoptic area and adjacent tissues surrounding the anterolateral third ventricle (Buggy *et al.*, 1979). The disparity between the effectiveness of icv sodium and equiosmolar sucrose suggests to other investigators (e.g., Osborne *et al.*, 1987) that both sodium and osmoreceptor mechanisms may contribute to the regulation of water intake.

Intraventricular infusions of 1 *M* NaCl, dissolved in CSF, do not reduce the salt appetite of adrenalectomized rats or rats pretreated with desoxycorticosterone (DOCA), angiotensin, or a combination of DOCA and angiotensin (Epstein *et al.*, 1984). Conversely, significant decreases in CSF sodium concentration, due to icv injections of hypertonic sucrose or isotonic or hypertonic mannitol, fail to elicit sodium appetite in the rat (Epstein *et al.*, 1984; Osborne *et al.*, 1983, 1987). These observations indicate that the concentration of sodium in CSF does not regulate sodium intake in the rat.

In the dog, there is as yet no evidence for sodium receptors. Equiosmolar icv injections of hypertonic sucrose or sodium chloride produce comparable effects on drinking as well as vasopressing release (Thrasher *et al.*, 1980a,b).

In rats (Epstein, 1978), dogs (Thrasher *et al.*, 1980a,b), and sheep (McKinley *et al.*, 1978) intravenous injections of urea or glucose (which did not elicit drinking) have been reported to produce elevations in CSF sodium that are comparable to those produced by equiosmotic loads of sodium or sucrose, which did elicit drinking.

In the pigeon, cellular thirst also appears to rely on osmoreceptor mechanisms, although a certain amount of NaCl must be present in cerebrospinal fluid. Intravenous injections of NaCl, sucrose, or mannitol elicit copious drinking, while hypertonic urea or glucose has little effect even though urea (as well as NaCl) produced a marked elevation of CSF sodium. Only NaCl also elicits drinking when administered icv in this species, suggesting the operation of a sodium receptor mechanism. However, when small amounts of NaCl are added to an icv injection of sucrose, drinking is promptly elicited. (Fitzsimons *et al.*, 1981; Thornton, 1984).

Brain Osmoreceptors

Electrophysiology
It has long been known that systemic injections of hypertonic solutions modify the firing rate of cells in the preoptic region (Verney, 1947; Von Euler, 1953; Cross and Green, 1959; Nicolaidis, 1969a,b; Novin and Durham, 1969).

Most of the responsive cells are in the region of the supraoptic and paraventricular nuclei. There is good evidence that these are the neurosecretory cells that produce antidiuretic hormone (ADH), also called vasopressin, and control its release from the pituitary. Many of these neurons respond to iontophoretic applications of vasopressin (Thornton et al., 1985).

In addition to its well-understood role as a stimulant for renal conservation of water, vasopressin may influence water intake directly. Microinjection of vasopressin into the third ventricle of dogs has been shown to elicit drinking (Szczepanska-Sadowska et al., 1982). The icv administration of various vasopressin antagonists delays and suppresses drinking response to hypertonic saline challenges (Szczepanska-Sadowska et al., 1986). A physiological role for this mechanism is indicated by the observation that the concentration of vasopressin in CSF changes in parallel with the osmolality of body fluids (Szczepanska-Sadowska et al., 1983; 1984).

In the rat, osmosensitive cells have also been found in portions of the preoptic region not known to be directly involved in the control of ADH secretion. For instance, Weiss and Almli (1975b) have reported that subcutaneous injections of hypertonic saline modified the activity of nine of 10 spontaneously active cells in the preoptic region. Similar effects on single- or multiple-unit activity in the lateral preoptic region (LPO) have been reported by other investigators (Blank and Wayner, 1975; Malmo and Mundl, 1975; Hatton, 1976; Hayward and Vincent, 1970).

Malmo and Malmo (1979), using multiple-unit recordings, have added the important observation that neurons in the LPO are equally sensitive to intracarotid infusions of hypertonic saline and hypertonic sucrose—firm support of the interpretation that osmoreceptor rather than sodium receptor mechanisms are activated by the injections.

Nicolaidis (1968, 1969a,b) has reported that some neurons in the preoptic area respond to hypertonic saline on the tongue as well as to intravenous injections. Some of the preoptic neurons that respond to systemic injections of hyper- or hypotonic saline are also activated by drinking (Sessler and Salhi, 1981; Vincent et al., 1972)

Neurons that increase their firing rate when hypertonic saline is injected systemically have also been found in the dorsolateral hypothalamus of cats (Emmers, 1973) and monkeys (Vincent et al., 1972). In the monkey, these cells decreased their firing rate when the animals drank water (Vincent et al., 1972). Oomura and colleagues (Oomura et al., 1969) have reported that some cells in the lateral hypothalamus of the rat appeared to be selectively activated by iontophoretic applications of sodium.

Microinjections

A second line of evidence for osmosensitive thirst mechanisms in the preoptic region comes from experiments that have demonstrated drinking in sated rats

(Blass and Epstein, 1971; Peck and Blass, 1975; Blass, 1974) and rabbits (Peck and Novin, 1971) following microinjections of hypertonic saline or sucrose (but not urea) into the lateral preoptic region and caudally adjacent zona incerta (Fig. 3.5). Microinjections of water into this region reduced the drinking response to systemic injections of hypertonic saline apparently specifically (Blass and Epstein, 1971). More recently, drinking has been reported in the rat following microinjections of hypertonic saline in the tissues of the anterior ventral third ventricle (AV3V) and particularly the organum vasculosum of the lamina terminalis (OVLT). It is interesting to note that both have been implicated in the drinking response to centrally applied angiotensin (Buggy, 1977; Buggy and Fisher, 1976; Buggy et al., 1979).

These microinjection experiments have been the subject of some controversy (Andersson, 1973; Peck, 1973; Peck and Blass, 1975), because the osmolality of the injected solutions was outside the physiological range of normal body fluids and well above the 1.5–2.0% increase shown to elicit drinking after systemic injections (see above). Peck and Blass (1975) have argued that dilution, occurring as a consequence of diffusion through the tissues immediately surrounding

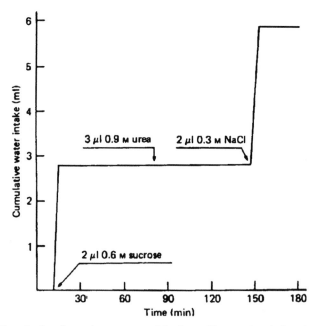

Fig. 3.5. Water intake of a rat in response to injections of hypertonic solutions into the lateral preoptic area. From: Blass, E. M., and Epstein, A. N. (1971). A lateral preoptic osmosensitive zone for thirst in the rat. *J. Comp. Physiol. Psychol.* **76**, 378–394. Reproduced with permission of the authors and the American Psychological Association.

the cannula implants, may have reduced the effective concentration of the injected solutions before they reached responsive osmosensitive cells. However, the possibility of nonspecific activation of thirst-related but not necessarily osmosensitive neurons cannot be excluded from consideration at this time.

A second problem that is not resolved by the available evidence is the possibility that the effective LPO injections may have acted upon the ependymal or circumventricular receptors, which Andersson (1978) has postulated on the basis of his observation that icv injections of hypertonic saline elicit drinking.

It is also curious that osmosensitive injection sites have been difficult to find even though most investigators have used relatively large (2 μl) injection volumes that undoubtedly resulted in extensive diffusion. Peck and Novin (1971), for instance, found evidence for osmoreceptors (positive responses to both sucrose and saline but not urea) at only six of 600 injection sites in the rabbit (positive responses to saline but not sucrose were more common in this study). In the rat, the success rate has generally been higher, especially when bilateral injections have been used (Blass and Epstein, 1971), but most investigators (Peck and Blass, 1975; Blass, 1974) report a proportion of negative placements that is puzzling when one considers the fact that the volume of the injection roughly equals the size of the entire target area in the LPO.

Lesions and Electrical Stimulation

Large lesions involving the lateral preoptic area of rats (Blass and Epstein, 1971; Almli and Weiss, 1974; Coburn and Stricker, 1978) and *rabbits* (Peck and Novin, 1971) have been reported to produce persisting impairments in the animal's ability to drink in response to experimentally induced cellular dehydration. In most animals, this is accompanied by impaired responses to polyethylene glycol-induced vascular hypovolemia (an extracellular thirst stimulus), but some investigators have reported apparently selective deficits in drinking to cellular dehydration (Blass and Epstein, 1971; Coburn and Stricker, 1978). Recent experiments have suggested, however, that this specificity may be influenced by the testing procedure. When a range of cellular and extracellular thirst stimuli was used, both types of thirst appeared to be impaired after iontophoretic injections of the neurotoxin kainic acid (KA) into the LPO of rats (McGowan *et al.*, 1988b). The KA-treated animals drank normally, or nearly so, in response to low concentrations of hypertonic saline or polyethylene glycol. However, when high concentrations were used, their response to polyethylene glycol (PG) as well as to salt loads was impaired. This does not, of course, diminish the potential significance of this region as a major target for information about the organism's state of cellular hydration. It suggests, instead, that it may also integrate this information with other thirst-related inputs and exert a more general influence of thirst than had been envisioned in the past.

It also seems unlikely that the lateral preoptic area is the only sensor for cellular thirst. Rats with large LPO lesions are not incapable of responding to cellular dehydration. In the first hours following a salt load, such animals attempt to deal with the problem mainly by increasing renal salt excretion. A delayed increase in water intake is seen, particularly at night when the nocturnal rat consumes 70–80% of its daily intake (Coburn and Stricker, 1978). Rats with LPO lesions also increase their water intake promptly when salt is added to their diet or hypertonic saline is administered intravenously (Coburn and Stricker, 1978).

These observations have led Coburn and Stricker (1978) to suggest that the effects of LPO lesions on water intake may be due to an interruption of fibers of passage, particularly catecholaminergic components of the medial forebrain bundle, which are part of a nonspecific arousal or activation system. According to this interpretation, LPO lesions reduce the normal drinking response to salt loads, not because mechanisms specifically related to cellular thirst are destroyed but because the animal cannot adequately cope with the stress of the experimental treatment.

The demonstration by McGowan *et al.* (1988b) that iontophoretic application of the neurotoxin kainic acid (which destroys nerve cell bodies without affecting fibers of passage) into the LPO of rats impairs drinking responses to cellular as well as extracellular (polyethylene glycol and angiotensin II) stimuli indicates that an interruption of fibers of passage may not be responsible for the effects of LPO lesions on water intake.

General disturbances in fluid regulation have also been reported (Almli *et al.*, 1976) after large LPO lesions were made in 10-day-old infant rats. When tested as juveniles or adults, these rats were hyperdipsic under ad libitum conditions and when tested after water deprivation or polyethylene glycol-induced hypovolemia. However, they showed impaired responses to cellular dehydration. It is not clear whether a disturbance of antidiuretic hormone release may contribute to this peculiar syndrome.

A different, although possibly not entirely unrelated, syndrome has been reported after much smaller lesions involving only the medial-most region of the anterior preoptic area—the area surrounding the anteroventral aspects of the third ventricle (AV3V) (Buggy and Johnson, 1977a,b; Johnson and Buggy, 1978; Lind and Johnson, 1981, 1982a,b,c). Rats with such lesions were adipsic for a number of days after surgery but recovered essentially normal ad libitum water intake. However, these animals retained a seemingly permanent deficit in their ability to drink in response to cellular dehydration as well as to most extracellular thirst stimuli.

It is possible that some or all of these effects may reflect damage to medial components of the MPO rather than cells lining the third ventricle itself. McGowan *et al.* (1988a) have reported that kainic acid-induced neuronal depletion from the MPO significantly reduced the drinking response to cellular as well as extracellular (PG and isoproterenol) thirst stimuli administered at high doses. Ad libitum water intake or the drinking response to low doses of hypertonic saline or PG was not affected in this series of experiments. Electrolytic lesions restricted to the ependymal lining of the anterior third ventricle and immediately adjacent tissues had no significant effects on ad libitum water intake or the response to any of the dipsogens tested.

A significant attenuation of drinking responses to increased plasma sodium has also been reported in dogs (Thrasher *et al.*, 1980a,b) and sheep (McKinley *et al.*, 1980; 1982) with lesions in the region of the AV3V and the adjacent organum vasculosum of the lamina terminalis (OVLT). These species appear to depend less than the rat on the mechanisms contained in this region, however, since their ad libitum water intake is not significantly modified by the lesion.

Lesions in the rostromedial zona incerta (ZI) just caudal to the dorsal aspects of the preoptic region produce a complete loss or extremely severe impairment of responding to subcutaneous (sc), ip, or iv injections of a wide range of doses of hypertonic saline in the rat (Grossman and Grossman, 1978; McDermott and Grossman, 1980a,b; Rowland *et al.*, 1979; Walsh and Grossman, 1976, 1978; Walsh *et al.*, 1977) (Fig. 3.6). Evered and Mogenson (1976) have reported intact drinking to hypertonic saline in rats with caudal ZI lesions, but the results of this experiment are difficult to interpret since the minuscule dose of salt administered in their test elicited only negligible water intake in controls as well.

Rats with rostromedial ZI lesions do retain the ability to excrete an exogenous salt load gradually (Rowland *et al.*, 1979). They do not, however, supplement this ability by delayed increased drinking even when iv infusions of saline are administered (Rowland *et al.*, 1979), as rats with LPO lesions have been reported to do (Coburn and Stricker, 1978).

Rats with rostromedial ZI lesions drink essentially normal or slightly less than normal quantities of water when it is available ad libitum, and respond normally to water deprivation if dry food is available during the deprivation period. They are, however, adipsic when food deprived and show variable deficits in responding to extracellular thirst stimuli. Drinking after exposure to icv or iv angiotensin or ip isoproterenol is abolished (Walsh and Grossman, 1978; Rowland *et al.*, 1979), while the response to hypovolemia induced by sc formalin or polyethylene glycol is normal or nearly so (Grossman and Grossman, 1978; Walsh and Grossman, 1976, 1978) (see Grossman, 1984, 1986, for review).

The effects of rostromedial zona incerta lesions on water intake appear to be due to the destruction of cellular components of the region, since the basic syndrome (including impaired responsiveness to hypertonic saline) has been reproduced by iontophoretic application of the neurotoxin kainic acid to the region, which resulted in extensive cellular depletion but no demonstrable destruction of fibers of passage (Brown and Grossman, 1980). That nigrostriatal projections, in particular, are not involved in the ZI lesion syndrome has been

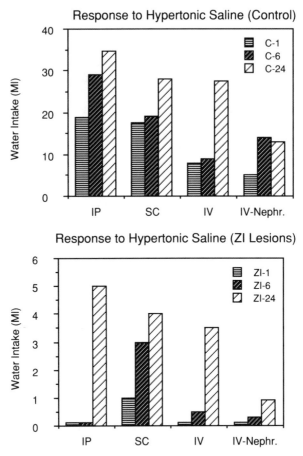

Fig. 3.6. Water intake for intact controls (top) and rats with rostromedial zona incerta lesions (bottom) 1, 6, and 24 h after injections of hypertonic saline. Five milliliters of 1 M NaCl solution was administered ip and sc. The iv infusion consisted of 1.5 ml of 2 M NaCl solution administered over 45 min. The iv infusion was repeated 2 h after nephrectomy. Data from: (1) Grossman, S. P., and Grossman, L. (1978). Parametric study of the regulatory capabilities of rats with rostromedial zona incerta lesions: Responsiveness to hypertonic saline and polyethylene glycol. *Physiol. Behav.* **21**, 432–440. And (2) Rowland, N., Grossman, L., and Grossman, S. P. (1979). Zona incerta lesions: Regulatory drinking deficits to intravenous NaCl, angiotensin but not to salt in the food. *Physiol. Behav.* **23**, 745–750.

demonstrated in experiments showing no loss of dopamine from the striatum following behaviorally effective electrolytic lesions (Walsh *et al.*, 1977).

Lesions in lateral and caudal portions of the zona incerta or adjacent tissues have been reported to produce varying degrees of hypodipsia that appears to be related to motor deficits involving the tongue (Evered and Mogenson, 1976).

Rats with such lesions also show typically small deficits in responding to various thirst stimuli that are difficult to interpret in view of these motor disturbances.

Electrical stimulation of the zona incerta has been reported to specifically and uniquely elicit drinking (in contrast to stimulation of electrode sites in the immediately adjacent lateral hypothalamus, which gave rise only to feeding responses in these studies) (Olds *et al.*, 1971; Huang and Mogenson, 1972).

Review and Conclusions

Systemic injections of solutions that contain osmotically active solutes that are excluded from cells or traverse the cell membrane only with difficulty elicit drinking and stimulate hormonal mechanisms that promote the retention of water and excretion of salts by the kidney. Both effects are due to cellular dehydration rather than an increase in the absolute osmotic pressure of the blood per se.

There are marked individual as well as species differences with respect to the relative importance of the two responses to salt loads. Some animals (and species) rely mainly on drinking and the resulting dilution of plasma; others deal with the problem primarily by excreting the salt in highly concentrated urine.

When the contribution of the kidney is prevented by nephrectomy, animals drink almost precisely enough water to restore the tonicity of their body fluids to normal levels. The complementary experiment, surprisingly, does not demonstrate a similarly precise regulation. When one administers a salt load and prevents the animal from drinking until the excess salt has been excreted, animals nonetheless drink substantial quantities of water. The cause of this drinking is not understood.

It is likely that both the behavioral (i.e., drinking) and renal (water conservation and solute excretion) responses to salt loads are due to the activation of osmoreceptors in most species (the goat and possibly the sheep being the principal known exceptions). These cells are thought to be sensitive to changes in their size or volume (or, possibly, to the movement of water across their membrane).

Although osmoreceptors have been found in several peripheral organs, including the liver, it is believed that both thirst and kidney-related osmoreceptors reside in the brain. The results from several experimental paradigms (including single-cell electrophysiology; microinjections and electrolytic as well as neurotoxin-induced lesions) agree in demonstrating ADH (vasopressin) related osmoreceptors in the supraoptic and paraventricular nuclei of the preoptic area. Thirst-related osmoreceptors have been identified in the lateral preoptic region, anteroventral third ventricle and organum vasculosum of the lamina terminalis.

Chapter 4

Extracellular Thirst I: Hypovolemia, Hyponatremia, and Hypotension

Hypovolemia

Humans and other complex animals cannot survive unless blood volume and pressure remain within narrow limits that guarantee an uninterrupted supply to all parts of the body. We cannot, in the context of our discussion of thirst and salt appetite, describe the intricate physiological mechanisms that regulate the pumping action of the heart and the distensibility of the arterial and venous blood vessels. We shall concentrate, instead, on the neural and endocrine processes that conserve and replenish plasma when fluid intake fails to keep up with obligatory water loss.

Fluid is constantly lost from plasma through evaporation from skin and lungs, sweat secretion, and waste removal in urine and feces. Initially, vascular volume and composition are maintained by the withdrawal of fluid and electrolytes from interstitial spaces. Eventually, the extracellular environment becomes sufficiently concentrated that osmotic pressure begins to extract fluid from the cellular fluid compartment. This gives rise to cellular dehydration thirst.

Unless water is obtained promptly, cells become increasingly unable to give up water, and blood volume (and pressure) decreases. This vascular hypovolemia is the cause of neural as well as hormonal events, which add a second powerful "extracellular" thirst stimulus. Water deprivation that continues for a significant period of time always results in a combination of cellular and extracellular thirst.

Under some unusual conditions, hypovolemic thirst occurs in the absence of cellular dehydration. It has long been known, for instance, that a sudden loss of blood, due to injury or to excessive fluid loss from the GI tract as a result of diarrhea, produces intense thirst (see Wolf, 1958, or Fitzsimons, 1979, for a review of the classic literature). Cellular dehydration cannot be responsible for this thirst because the loss of isotonic plasma does not alter the osmotic pressure of the extracellular fluid and thus does not cause an efflux of water from cells.

The mechanisms responsible for extracellular thirst have only relatively re-

43

cently become the object of systematic experimental attention. We therefore do not yet have as clear a picture as we do in the case of cellular dehydration thirst, particularly because there may be several extracellular thirst mechanisms that may be able to function independently under some circumstances.

It is well established that a 10–15% decrease in plasma volume elicits drinking as well as elevated plasma antidiuretic hormone (ADH), which decreases urine flow in the rat (Fitzsimons, 1961b; Stricker, 1966) as well as the dog (Szczepanska-Sadowska, 1973).

In addition to bleeding (Fitzsimons, 1961b), several different techniques have been used to deplete plasma volume experimentally. These include depletion of plasma sodium (which results in osmotic gradients that force extracellular fluid into cells) (Holmes and Cizek, 1951; Swanson et al., 1935; Falk, 1961) and injections of highly concentrated colloids that sequester plasma in intraperitoneal (Fitzsimons, 1961a) or subcutaneous (Stricker, 1966) edemas. It has also been found that surgical procedures that lower blood pressure in the heart and/or kidney without actually inducing hypovolemia produce thirst (Fitzsimons, 1964, 1969a). Beta-adrenergic drugs that have pronounced hypotensive effects, such as isoproterenol, also are powerful dipsogens in many species (Lehr et al., 1967; Peskar et al., 1970).

There is considerable experimental evidence that extracellular thirst may be mediated by neural as well as hormonal mechanisms. A fall in blood volume (and pressure) modulates the activity in the low-ressure chambers of the heart and associated veins of stretch and pressure receptors that exert tonic influences on brain ADH secretion (Linden and Kappagoda, 1982). Fitzsimons (1979) has suggested that similar receptor mechanisms may also transmit to the brain signals that activate mechanisms concerned with extracellular thirst.

Mechanical stimulation of these receptors by means of inflating balloons implanted into the junction of the pulmonary vein and left atrium of the heart of dogs has been shown to decrease ad libitum water intake as well as drinking after the beta-adrenergic agonist isoproterenol (Fitzsimons and Moore-Gillon, 1980a). In rats, the inflation of balloons implanted into the junction of the superior vena cava and right atrium of the heart has been shown to decrease ad libitum as well as deprivation-induced water intake as well as the response to various extracellular thirst stimuli (Kaufman, 1984, 1986b).

Vascular hypovolemia or hypotension also release renin from the kidney. Renin acts on circulating substrate (angiotensinogen) to form angiotensin I which, in turn, is converted into angiotensin II. The latter is the most potent dipsogen (thirst-inducer) known to humans. Angiotensin may affect thirst (as well as ADH secretion) by acting directly on the brain but may also modulate the sensitivity of vascular stretch or pressure receptors in the great veins and/or atria of the heart. There is much evidence, as we shall see, that the renin–angiotensin system may be responsible for extracellular thirst under many circumstances.

However, other mechanisms must be available since plasma hypovolemia can elicit drinking in nephrectomized as well as adrenalectomized rats (Fitzsimons, 1961b, 1969b).

Hemorrhage

Thirst after hemorrhage is a commonly reported clinical observation. The phenomenon has been curiously difficult to demonstrate experimentally, possibly because the thirst system that is responsive to extracellular hypovolemia responds only to relatively large fluid losses, which are sufficiently debilitating to interfere with behavioral regulation.

In the rat, the removal of 10–15% of the total blood supply has been reported to elicit drinking in normal as well as in nephrectomized animals (Fitzsimons, 1961b; Oatley, 1964) and to increase water intake after salt loads (Oatley, 1964) or deprivation (Fitzsimons and Oatley, 1968). The amount of water consumed is directly proportional to the amount of blood removed over a significant range of values (Russell et al., 1975) (Fig. 4.1).

In the dog, there is a puzzling report that the removal of 20–40% of the total blood volume did not induce drinking or enhance the effects of a salt load (Holmes and Montgomery, 1953). More recent reports have presented evidence of significant drinking and facilitated osmotic thirst after 15% or more of the normal blood volume was removed (Szczepanska-Sadowska, 1973; Kozlowski and Szczepanska-Sadowska, 1975; Ramsay and Thrasher, 1986).

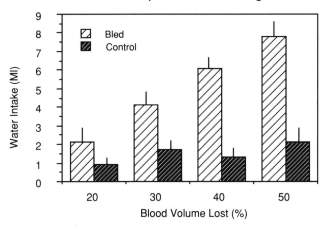

Fig. 4.1. Water intake during 5 h following hemorrhage in rats. After: Russell, P. J. D., Abdelaal, A. E., and Mogenson, G. J. (1975). Graded levels of hemorrhage, thirst and angiotensin II in the rat. *Physiol. Behav.* **15**, 117–119. With permission of the authors and Pergamon Press.

In humans, there are many anecdotal clinical reports of thirst after blood loss (see Wolf, 1958), but an experimental investigation of the phenomenon failed to find consistent evidence of thirst in blood donors who had 500 ml (approximately 10% of total blood volume for a 150-pound person) removed by venous puncture (Holmes and Montgomery, 1951, 1953).

Hyponatremia

Historically, the first indication that cellular dehydration cannot account for thirst under all conditions came from clinical and experimental reports of increased thirst after sodium chloride deprivation, which dilutes the extracellular fluid and causes a movement of water into cells (Elkinton and Squires, 1951; Strauss, 1957).

More recent experiments have used peritoneal or intravenous dialysis to remove sodium from the extracellular fluids. In these experiments, an isotonic glucose solution is injected and allowed to equilibrate with extracellular fluid, before a comparable quantity of fluid, containing sodium chloride and other electrolytes, is removed. The procedure results in a rapid removal of sodium and other electrolytes from extracellular fluid. This, in turn, causes water to move into cells and thus produces extracellular hypovolemia (Fig. 4.2).

In the rat, salt-deficient diets increase water intake reliably (Swanson *et al.*, 1935; Radford, 1959). Intraperitoneal glucose dialysis also increases water intake and elicits a preference for a hypertonic (3%) saline solution (Falk, 1965a,b) (Fig. 4.3).

Significant plasma sodium depletions have been recorded within 30 min after the injection of a hypertonic load, but the preference for hypertonic saline develops only after a delay of as much as 12–24 h (Ferreyra and Chiaraviglio, 1977). The salt appetite persists for several days in spite of the fact that quantities of sodium far in excess of the amount removed in the dialysis are ingested within the first 24 h of the dialysis (Falk, 1966; Ferreyra and Chiaraviglio, 1977). Even extremely large intraperitoneal salt loads do not abolish the excessive ingestion of hypertonic saline after dialysis (Falk and Lipton, 1967).

Continuous intracerebroventricular (icv) infusions of isotonic artificial cerebrospinal fluid (CSF) during the 24 h after peritoneal dialysis have been reported to decrease the intake of hypertonic saline significantly (Chiaraviglio and Pérez-Guaita, 1986). Intracerebroventricular infusions of a hypertonic saline solution containing the same total amount of salt during the first 8 h of the dialysis (when sodium depletion is maximal) had no effect on saline intake. Similar infusions of hypertonic saline administered 16–24 h after the onset of the dialysis produced the most severe inhibitory effects on salt appetite in these experiments.

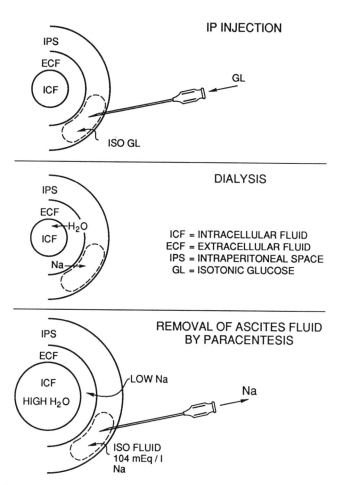

Fig. 4.2. Water and electrolyte changes produced by intraperitoneal dialysis. From: Falk, J. L., and Tang, M. (1980). Rapid sodium depletion and salt appetite induced by intraperitoneal dialysis. *In*: "Biological and Behavioral Aspects of Salt Intake" (M. R. Kare, M. J. Fregly, and R. A. Bernard, eds.), pp. 205–220. Academic Press, New York. Reproduced with permission of the authors and Academic Press.

In the dog (Cizek *et al.*, 1951) and rabbit (Huang, 1955), peritoneal glucose dialysis increases water intake after an initial period of general depression that may last 24–48 h.

A classic experiment by McCance (1936a) found that human subjects depleted of sodium by a salt-deficient diet and repeated sweat-inducing heat treatments complained of unusual taste sensations that some of the subjects identified as thirst, although the sensations were not alleviated by the ingestion of water.

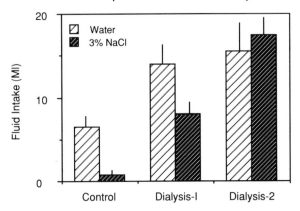

Fig. 4.3. Water and hypertonic saline intake on a 1-h test following intraperitoneal dialysis. The second dialysis test was given 2 days after the first and resulted in significantly greater saline intake. Water intake was not significantly different on the two dialysis tests. After: Falk, J. L. (1965a). Water intake and NaCl appetite in sodium depletion. *Psych. Reports* **16**, 315–325. With permission of the author and the American Psychological Association.

Experimental Edema

That the thirst induced by hyponatremia (above) is not due to cellular overhydration, as some investigators have suggested (Wolf, 1950, 1958), was demonstrated by Stricker (1969), who found that intragastric injections of distilled water that increased cellular as well as extracellular hydration did not elicit drinking in rats.

That vascular hypovolemia itself might be the essential stimulus had been suggested earlier by Fitzsimons's (1961b) observation that intraperitoneal injections of hyperoncotic concentrations of the colloid polyethylene glycol (PG) significantly increased water intake in rats.

Polyethylene glycol disrupts the Starling equilibrium of capillaries and withdraws isotonic protein-free plasma from the circulation. Intraperitoneal (Fitzsimons, 1961b) or subcutaneous (Stricker, 1966, 1968) injections of PG sequester fluid in an edema formed at the site of injection. The more concentrated the injection, the higher its oncotic pressure and the larger the edema. The decreased vascular volume equilibrates with interstitial fluid so that a general depletion of extracellular fluid results. Because the osmolality of extracellular fluid is not affected, cellular hydration remains unchanged. (Fitzsimons, 1961b; Stricker, 1968; Stricker and MacArthur, 1974).

It has been suggested that transient changes in osmotic pressure (Stricker,

1969; Almli, 1971; Weiss and Almli, 1975a) or sodium depletion (Tang, 1976) (sodium, as well as water, is sequestered in the edema and thus becomes unavailable to the organism) may contribute to the drinking response to PG, particularly during the first hours after the injection when the edema is formed. However, it is well established that hypovolemia *per se* is the principal cause of the effect of PG on water intake.

An hour or two after the injection of PG, rats begin to drink and conserve water as well as sodium by reducing urine flow (Stricker, 1966, 1968; Cort, 1952; Fitzsimons, 1961b), at least in part because of increased secretion of antidiuretic hormone (Dunn *et al.*, 1973) and aldosterone (Stricker *et al.*, 1979). The animals continue to drink for about 24 h, consuming a significant amount of water, which is proportional to the quantity of extracellular fluid sequestered in the edema (Stricker, 1968; Leenen and Stricker, 1974).

Only a small percentage of the ingested water remains in the circulation because water dilutes plasma and thus creates osmotic pressure gradients that cause the movement of water into the intracellular compartment. When only water is available, rats stop drinking after 8–12 h, in spite of continuing vascular hypovolemia and a general dilution of body fluids that may reach 8–10% (Stricker, 1969, 1971a). The cessation of drinking after PG is presumably due to osmotic dilution (Stricker, 1969, 1971b).

The increased water intake after PG is fully present in nephrectomized rats, indicating the effect is not mediated by the renin–angiotensin system (Fitzsimons, 1961b; Stricker, 1973).

When saline is available in addition to water, rats drink mostly water during the first 5–6 h after subcutaneous injections of PG, even though sodium is needed for the restoration of the vascular fluid volume. During the following 12–18 h they ingest significant quantities of saline (even in concentrations that are sufficiently hypertonic to be mildly aversive under normal circumstances), but continue to ingest enough water so that the total fluid ingested remains hypotonic (Stricker, 1981) (Fig. 4.4).

The animals retain most of the sodium ingested during this second phase and eventually reverse the hyponatremia of the extracellular fluid. This draws water out of cells and helps to restore a normal vascular fluid volume (Jalowiec and Stricker, 1970a,b). Sodium intake continues after plasma volume has been replenished, increased excretion by the kidney taking care of the overshoot (Stricker and Jalowiec, 1970; Jalowiec and Stricker, 1970b; Stricker, 1981).

The osmolality and volume of the body's fluids, indeed, cannot return to normal levels until enough salt is ingested to reverse the dilution of the cellular (and extracellular) fluids that occurs during the initial phase of hypovolemic thirst when only water is ingested. But why is the sodium appetite so delayed, and what, precisely, triggers it? Vascular dilution (or the accompanying cellular overhydration) could be the event that terminates water drinking after hypo-

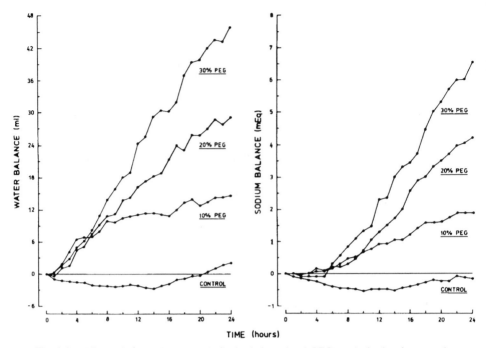

Fig. 4.4. Effects of sc injections of 5 ml of polyethylene glycol (PEG) on the intake of water and a 0.5 M NaCl solution. The data are expressed as water and sodium "balance" (intake minus urinary loss). From: Stricker, E. M. (1981). Thirst and sodium appetite after colloid treatment in rats. *J. Comp. Physiol. Psychol.* **95**, 1–25. Reproduced with permission of the author and the American Psychological Association.

volemia. Could it also provide the critical stimulus for salt appetite? The answer is not entirely clear at this time.

When both water and saline are withheld during the first 8 h after the onset of extracellular hypovolemia, so that vascular dilution and cellular overhydration do not develop, little saline or water is ingested when first offered even though salt appetite is normally well established at this time (Stricker and Wolf, 1966). Yet, when both water and saline are withheld for 24 h in the same experiment, rats avidly drink a mixture of both that produces the isotonic fluid needed to restore the volume and composition of their body fluids.

When an acute sodium loss is added to vascular hypovolemia, as a consequence of sc injections of formalin, which damages cellular and capillary membranes at the injection site, rats develop a salt appetite much more rapidly than after PG treatments that result in comparable effects on vascular volume.

When both water and saline are withheld for 8 h after the formalin injection, hypertonic saline is consumed avidly when first offered. This is quite different from the PG-treated rat, which presumably suffers from comparable hypovolemia without the acute sodium loss produced by formalin. One might conclude that hyponatremia is the critical stimulus for salt appetite in these studies, but acute osmotic dilution produced by water loads did not elicit salt appetite in the same experiments (Stricker, 1966; Stricker and Wolf, 1966; Jalowiec and Stricker, 1970a).

The evidence for hypovolemia itself is similarly conflicting. High doses of PG produce a volume deficit of ~25% 6 h after the injection when salt appetite first becomes prominent. Is it possible that this represents a threshold? Stricker (1968) demonstrated that far lower doses of PG produce significant salt appetite even though they never produce comparable plasma deficits. Moreover, volume deficits develop more rapidly after higher concentrations of PG yet the onset of sodium appetite appeared to be unrelated to concentration (Stricker and Jalowiec, 1970; Stricker, 1980). Very high doses of PG have, in fact, been reported to increase water drinking without producing a delayed sodium appetite (Stricker, 1971b; 1973).

Stricker (1981) has suggested that salt appetite after PG might be delayed because hypovolemic thirst initially overrides the early manifestations of salt appetite. This hypothesis accounts for the typical pattern of ingestion by proposing the following interplay of influences: The ingestion of water during the first 5 h after PG results in rapid osmotic dilution and a consequent reduction of hypovolemic thirst. This permits the behavioral manifestation of salt appetite. The resulting ingestion of hypertonic saline, in turn, reduces osmotic dilution and reinstates hypovolemic thirst. The animal then "cycles" between draughts of saline and draughts of water, the proportion between the two fluids being a function of the tonicity of the saline solution. Sodium appetite becomes more and more prominent as the original stimulus for thirst, vascular hypovolemia, is gradually eliminated.

The hypothesis is supported by the observation (Stricker, 1981) that rats maintained on a salt-deficient diet prior to PG treatments drank saline promptly, skipping most of the first stage of water ingestion normally seen after this treatment. The pattern of salt and water ingestion in these experiments was affected by the duration of the preinjection salt deprivation in a manner consistent with the proposed interpretation.

These findings are compatible with Denton's (1966) earlier suggestion that salt appetite may be result of activation of receptors in the brain that monitor the availability of salt in extracellular fluid (see also Stricker, 1981).

Caval Ligation

Ligation of the abdominal inferior vena cava, which carries about 30% of the venous return to the heart, decreases arterial blood pressure and elicits drinking in the rat (see Fig. 4.5). The procedure also sharply reduces urine volume as well as urine sodium and potassium excretion (Fitzsimons, 1964, 1969a). Although

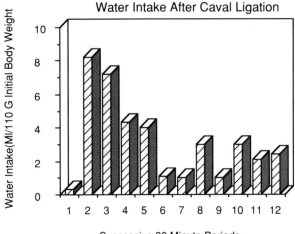

Fig. 4.5. Water intake during 6 h following caval ligation above the renal veins in the rat. After: Fitzsimons, J. T. (1969a). The role of renal thirst factor in drinking induced by extracellular stimuli. *J. Physiol.* **201**, 349–368. With permission of the author and the Physiological Society, Oxford, England.

the increased water intake and decreased urine flow result in a considerable dilution of the body fluids, rats given a choice of water or 1.8% saline select water during the initial 6-h period following caval ligation.

The kidneys appear to play a major role in the development of thirst after caval ligation, since the effect is markedly reduced after nephrectomy (Fitzsimons, 1964, 1969a). Unfortunately, this potentially very important observation is difficult to interpret because the behavioral competence of the nephrectomized animal is compromised by general malaise as well as a redistribution of fluids throughout the body.

Partial occlusion of the thoracic inferior vena cava also produces drinking, ADH secretion, and urine retention in dogs. The effect is decreased by systemic or central injections of the competitive angiotensin blocker saralasin (Thrasher *et al.*, 1982c, 1983; Ramsay *et al.*, 1975). Similar effects can be produced by inflation of a balloon inside the inferior vena cava. The response to balloon inflation is reduced but not abolished by saralasin (Fitzsimons and Moore-Gillon, 1979, 1980b).

A selective fall in the pressure of the renal arteries, produced by partial constriction of either the abdominal aorta above the renal arteries or the renal arteries themselves, elicits copious drinking, lasting for several hours, and reduces urine flow and electrolyte excretion. The effects are reduced after nephrectomy and appear similar to those seen after caval ligation (Fitzsimons, 1969a).

The fact that the effects of caval ligation are reduced by nephrectomy as well as systemic or central injections of the competitive angiotensin blocker saralasin indicates that angiotensin may be responsible, at least in part, for the increased water intake. However, other, possibly neural mechanisms also are likely to contribute, since neither nephrectomy nor saralasin eliminates the effects of caval ligation completely.

Occlusion of the abdominal aorta between the renal arteries causes the left kidney to secrete excessive amounts of renin. This is presumably responsible for the increased intake of water and hypertonic saline seen in this preparation, since the effects are abolished by nephrectomy (Rojo-Ortega and Genest, 1968; Costales *et al.*, 1984). It is interesting to note that bilateral ligation of the ureters themselves also increases plasma renin activity and drinking, an effect that does not appear to be due to anuria itself since the nephrectomized rat does not overdrink (Fitzsimons, 1986).

Beta-Adrenergic Thirst

Beta-adrenergic drugs are powerful hypotensive agents, which decrease blood pressure by a direct action on smooth muscle. They also act on renal receptors, and the two effects add to release renin (Ganong, 1972). In the rat and dog, isoproterenol (also called isoprenaline), the most commonly used beta-adrenergic drug, elicits copious drinking and antidiuresis (Lehr *et al.*, 1967; Falk and Tang, 1973; Falk and Bryant, 1973; Fitzsimons and Szczepanska-Sadowska, 1973; Ramsay, 1978) (Fig. 4.6). Goats (which also do not drink in response to

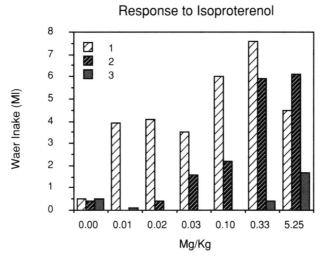

Fig. 4.6. Water intake 1, 2, and 3 h after various doses of isoproterenol. Data from: Lehr, D., Mallow, J., and Kurkowski, M. (1967). Copious drinking and simultaneous inhibition of urine flow elicited by beta-adrenergic stimulation and contrary effect of alpha-adrenergic stimulation. *J. Pharm. Exptl. Therap.* **158**, 150–163.

renin or angiotensin) (Anderson and Westbye, 1970) appear to be unresponsive to isoproterenol (Olsson and Rundgren, 1975).

Propranolol, a beta-adrenergic blocking agent, prevents the dipsogenic as well as renin-releasing activity of beta-adrenergic agonists such as isoproterenol (Lehr *et al.*, 1967; Gutman *et al.*, 1971; Meyer *et al.*, 1971b, 1973).

Isoproterenol-induced drinking is significantly attenuated during the inflation of a balloon that is chronically implanted at the junction of the pulmonary vein and left atrium of the heart (Fitzsimons and Moore-Gillon, 1980a).

There are several reports that nephrectomy abolishes the drinking response to isoproterenol in the rat (Houpt and Epstein, 1971; Meyer *et al.*, 1971a,b) as well as the dog (Rolls and Ramsay, 1975). However, more recent investigations have indicated that removal of the kidney does not block the drinking response to isoproterenol completely in the rat (Rettig *et al.*, 1981) or the dog (Szczepanska-Sadowska and Fitzsimons, 1975; Ramsay, 1978; Ramsay and Thrasher, 1986).

Ramsay and Thrasher (1986) have suggested that nephrectomy may abolish drinking in response to low doses of beta-adrenergic drugs, which release renin but have relatively small effects on blood pressure. Higher doses, which produce major effects on blood pressure, would be expected to strongly stimulate the cardiovascular stretch receptor and thus activate an extrarenal mechanism that is responsible for the effectiveness of the drug in nephrectomized animals.

Stricker (1978a) has argued that the failure of the nephrectomized rat to respond to isoproterenol under many circumstances might reflect general malaise and lack of behavioral competence due to an inability to maintain blood pressure within acceptable limits. In support of this interpretation, Stricker and associates (Hosutt *et al.*, 1978) demonstrated that nephrectomized rats that did not drink in response to isoproterenol did so when blood pressure was increased by the administration of pressor agents such as epinephrine.

The relationship between beta-adrenergic thirst, renin release, and neural responses to decreased blood pressure levels is complex and not yet fully elucidated. Clonidine, an alpha-adrenergic agonist that decreases blood pressure and inhibits renin release (Laubie and Schmitt, 1977; Pettinger *et al.*, 1976), attenuates the dipsogenic action of isoproterenol (Fregly and Kelleher, 1980; Fregly and Rowland, 1986). The alpha-2-adrenergic antagonists yohimbine and tolazoline have been reported to facilitate the drinking response to isoproterenol at doses that did not affect ad libitum drinking (Fregly *et al.*, 1983; Fregly and Rowland, 1986). The alpha-adrenergic receptor blocker phentolamine, which lowers blood pressure and increases plasma renin (Meyer and Herttig, 1973, 1975), induces drinking, much like isoproterenol (Meyer *et al.*, 1973).

Matters are further complicated by a report that several direct-acting hypotensive drugs do not elicit drinking even though they increase renin activity (Falk *et al.*, 1973). Moreover, propranolol, which antagonizes the dipsogenic effects of beta-adrenergic drugs, does not interfere with the hypotensive action of some compounds (Falk *et al.*, 1973).

Attempts to relate beta-adrenergic thirst to the renin–angiotensin system more directly also have produced mixed results. Isoproterenol-induced drinking in the rat is significantly reduced by iv infusions of antiserum to angiotensin II (Abdelaal *et al.*, 1974). However, iv infusions of the competitive angiotensin receptor blocker sarcosine-1-alanine-8-angiotensin II (saralasin), which blocks the drinking response to renin or angiotensin, have been reported not to attenuate the drinking response of rats to isoproterenol or other hypotensive agents (Tang and Falk, 1974). Conflicting positive results have been observed in dogs (Rolls and Ramsay, 1975). As yet, this story does not have a happy ending. Schwob and Johnson (1975) have reported inhibitory effects of intracranial injections of saralasin on beta-adrenergic drinking in the rat.

The pattern of results observed in the rat suggests that beta-adrenergic thirst may be mediated by a central effect of angiotensin, since saralasin does not readily cross the blood–brain barrier (Hoffman and Phillips, 1976c). This interpretation does not, however, account for reports of enhanced isoproterenol drinking after sc injections of SQ 20881, an inhibitor of the enzyme that converts inactive angiotensin I to the dipsogenic angiotensin II (Lehr *et al.*, 1973, 1975). The facilitatory effect of SQ 20881 was reduced or abolished by nephrectomy, indicating that it was mediated by angiotensin of renal origin. In contrast to the effectiveness of intracranial saralasin (above), it was found that intraventricular injections of the converting-enzyme inhibitor SQ 20881 reduced the drinking response to systemically administered renin but failed to reduce isoproterenol-induced drinking in these experiments.

Although the effects of isoproterenol on blood pressure, renin release, and drinking are temporally associated (Leenen and McDonald, 1974), there is no clear quantitative or temporal relationship between the effects of various other hypotensive agents on plasma renin activity and the drinking response to them (Leenen *et al.*, 1975).

Isoproterenol has been reported not to elicit salt appetite in short-term experiments (Fitzsimons and Wirth, 1978). Long-term observations, which might be important in view of the generally delayed salt appetite seen after other extracellular challenges, have not yet been performed.

Mechanical Stimulation of Atrial Receptors

Kaufman (1984, 1986a,b) has reported a significant decrease in (a) ad libitum water intake, (b) water intake after 24 h of deprivation, (c) drinking in response to polyethylene glycol or (d) to isoproterenol, as well as (e) sodium appetite, in rats after the inflation of balloons surgically implanted into the superior vena cava at the junction with the right atrium of the heart. The balloon inflation did not reduce drinking in response to osmotic stimuli. It also had very little influence on plasma renin activity and did not prevent the normal increase of plasma renin after polyethylene glycol (PG) or isoproterenol, suggesting that the observed inhibitory effects on the drinking response to various extracellular stimuli were mediated by direct stimulation of neural receptors rather than activation of the renin–angiotensin system.

Inflation of right-atrial/superior vena cava balloons 17 h after the administration of PG reduced the sodium intake of rats previously maintained on a salt-deficient diet. However, when the balloons were deflated after 2 h, the experimental animals increased their saline intake so that at the end of a 6-h test no significant differences between the experimental and control groups remained (Kaufman, 1986a).

Rats that developed a salt appetite after being maintained on a low-salt diet and treated with the mineralocorticoid DOCA for 8 consecutive days also drank less of a hypertonic saline solution during the inflation of right-atrium/super vena cava balloons. These results further support the hypothesis that the effects of the balloon procedure reflect direct stimulation of neural receptors, since long-term DOCA treatments are known to result in a return to normal sodium levels and a suppression of the renin–angiotensin system (the so-called "mineralocortical escape") (Kaufman, 1986a).

In dogs, inflation of a balloon implanted into the pulmonary vein near its junction with the left atrium also has been reported to reduce ad libitum water intake as well as the drinking response to the beta-adrenergic agonist isoproterenol, presumably because stretch receptors sensitive to increases in blood pressure were stimulated by the procedure (Fitzsimons and Moore-Gillon, 1980a).

Atrial Natriuretic Factor

In 1981, deBold and associates (deBold et al., 1981) reported the discovery of a hormone, now called atrial natriuretic factor (ANF) or atriopeptin, which appears to play a significant, if as yet incompletely understood, role in the regulation of blood pressure and extracellular body fluid regulation (Fig. 4.7).

The polypeptide hormone exerts a potent, rapid but short-lived diuretic and natriuretic effect (deBold et al., 1981) accompanied by regional vasorelaxation (Winquist, 1986), hypotension (Currie et al., 1983), and an inhibition of aldosterone (Atarashi et al., 1984; Elliott and Goodfriend, 1986), renin (Freeman et al., 1985), and vasopressin (Samson, 1985) secretion (see deBold, 1986, for review).

Although there has been a great deal of interest in ANF and much progress in identifying the structure of its component peptides, their receptors, and genetic code, our knowledge of its normal functions in intact organisms is, as yet, unsystematic and quite incomplete (see Blaine, 1986, for review).

deBold's pioneering experiments (deBold et al., 1981) demonstrated that ex-

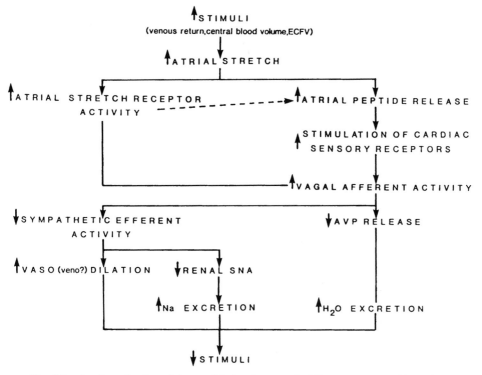

Fig. 4.7.   A schematic view of the possible involvement of ANF in the control of body fluid balance. From: Gellai, M., Allen, D. E., and Beeuwkes R. (1986). Contrasting views on the action of atrial peptides: lessons from studies of conscious animals. *Fed. Proc.* **45**, 2387–2391. Reproduced with permission of the authors and The Federation of American Societies for Experimental Biology.

tracts of rat atrial tissue produced a marked natriuresis and diuresis in rats. Subsequent research has shown that extracts from the atria of water-deprived rats (Johnson, 1985) or salt-loaded animals (Ackerman and Irizawa, 1984) have higher natriuretic activity than extracts from control animals. Prolonged water deprivation has also been reported to reduce the amount of immunoreactive atriopeptin in plasma while increasing cardiac atriopeptin stores (Takayanagi *et al.*, 1985).

When these extremely water-deprived animals were challenged with hypertonic saline (1.8% NaCl in the drinking water), cardiac stores of atriopeptin decreased and plasma levels rose (Takayanagi *et al.*, 1985). Rats fed a high-salt diet for 2 weeks had significantly lower levels of cardiac atriopeptin than controls. Rats maintained on a low-salt diet had elevated levels (Manning *et al.*, 1985).

Acute hypervolemia releases atriopeptin (Pettersson *et al.*, 1985) and results in transient natriuresis and diuresis (Veress and Sonnenberg, 1984). A causal relationship between the increased atriopeptin release and the renal response to hypervolemia is indicated by experiments that have shown that the natriuretic and diuretic response to acute volume expansion is greatly attenuated by right-atrial appendectomy (which removes the source of endogenous atriopeptin without interfering with the effects of exogenous atriopeptin) (Veress and Sonnenberg, 1984).

There is a strong correlation between increased right-atrial pressure and atriopeptin release (Lang et al., 1985), and there is evidence of vasopressin-induced release that appears to be specifically related to the pressor activity of the hormone (Manning et al., 1985). The interaction between atriopeptin and vasopressin is, however, complex, since the atrial factor has been reported to reduce the increase in plasma vasopressin normally seen after dehydration or hemorrhage (Samson, 1985).

Lowered atrial pressure may produce opposite, inhibitory effects on this system, since ligation of the thoracic inferior vena cava has been shown to abolish basal urine output of sodium as well as the natriuretic response to exogenous atriopeptin (Freeman et al., 1985).

Atrial natriuretic factor has been reported to inhibit basal aldosterone synthesis (Atarashi et al., 1984; Kudo and Baird, 1984; Goodfriend et al., 1984) as well as the secretion normally stimulated by angiotensin, potassium, ACTH, and prostaglandin E_2 (Atarashi et al., 1984; Kudo and Baird, 1984).

This brief review of the recent literature on ANF clearly indicates that the hormone can affect hormonal and hemodynamic mechanisms that play a major role in the regulation of extracellular body fluids. It is, however, premature to conclude that it does so under normal circumstances. Although many investigators in the field enthusiastically pursue the hypothesis that ANF may be a major influence on extracellular fluid regulation and, indeed, provide a "counterbalance to the renin–angiotensin system" (Blaine, 1986), the meager data so far available do not yet support this conclusion. Indeed, it has recently been suggested that ANF may play a rather modest local modulator role in controlling atrial stretch and that it may be released in sufficient quantities to assume hormonal functions at distant (e.g., renal, adrenal) sites only as a result of "extreme provocation" such as pharmacological doses of vasopressin or extreme atrial distension or volume expansion (Gellai et al., 1986). Far more research is clearly needed before we can determine whether ANF is indeed an important variable in extracellular thirst.

Review and Conclusions

A 10–15% decrease in plasma volume elicits drinking and decreases urine flow (mainly because of increased ADH secretion). A pronounced salt appetite develops after a delay of 6–8 h. These effects have been experimentally produced in several species, including rats and dogs. There are also clinical reports of thirst after blood loss in humans. The effects of extracellular hypovolemia cannot be due to cellular dehydration because the loss of isotonic plasma does not result in significant persisting perturbations of osmotic relationships between cellular and extracellular fluids.

Vascular hypovolemia causes the release of renin from the kidney. Renin acts on substrate in blood to form angiotensin I, which in turn is converted to angiotensin II. Angiotensin II (A-II) is a powerful dipsogen. Nephrectomy, as well as the administration of drugs that inhibit the formation of A-II or block its action at the receptor, reduces the drinking response to many extracellular thirst stimuli. Renin may exert its effects by acting directly on thirst-related cells in the brain or indirectly by modulating the sensitivity of stretch receptors in the atria of the heart and the great veins leading to it. (The role of the renin–angiotensin system is discussed in greater detail in Chapter 5.)

The fact that the response to extracellular thirst stimuli is not abolished by nephrectomy or pharmacological blockade of the renin–angiotensin system (although it is significantly reduced under many circumstances) indicates that an alternate or additional mechanism must exist. There is much evidence that stretch or pressure receptors in the in the atria of the heart may provide a neural channel of information about blood volume and pressure to the brain.

It is not necessary to actually remove extracellular fluid from the body in order to produce a state of extracellular hypovolemia. A transfer of fluid from the extracellular to the cellular compartment can be achieved by depleting plasma of sodium either chronically by a salt-deficient diet or acutely by intraperitoneal dialysis with isotonic glucose. The resulting loss of salt from plasma produces osmotic forces that cause the movement of water into the relatively more concentrated cellular compartment. As one might predict, thirst and a delayed sodium appetite result.

Thirst and delayed sodium appetite are also produced when extracellular fluid is sequestered in an edema. Although still inside the body, the fluid is no longer available for circulation. The most commonly used procedure for producing such an edema experimentally is to inject polyethylene glycol (PG) ip or sc. This compound exerts strong oncotic pressures, which result in the movement of isotonic fluid from plasma into the region of the injection where it is retained.

Extracellular thirst can also be produced by experimental procedures that lower blood pressure. This can be achieved surgically by ligating the inferior vena cava, which carries about 30% of the venous return to the heart.

Also effective are some (although apparently not all) hypotensive drugs. The most commonly used drug is isoproterenol, a beta-adrenergic compound that elicits copious drinking and antidiuresis in many species, including rats and dogs. Propranolol, a beta-adrenergic blocking agent, prevents the dipsogenic effects of isoproterenol.

Nephrectomy reduces or abolishes beta-adrenergic drinking under some but not all circumstances. It has been suggested that nephrectomy may abolish drinking in response to low doses of beta-adrenergic drugs, which release renin but have relatively small effects on blood pressure. Higher doses, which produce major effects on blood pressure and would be expected to strongly stimulate cardiovascular stretch receptor, may activate an extrarenal neural mechanism that is responsible for the effectiveness of the drug in nephrectomized animals.

The failure of the nephrectomized rat to respond to isoproterenol under many circumstances may also be caused by a lack of behavioral competence due to an inability to maintain blood pressure within acceptable limits.

Stimulation of receptors in the atria and great veins as a result of the inflation of a balloon inserted into the junction of the superior vena cava with the right atrium has been reported to produce a significant decrease in (a) *ad libitum* water intake, (b) water intake after 24 h of deprivation, (c) drinking in response to polyethylene glycol or (d) to isoproterenol, as well as (e) sodium appetite.

Increased pressure in the right atrium of the heart releases atrial natriuretic factor (ANF) or atriopeptin, which appears to play a significant role in the regulation of blood pressure and extracellular body fluid volume and composition. The polypeptide hormone exerts a potent, rapid but short-lived diuretic and natriuretic effect, and produces regional vasorelaxation, hypotension, and inhibition of aldosterone, renin, and vasopressin secretion. The nature of the relationship between this hormonal response to increased right-atrial pressure and various extracellular dipsogens remains to be elucidated.

Chapter 5

Extracellular Thirst II: The Renin–Angiotensin System

Introduction

All "extracellular" thirst stimuli reduce blood volume and/or pressure by (a) removing extracellular fluid from the body (hemorrhage), (b) sequestering it in a peritoneal or subcutaneous edema (polyethylene glycol, formalin), (c) preventing its normal circulation (ligation of thoracic or abdominal vena cava or renal arteries), or (d) dilating blood vessels (beta-adrenergic agonists).

There is much evidence that these changes in blood volume and/or pressure are sensed by neural receptors in the great veins and low-pressure chambers of the heart. Signals from these receptors reach the brain via vagal and sympathetic afferents. It is almost certain that this provides thirst-related brain mechanisms with important information about the status of the organism's extracellular fluid balance.

However, extracellular thirst stimuli also activate hormonal mechanisms, which act on peripheral as well as central mechanisms to produce vasoconstriction and renal conservation of water and sodium as well as thirst. Although other hormones [such as aldosterone and glucocorticoids from the adrenal gland, and vasopressin (antidiuretic hormone) from the hypothalamo-pituitary axis], play a significant role in the organism's hormonal response to extracellular thirst stimuli, the principal and in many respects primary mechanism is the renin–angiotensin system.

The proteolytic enzyme renin is manufactured, stored, and released by secretory cells in the kidney. Renin is released when the perfusion pressure of the renal vascular bed drops or the concentration of sodium in the macula dentata of the kidney falls. The renin-secreting cells are innervated by beta-adrenergic neurons. Renin is consequently also released in response to sympathetic stimulation, irrespective of changes in renal blood flow or ion concentration. Much evidence suggests that volume receptors in the thoracic veins and atria of the heart may be an important source of sympathetic neural input to the renin-secreting cells. Changes in the volume and/or perfusion pressure of the general circulation thus may have several inputs to the renal renin–angiotensin system.

Renin and its precursors are physiologically inactive and have a relatively short half-life in the circulation (15–20 min in the rat, 45–80 min in the dog) (Laragh and Sealy, 1973). After its release into the general circulation, renin acts on its substrate angiotensinogen to produce angiotensin I (A-I), which is also physiologically inactive. Angiotensin I is converted into the physiologically active angiotensin II (A-II) by angiotensin-converting enzyme. This reaction takes place mainly in the lungs. Angiotensins I and II are inactivated in a single passage through the circulation and their half-lives, therefore, are short. The principal biologically active degradation product of A-II is angiotensin III, which has dipsogenic, pressor, and aldosterone-stimulating effects in some species (Wright et al., 1984; Blair-West et al., 1971; Türker, 1986).

The principal function of the renin–angiotensin system is the behavioral and renal control of blood volume. Angiotensin has pronounced dipsogenic properties, which will be the principal subject of the following discussion. It also plays a major role in the control of the synthesis and release of aldosterone and corticosterone from the adrenal gland (which increases reabsorption of sodium and water by the kidney) (Peart, 1969) as well as vasopressin (antidiuretic hormone) from the hypothalamo-pituitary system (which decreases urine flow) (Mouw et al., 1971; Shade and Share, 1975). In addition, angiotensin has powerful vasomotor effects, acting directly as a vasoconstrictor on vascular smooth muscles and indirectly by stimulating peripheral sympathetic nerves and brain mechanisms that influence vasomotor functions.

Although angiotensin exerts important influences on these hormonal and neural functions, other mechanisms also operate, particularly in their long-term control (Blair-West et al., 1973; Cadnapaphornchai et al., 1975; McCaa et al., 1975). Removal or blockade of the renin–angiotensin system therefore does not abolish regulatory influences over blood volume and pressure entirely.

The Role of Angiotensin in Thirst

Just how the dipsogenic properties of angiotensin fit into this general picture is not yet entirely clear. Fitzsimons (1966, 1969a, 1970a,b, 1979) has suggested that angiotensin may play a major role in mediating the effects of hypovolemia and hypotension on thirst. He proposed that the dipsogenic effects of angiotensin may be mediated by at least two distinct mechanisms. Increased renin release may heighten the sensitivity of vascular stretch receptors in the great veins and low-pressure atria of the heart. This would amplify the effects of hypovolemia or hypotension on a neural pathway that appears to inform the central nervous system of the need to replenish extracellular fluid. The second mechanism postulated by Fitzsimons assumes a direct action of angiotensin on thirst-related angiotensin receptors in the brain.

The hypothesis that the renin–angiotensin system plays an important role in the regulation of water intake as well as water and sodium conservation is attractive because all "extracellular" thirst stimuli release renin (e.g,. Stricker, 1973; Fitzsimons, 1973, 1979). It has nonetheless been questioned because:

1. The correlation of thirst or water intake and plasma renin or angiotensin activity is not always as good as one might expect.
2. Doses of exogenous angiotensin that appear high when compared to normal plasma values often elicit only disappointingly small increases in water intake.
3. Nephrectomy, which effectively removes the source of endogenous renin, produces little effect on the drinking response to some extracellular thirst stimuli.
4. Drugs that prevent the conversion of the physiologically inactive angiotensin I to the dipsogenic angiotensin II do not completely block extracellular thirst.
5. Drugs that block angiotensin receptors are similarly ineffective under some circumstances.
6. Angiotensin does not cross the blood–brain barrier and could thus act only on certain circumventricular organs known to permit relatively easy access of blood-borne substances to neural tissue. Evidence for a separate brain renin–angiotensin system exists (Ganong, 1984), but its functional significance is controversial and plausible mechanisms for its interaction with plasma angiotensin have yet to be elucidated.

As we examine each of these questions in some detail below, it is useful to keep in mind that the renin–angiotensin system almost certainly never carries the entire burden of control over extracellular fluid volume and pressure under normal physiological circumstances. Water deprivation, undoubtedly the most common cause of primary thirst, elicits cellular dehydration signals that probably contribute prepotent signals for drinking, at least in the short term. Even unusual circumstances that give rise to primary hypovolemia and/or hypotension without cellular dehydration almost certainly activate neural mechanisms. These may well be able to function effectively without the assistance of the renin–angiotensin system except under extreme conditions such as those often existing in laboratory experiments designed to elucidate the mechanisms controlling extracellular thirst.

Far from questioning the importance of the renin–angiotensin system in thirst, these comments are designed to emphasize the fact that it operates within the framework of a complex system of multiple neural and hormonal influences, which interact to accomplish the intricate tasks of regulating the volume and composition of body fluids. The fact that its influence may not always be readily apparent under some experimental conditions should not be interpreted lightly to indicate its failure to contribute importantly under normal physiological circumstances.

The Dipsogenic Properties of Renin and Angiotensin

It has long been known that ip injections of renal extracts increase water intake in intact as well as nephrectomized animals (Nairn *et al.*, 1956; Asscher and Anson, 1963; Fitzsimons 1969a). More recently, it has been shown that the active principle in these extracts is renin and, more specifically, its product, angiotensin II (Fig. 5.1)

Systemic administration of renin and/or angiotensin has been shown to be an effective dipsogen in many species, including mammals such as the rat (Fitzsimons and Simons, 1968, 1969), rabbit (Fitzsimons, 1975), cat (Cooling and Day, 1975), and dog (Tripodo *et al.*, 1976), as well as birds such as the pigeon (Evered and Fitzsimons, 1976a,b) chicken (Snapir *et al.*, 1976), and sparrow (Wada *et al.*, 1975). The phenomenon of angiotensin-induced drinking has also been reported in such unusual laboratory animals as eel (Hirano *et al.*, 1978), iguana (Fitzsimons and Kaufman, 1977), and euryhaline killifish (Malvin *et al.*,

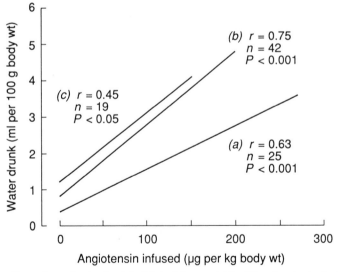

Fig. 5.1. Regressions of water drunk in 6 h by (*a*) normal rats, (*b*) nephrectomized rats, and (*c*) nephrectomized/adrenalectomized rats on the total amount of angiotensin infused. The right-hand limit of each regression line indicates the highest dose administered to that group. From: Fitzsimons, J. T. (1979). "The Physiology of Thirst and Sodium Appetite." Cambridge: Cambridge University Press. Reproduced with permission of the author and Cambridge University Press.

1980). A few species have been found to respond poorly or not at all to systemic renin–angiotensin, including *mongolian gerbils* (Wright *et al.*, 1984), goats (Andersson and Westbye, 1970), and sheep (Abraham *et al.*, 1975).

Intracranial injections of angiotensin, in doses too small to produce systemic effects, have been shown to be dipsogenic in every species tested to date (including some, such as the goat, sheep, and gerbil, that do not drink in response to systemic angiotensin). The long list includes mammals such as the rat (Booth, 1968; Epstein *et al.*, 1969), gerbil (Block *et al.*, 1974), cat (Sturgeon *et al.*, 1973), monkey (Setler, 1971), goat (Andersson and Westbye, 1970), sheep (Abraham *et al.*, 1975), and opossum (Elfont *et al.*, 1980), as well as birds such as the pigeon (Evered and Fitzsimons, 1976a,b), sparrow (Wada *et al.*, 1975), chicken (Snapir *et al.*, 1976), and duck (de Caro *et al.*, 1980a,b). In rat pups, icv angiotensin is dipsogenic as early as the second day of life when most other thirst stimuli are as yet ineffective (Misantone *et al.*, 1980; Ellis *et al.*, 1984).

Intracerebroventricular angiotensin injections appear to produce specific effects on thirst-related motivational systems, since angiotensin elicits drinking as well as water-rewarded instrumental behaviors such as bar-pressing (Rolls *et al.*, 1972) but has no effect on or even decreases deprivation-induced food intake (McFarland and Rolls, 1972). Gastric preloads of water or isotonic saline reduce the drinking response to icv angiotensin II in a dose-dependent manner, water being twice as effective as saline (Rolls and McFarland, 1973).

Are Physiological Doses of Angiotensin Dipsogenic?

Many of the early investigations of the dipsogenic properties of renin or angiotensin used doses, both systemically and centrally, that proved to be far beyond the normal physiological range, and the significance of the phenomenon has consequently been questioned.

Stricker (1977, 1978a; Stricker *et al.*, 1976), for instance, reported that ip injections of renin produced far less drinking than extracellular thirst stimuli such as polyethylene glycol or isoproterenol, which elevated plasma renin activity to comparable levels.

Stricker argued that the effects of exogenous renin and angiotensin, while statistically significant, were too small to have practical significance. According to his calculations, renin- or A-II-induced drinking can dilute body fluid by no more than 1 or 2%, an amount that would not come close to restoring blood volume or pressure under most circumstances. Stricker proposed that the renin-angiotensin system might play merely a "permissive" role in thirst by maintaining blood pressure within a range that allows the animal to make appropriate behavioral responses (such as seeking and consuming water) to extracellular thirst stimuli.

Hosutt *et al.* (1978) supported this interpretation by showing that nephrectomized rats, which did not drink in response to isoproterenol, did so when
pressor agents such as epinephrine were administered to restore blood pressure.
Atkinson *et al.* (1979) similarly reported that low doses of renin that did not elicit
drinking in nephrectomized rats did so when administered together with isoproterenol. Atkinson suggested that isoproterenol cannot be dipsogenic unless a
small quantity of renin/angiotensin is present in plasma.

Plasma renin may not provide a good measure of A-II activity, particularly
under experimental conditions that deplete essentially all endogenous renin (e.g.,
nephrectomy) or result in plasma levels that may exceed the normal capabilities
of the system. The concentration of angiotensin II is influenced by the availability of angiotensinogen (which converts renin into A-I) and angiotensin-
converting enzyme (which converts the physiologically inactive A-I into the
dipsogenic A-II). The ability of the renin–angiotensin system to display up- or
down-regulation under abnormal circumstances remains to be explored.

When plasma levels of A-II were measured directly by radioimmunoassay
(Mann *et al.*, 1980) in nephrectomized as well as intact rats, doses of A-II known
to produce reliable drinking responses in this species (Hsaio *et al.*, 1977) were
found to produce plasma A-II concentrations that were lower than those seen
after 14 or 48 h of water deprivation, caval ligation, dipsogenic doses of
isoproterenol, or polyethylene glycol-induced hypovolemia (Johnson *et al.*,
1981b; Mann *et al.*, 1980) (Fig. 5.2).

More recently, Wright *et al.* (1987) have reported significant positive correlations between plasma angiotensin levels and drinking after PG or isoproterenol in
rats and gerbils. The water intake resulting from sc injections of hypertonic
saline was not accompanied by detectable changes in plasma angiotensin.

In the dog, Fitzsimons *et al.* (1978b) obtained prompt and significant drinking
after iv infusions calculated to produce increases in arterial concentration within
the physiological range. Angiotensin infused into one carotid artery was even
more effective (presumably because of a direct action on central mechanisms),
even though it did not produce a measurable increase in blood pressure.

Robinson and Evered (1986) have recently argued that the drinking response
to exogenous renin or angiotensin may be small in the intact animal not because
A-II is a merely "permissive" component of extracellular thirst as Stricker (1977,
1978a) has suggested, but because hypertensive reactions in the intact animal
may interfere with consummatory behavior.

According to this argument, endogenous renin is normally released only in
response to extracellular thirst stimuli that cause hypovolemia and/or hypotension. The release of renin helps to restore normal blood pressure under these
circumstances, and this may facilitate behavioral responses such as searching for
and ingesting water. However, when renin or angiotensin is administered to

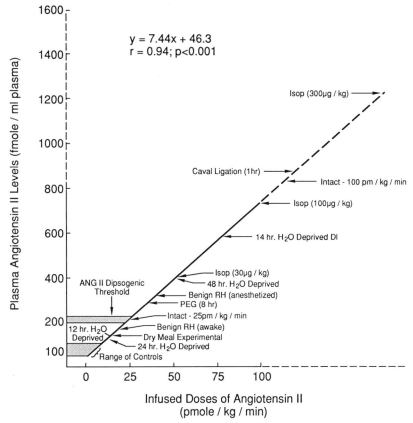

Fig. 5.2. Regression line of the relationship between doses of angiotensin II in the dipsogenic range (25 and 100 pmol/kg/min infused for 60 min) and plasma levels of angiotensin II. Also shown are the plasma angiotensin levels measured after various dipsogens. Abbreviations: DI, diabetes insipidus; RH, renal hypertension; PEG, polyethylene glycol; Isop, isoproterenol. From: Johnson, A. K., Robinson, M. M., and Mann, J. F. E. (1986). The role of the renal renin-angiotensin system in thirst. *In*: "The Physiology of Thirst and Sodium Appetite" (G. deCaro, A. N. Epstein, and M. Massi, eds.), pp. 161–180. Plenum Press, New York. Reproduced with permission of the authors and Plenum Press.

normotensive animals, hypertension results and this interferes with the behavioral responses to the dipsogenic actions of the renin–angiotensin system.

In support of this argument, Robinson and Evered (1986) demonstrated that low doses of angiotensin that produced plasma levels comparable to those seen after only 12 h of water deprivation caused copious drinking when administered in conjunction with vasodilators such as isoproterenol, diazoxide, or minoxidil (Fig. 5.3). (The angiotensin-converting-enzyme inhibitor captopril was concur-

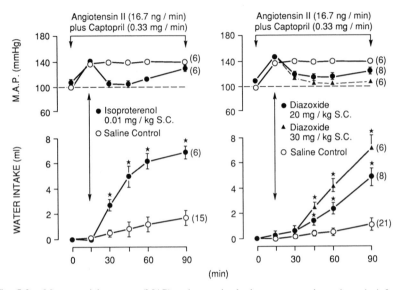

Fig. 5.3. Mean arterial pressure (MAP) and water intake in response to iv angiotensin infusions (combined with captopril, which prevents the endogenous synthesis of A-II). Significant drinking was observed when the pressor response to angiotensin was prevented by isoproterenol or another vasodilator diazoxide (administered at the large arrow). The dose of captopril used was sufficient to block the drinking response to the vasodilators administered alone. After: Robinson, M. M., and Evered, M. D. (1986). Angiotensin II and arterial pressure in the control of thirst. *In*: "The Physiology of Thirst and Sodium Appetite" (G. deCaro, A. N. Epstein, and M. Massi, eds.) pp. 193–198. Plenum Press, New York. With permission of the authors and Plenum Press.

rently infused in these experiments in doses sufficient to block the dipsogenic properties of the vasodilators themselves, which depend upon the release of renin from the kidney and its conversion to A-II.)

In humans, Rolls *et al.* (1986) have reported that only four of 10 male subjects increased their water intake after iv infusions of A-II that produced plasma levels "far in excess" of those seen under physiological conditions. There were no differences in plasma A-II between the four men who increased their water intake after the infusion and the remaining six who did not. Moreover, 24 h of fluid deprivation did not reliably elevate plasma A-II levels in this study, a result that calls into question the significance of an earlier report of reliable effects of fluid deprivation on plasma renin activity in human subjects (Maebashi and Yoshinaga, 1967).

In sheep, it has been reported (Abraham *et al.*, 1975) that iv, intracarotid, or icv injections of A-II failed to elicit drinking when administered in doses that produced blood or CSF levels comparable to those seen after various thirst-inducing experimental procedures. Higher "pharmacological" doses were dipsogenic in this investigation.

Since comparable studies, using only doses known to produce effects within the normal physiological range, have not yet been conducted in many of the species known to drink in response to renin or angiotensin, the significance of the apparent species generality of the effect remains to be established.

Facilitation of Responses to Cellular and Extracellular Thirst Stimuli

Angiotensin has been reported to facilitate drinking in response to various extracellular thirst stimuli as well as cellular dehydration.

Nephrectomized rats that drink little in response to caval ligation displayed nearly normal drinking when iv infusions of angiotensin were combined with the ligation procedure (Fitzsimons and Simons, 1969). Drinking did not appear to be due solely to the angiotensin infusion, since rats given angiotensin in conjunction with caval ligation drank more than controls that received only angiotensin (Fig. 5.4).

Systemic injections of angiotensin have also been reported to enhance the drinking response of rats, dogs, and iguanas to hypertonic saline (Fitzsimons and Simons, 1969; Kozlowski et al., 1972; Fitzsimons and Kaufman, 1977). This suggests a general facilitatory effect on thirst mechanisms not confined to extracellular stimuli.

That this may involve a direct action of angiotensin on the brain is indicated by

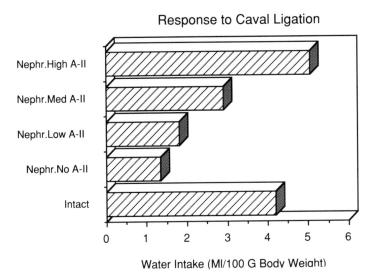

Response to Caval Ligation

Water Intake (Ml/100 G Body Weight)

Fig. 5.4. The effect of iv infusions of low (20–39 μg/kg), medium (40–79 μg/kg), and high (80–163 μg/kg) doses of angiotensin II on the water intake of nephrectomized rats after caval ligation. After Fitzsimons and Simons (1969).

the observation that intracranial injections of angiotensin also increase the drinking response to hypertonic saline, PG-induced hypovolemia, and intracranial carbachol (Fitzsimons 1970b; Severs *et al.*, 1974; Fitzsimons and Setler, 1975).

Extracellular Thirst after Blockade of the Renin–Angiotensin System

Renin and other components of the renin–angiotensin system have been found not only in the kidney but also in other tissues including the brain. The possible functional significance of extrarenal angiotensin is essentially unknown, although there has been much speculation about the functions of a brain iso-renin/angiotensin system (see Chapter 8).

It is generally accepted that the kidney is the sole significant source of circulating renin. Nephrectomy should completely eliminate this source and thus permit a direct evaluation of its role in extracellular thirst.

This seemingly logical argument unfortunately fails to take into account the fact that hypovolemia and hypotension not only release renin but also affect neural receptors that affect hemodynamic mechanisms directly as well as indirectly and probably provide a separate neural input to thirst-related brain mechanisms. This parallel neural pathway may be able to maintain normal or nearly normal drinking to some extracellular thirst stimuli even though the renin–angiotensin system normally participates in the organism's response to them. The survival of drinking responses to specific extracellular thirst stimuli in nephrectomized animals must thus be interpreted with caution.

Conversely, diminished or absent drinking in nephrectomized animals may reflect nonspecific debilitating effects of extracellular thirst stimuli that share the ability to deplete vascular volume and/or induce hypotension—conditions known to result in disorientation and to interfere with coordinated behavior in general.

The effect of nephrectomy on drinking responses to various extracellular thirst stimuli has nonetheless been investigated, and it is appropriate to summarize the relevant findings briefly (see related sections of Chapter 4, Extracellular Thirst Stimuli, p. 43, for additional detail).

Nephrectomy

Bilateral removal of the kidney has been shown to (a) abolish the drinking response to isoproterenol in the rat (Houpt and Epstein, 1971; Meyer *et al.*, 1971a) but not in the dog (Szczepanska-Sadowska and Fitzsimons, 1975), which drinks avidly; (b) severely attenuate but not abolish completely the increased water intake seen after caval ligation in the rat (Fitzsimons, 1969a); (c) reduce only slightly the drinking observed in rats after hemorrhage (Fitzsimons, 1961b);

(d) have no significant effect (Fitzsimons, 1961b; Fitzsimons and Stricker, 1971) or reduce only slightly (Blass and Fitzsimons, 1970) the drinking response to the hypovolemia induced by ip or sc injections of polyethylene glycol; and (e) have no significant effect on water intake after deprivation (Rolls and Wood, 1977), even though extracellular stimuli are thought to constitute a significant component of deprivation-induced thirst.

Drug-Induced Blockade

A number of investigators have attempted to elucidate the functions of the renin–angiotensin system by examining the effects of drugs that interfere with the conversion of A-I to A-II or the action of A-II on its receptor.

The results of these experiments should be viewed with caution. When administered systemically, these drugs have hypotensive effects that may be sufficiently severe to produce general behavioral depression, manifest in a reduced responsiveness to thirst in general, or, if less severe, may themselves act as extracellular thirst stimuli (Stricker, 1977, 1978a). The currently available drugs also have other "side effects" that may interfere with drinking in various nonspecific ways.

It has been argued that these problems can be circumvented by intracerebral injections of very small quantities, but this may be a questionable assumption in view of the fact that intracranial injections of angiotensin itself can produce increased blood pressure and vasopressin release (Severs et al., 1966, 1970; Ueda et al., 1972).

Antiserum to Angiotensin II
Intracerebroventricular injections of anti-A-II serum have been shown to inhibit the drinking response to subsequent icv injections of angiotensin II. Intravenous injections of antiserum also have been reported to block drinking after PG-induced hypovolemia or isoproterenol (Abdelaal et al., 1974a).

Competitive Angiotensin Receptor Blockers
The drug most commonly used to block angiotensin receptors is sarcosine-1-alanine-8-angiotensin II (saralasin or P113) (See Türker, 1986, for detail on 8-substituted analogues of angiotensin).

Intravenous injections of saralasin have been reported to inhibit drinking responses to iv renin or A-II in the rat (Vaughn et al., 1973; Tang and Falk, 1974; Summy-Long and Severs, 1974) without reducing drinking response to hypertonic saline (Summy-Long and Severs, 1974) or such extracellular thirst stimuli as various beta-adrenergic agonists (Tang and Falk, 1974), PG-induced hypovolemia (Summy-Long and Severs, 1974), or caval ligation (Rolls and Wood, 1977) (Fig. 5.5).

That an angiotensin receptor blocker should not interfere with cellular dehydration thirst is not surprising. However, the reported failures of such drugs to interfere with various extracellular thirst stimuli have been the cause of some concern in view of the widely accepted notion that the renin–angiotensin system is a major source of information about the status of extracellular, and particularly vascular, fluid.

Mann *et al.* (1978, 1981) have suggested that the reported failures may be due to the fact that low doses of saralasin may be ineffective because they interfere with the recovery of hypotension that is responsible for renin release in the first place without completely blocking drinking-related angiotensin receptors. Very high doses, on the other hand, have marked agonistic effects (Mann *et al.*, 1978) that stimulate rather than inhibit aspects of the renin–angiotensin system. In support of this hypothesis, Mann *et al.* (1981) demonstrated that slow iv infusions of saralasin did reduce drinking after vena cava ligation.

Intracerebral (icv as well as intraparenchymal) injections of saralasin inhibit drinking to iv as well as icv angiotensin in the rat (Fitzsimons, 1975; Fitzsimons *et al.*, 1978a; Felix *et al.*, 1986), dog (Lee *et al.*, 1981), and sheep (Abraham *et al.*, 1976) without inhibiting the response to systemic hypertonic saline (Summy-Long and Severs, 1974; Lee *et al.*, 1981; Abraham *et al.*, 1976) or deprivation-

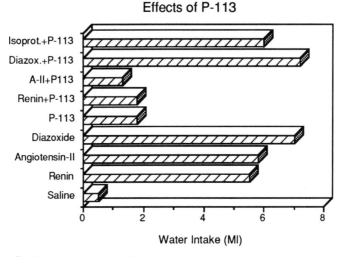

Fig. 5.5. Continuous iv infusions of the angiotensin-blocking analogue saralasin (P–113) significantly attenuate the drinking response to renin and angiotensin II but have no effect on the response to alpha-adrenergics such as isoproterenol or diazoxide. After: Tang, M., and Falk, J. L. (1974). Sar-Ala angiotensin II blocks renin-angiotensin but not beta-adrenergic dipsogens. *Pharm. Biochem. Behav.* **2**, 401–408. With permission of the authors and Pergamon Press.

induced water intake (Phillips and Hoffman, 1977; Lee *et al.*, 1981; Ramsay and Reid, 1975; Abraham *et al.*, 1975, 1976). In the rat, there is a report of delayed and reduced drinking after icv saralasin (Malvin *et al.*, 1977), but the data suggest that the effect may be due to nonspecific debilitation since the reduced intake appears to be due entirely to periods when drinking was abolished completely rather than a general reduction in the rate of ingestion.

In view of the controversy surrounding the failure of systemic saralasin to block drinking in response to various extracellular thirst stimuli, it is interesting to note that intracranial saralasin also has been reported not to interfere with isoproterenol-induced drinking in the rat (Schwob and Johnson, 1975) or the response to caval ligation in the dog (Lee *et al.*, 1981).

Intracerebroventricular injections of Sar-1-Ile-8-angiotensin II (SAR), another angiotensin receptor antagonist, have been reported to reduce salt appetite (as well as water intake) after icv angiotensin in sodium-depleted rats (Weiss, 1986).

Angiotensin-Converting Enzyme Inhibitors

Intracerebroventricular injections of SQ 20881, the first of the angiotensin-converting enzyme inhibitors to be used experimentally in this field have been reported to inhibit drinking responses to icv renin, synthetic renin substrate, and angiotensin I, but to enhance the response to A-II in rat (Fitzsimons, 1975; Fitzsimons *et al.*, 1978a; Severs *et al.*, 1973) and pigeon (Evered and Fitzsimons, 1976b).

Intrahypothalamic injections of SQ 20881 have been reported to inhibit, in a dose-dependent manner, the drinking response to intrahypothalamic renin (Burkhardt *et al.*, 1975) but to have no effect on the response to either A-I or A-II (Burkhardt *et al.*, 1975; Swanson *et al.*, 1973b; Bryant and Falk, 1973).

It has been suggested (Fitzsimons, 1979) that the negative results obtained in some of these experiments may reflect insufficient blockade of central angiotensin-converting enzyme stores, since the ratio of agonist to antagonist was consistently lower than in the investigations that have reported positive effects. The apparent failures may also reflect, at least in part, the possibly less effective intraparenchymal route of administration used in the investigations that failed to observe significant blockade of A-I drinking.

Subcutaneous or intramuscular injections of SQ 20881 have been reported to increase, rather than decrease, drinking in response to isoproterenol, caval ligation, PG-induced hypovolemia, or water deprivation (Lehr *et al.*, 1973; 1975; Summy-Long and Severs, 1974). Since the nonapeptide SQ 20881 does not readily cross the blood–brain barrier, it would appear that these are systemic effects, possibly due to the accumulation of high levels of A-I in the circulation, which may promote its access to regions of the brain where it can be converted into A-II (Lehr *et al.*, 1973).

That the observed facilitatory effect of SQ 20881 in these experiments is, indeed, likely to be renin-dependent is indicated by the observation that nephrectomy reduced or abolished it. Intracerebroventricular injections of SQ 20881 reduced the drinking response to renin, as expected, but had no effect on water intake after isoproterenol or caval ligation (Lehr *et al.*, 1973, 1975). A facilitatory effect on PG-induced hypovolemia was observed in one of these experiments (Summy-Long and Severs, 1974). Combined icv and systemic injections of SQ 20881 prevented the facilitatory effects seen after systemic injections alone but did not depress isoproterenol or PG drinking below baseline (Lehr *et al.*, 1975).

Most contemporary research in this area has used captopril, an angiotensin-converting enzyme inhibitor that is far more powerful than SQ 20882 (Horovitz, 1981). Its effects on extracellular thirst and sodium appetite can be understood (Epstein, 1983, 1986; Lehr *et al.*, 1973) when one considers the following: When low doses of captopril are administered systemically, it does not enter the brain in significant quantities (Cohen and Kurz, 1982). Peripherally, captopril prevents the conversion from A-I to A-II. This should abolish dipsogenic responses to renin as well as angiotensin I since these two substances are themselves inactive. The resulting loss of angiotensin II removes inhibitory feedback to the endogenous renin–secreting mechanisms and therefore facilitates renin release and A-I formation (Schiffrin *et al.*, 1981). The increased availability of A-I in turn promotes its transport into the brain where it is converted into A-II (since the converting-enzyme inhibitor is excluded from brain at low doses). The elevated brain levels of A-II should elicit water intake and salt appetite.

When high doses of captopril are administered systemically the converting-enzyme inhibitor enters the brain in significant quantities (Evered *et al.*, 1980; Cohen and Kurz, 1982). This prevents the conversion of A-I to A-II in brain as well as peripherally and inactivates the excess A-I, which is transported into brain as a consequence of the peripheral effects of captopril or other renin-releasing extracellular thirst stimuli.

In accordance with this model, we find that systemic injections of low doses of captopril elicit some drinking and enhance water intake in response to extracellular thirst stimuli (Elfont and Fitzsimons, 1983; Barney *et al.*,1980; Katovich *et al.*, 1979; Lehr *et al.*, 1973; Mann *et al.*, 1986). These facilitatory effects of low doses of captopril appear to be renin-dependent since they are abolished by nephrectomy (Fitzsimons, 1986).

The facilitatory effects of captopril are also abolished when the blood–brain barrier is surgically compromised (e.g., shortly after the implantation of an icv cannula) or captopril is administered icv in amounts known to block the A-I to A-II conversion centrally.

High systemic doses of captopril (or low systemic doses combined with small icv injections) attenuate water intake elicited by polyethylene glycol (Mann *et al.*, 1986) or partial occlusion of the abdominal aorta between the renal veins (which causes the left kidney, distal to the occlusion, to secrete abnormally large

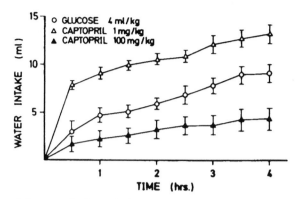

Fig. 5.6. Cumulative water intake beginning 5 h after sc injections of polyethylene glycol. The angiotensin-converting enzyme inhibitor captopril or its vehicle glucose were administered by gastric gavage 4 h after the PG injections. From: Mann, J. F. E., Eisele, S., Ganten, D., Johnson, A. K., Rettig, R., Ritz, E., and Unger, T. (1986). Angiotensin dependent thirst following polyethylene glycol treatment in the rat. *In*: "The Physiology of Thirst and Sodium Appetite" (G. deCaro, A. N. Epstein, and M. Massi (Eds.) pp. 199–203. Plenum Press, New York. With permission of the authors and Plenum Press.

amounts of renin) (Costales *et al.*, 1986; Vijande *et al.*, 1986; Fitzsimons, 1986) (Fig. 5.6).

Intracerebroventricular injections of captopril attenuate the drinking response to icv A-I without affecting drinking response to icv A-II (Moe *et al.*, 1984; Weiss, 1986). Continuous icv infusions of captopril in sodium-depleted (due to furosemide-induced natriuresis and a low-salt diet) rats have been reported to inhibited sodium intake in a dose-dependent manner without affecting ad libitum water (or food) intake (Weiss, 1986).

Peptide Effects Related to A-II

Several peptides have been shown to have dipsogenic properties that may be related to an interaction with the renin–angiotensin system. Among the first to be described and most extensively studied is insulin. When this pancreatic hormone is administered systemically in large pharmacological doses the water intake of rats is increased significantly (Novin, 1964; Booth and Brookover, 1968; Spitz, 1974), although it produces neither hypovolemia nor increased plasma osmolality (Waldbillig and Bartness, 1981). The effect appears to be independent of the hormone's well-known stimulatory effect on food intake.

The dipsogenic properties of insulin are abolished by nephrectomy and attenuated by icv injections of the competitive angiotensin receptor blocker saralasin (Costales *et al.*, 1986).

Large doses of compounds such as captopril or MK-421 that inhibit the conversion of the physiologically inactive A-I to the dipsogenic A-II have been reported to produce an apparently paradoxical enhancement of insulin drinking (Costales *et al.*, 1986). This may be due to the systemic accumulation of A-I, which enters the brain in large quantities where it is converted to A-II since the converting-enzyme inhibitors are thought to be excluded by the blood–brain barrier (Elfont and Fitzsimons, 1981).

Insulin-induced drinking is antagonized by peripheral histamine blockers, which have no significant effect on the rat's ability to respond appropriately to water deprivation (Kraly *et al.*,1983).

There is also a report (Lewis *et al.*, 1979) of prompt and copious drinking as well as delayed sodium appetite in water-replete rats after intracranial injections of nerve growth factor (NGF), a peptide that has been of much recent interest. The authors or this report point out that the pattern of drinking after icv injections of nerve growth factor appeared to be similar, in every respect, to that seen after icv A-II. The relationship between the two dipsogens remains to be studied further.

Review and Conclusions

The kidney releases renin when the perfusion pressure of the renal vascular bed drops or the concentration of sodium in the macula dentata of the kidney falls. Renin is also released in response to sympathetic stimulation, irrespective of changes in renal blood flow or ion concentration.

The principal function of the renin–angiotensin system is the behavioral and renal control of blood volume and pressure. Its influence on renal water and sodium absorption is mainly due to the action of angiotensin II on the synthesis and release of aldosterone and corticosterone from the adrenal gland and vasopressin from the hypothalamo-pituitary system. Blood pressure may be affected by a direct action of renin on the vasculature, a stimulating action on sympathetic nerves, and a direct or indirect action on brain mechanisms that contribute to the regulation of blood pressure. Angiotensin affects thirst, in part because of its influence on blood pressure and volume. It also may have a direct effect on brain mechanisms concerned with the regulation of extracellular fluid.This may be due to a modulating action on baroreceptors in the great veins and atria of the heart and/or a direct effect on circumventricular organs of the brain that control extracellular thirst.

That angiotensin plays an important role in thirst is supported by a large and generally consistent body of evidence, including the following:

1. Systemic injections of angiotensin or its precursors are dipsogenic in many species.
2. Intracranial injections of angiotensin, in doses too small to produce systemic effects, are dipsogenic in every species tested to date.

3. All extracellular thirst stimuli elicit renin secretion and thus increase plasma A-II.

Fitzsimons and others have proposed that extracellular thirst may be mediated, at least in part, by the release of renin from the kidney. Others (e.g., Stricker) have hypothesized that the renin–angiotensin system may play only a permissive role in extracelllular thirst by restoring blood pressure to levels which make it possible for the animal to drink.

The controversy arises because:

1. The correlation of thirst or water intake and plasma renin or angiotensin activity is not always as good as one might expect.
2. Doses of exogenous angiotensin that appear high when compared to normal plasma values or the amounts released in response to extracellular thirst stimuli often elicit only disappointingly small increases in water intake.
3. Nephrectomy, which effectively removes the source of endogenous renin, produces little effect on the drinking response to some extracellular thirst stimuli. (It abolishes the drinking response to isoproterenol in the rat but not in the dog ; severely attenuates but does not abolish completely the increased water intake seen in rats after caval ligation; reduces only slightly the drinking observed in rats after hemorrhage; and has little or no effect on drinking during PG- or formalin-induced hypovolemia. It also has no effect on deprivation-induced water intake, which is thought to have a significant extra-cellular component.)
4. Drugs such as saralasin that competitively block angiotensin receptors block the dipsogenic effects of angiotensin but do not reduce the drinking response to beta-adrenergic agonists, polyethylene glycol, or caval ligation.
5. Drugs such as SQ 20881 or captopril that prevent the conversion of the physiologically inactive angiotensin I to the dipsogenic angiotensin II do not completely block extracellular thirst. Indeed, at low doses they increase rather than decrease drinking responses to several extracellular thirst stimuli. (The effect may be due to an accumulation of A-I in the periphery, which could promote increased uptake into the brain where it is converted into A-II because the conversion blocker does not enter the brain—a logically sound explanation, but many of its assumptions remain to be demonstrated.)

Robinson and Evered have countered some of these arguments by suggesting that the drinking response to exogenous renin or angiotensin may be small in the intact animal not because A-II is a merely permissive component of extracellular thirst as Stricker has suggested, but because hypertensive reactions in the intact animal may interfere with consummatory behavior.

We will encounter additional complications when we discuss the effects of angiotensin and related compounds on the brain (Chapter 8). It is clear that we do not yet fully understand the normal physiological role of angiotensin in thirst, perhaps because the renin–angiotensin system never carries the entire burden of control over extracellular fluid volume and pressure under normal physiological circumstances. Water deprivation, undoubtedly the most common cause of primary thirst, elicits cellular dehydration signals that probably contribute prepotent signals for drinking, at least in the short term. Even unusual circumstances that give rise to primary hypovolemia and/or hypotension without cellular dehydration almost certainly activate neural mechanisms. These may well be able to function effectively without the assistance of the renin–angiotensin system except under extreme conditions such as those often existing in laboratory experiments designed to elucidate the mechanisms controlling extracellular thirst.

Chapter 6

Satiety

Patterns of Drinking

As we have seen, humans as well as other terrestrial mammals maintain the body's fluids and electrolytes within narrow tolerances, and this requires a frequent resupply of stores that are subject to constant obligatory losses. In the artificial laboratory situation where food and water are available ad libitum, the problem is solved simply (at least by the rat, which has been the favorite subject of study) by feeding-associated drinking, which tends to anticipate need and exceeds actual requirements. In this circumstance, the animal becomes a "kidney regulator," consuming more water (as well as sodium in its salty diet) than needed and fine-tuning the system largely by excretion. Modern man tends to follow that example, although the ingestion of fluids is not as tightly tied to meals as it is for the rat.

In more natural habitats where food and water are available only intermittently and rarely concurrently, and drinking may involve exposure to predators, we see a much closer relationship between ingestive behavior and need. When thirst occurs in response to deprivation, many species, including dogs, rabbits, donkeys, camels, sheep, mule, and deer, promptly drink an amount of water that is just about equal to the water deficit they incurred. Others, such as humans, horse, guinea pig, and rat, do not fully compensate before pausing and sustain voluntary dehydration until they eventually consume enough water to cover actual need (Adolph, 1943, 1950, 1964) (Fig. 6.1).

Most of the species that compensate promptly for their actual water needs as soon as water becomes available after a period of deprivation drink very quickly and stop before the ingested water can be absorbed and thus restore cellular and extracellular fluid needs. These animals appear to be able to recognize the magnitude of their fluid deficit and somehow measure the ingested fluid orally and/or gastrically so that they can stop drinking when the appropriate amount of water is ingested even though only little has been absorbed from the intestine.

The dog, for instance, drinks enough water within 2–3 min to compensate

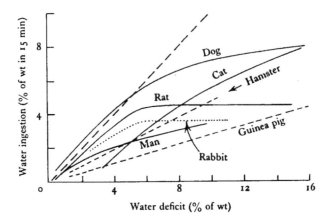

Fig. 6.1.   Relation between initial water ingestion and water deficit in seven species. With high probability, each of the curves is different. Note that all of the curves except for that of the dog fall below the upper dashed line, which represents restoration of the fluid balance. From: Fitzsimons, J. T. (1979). "The Physiology of Thirst and Sodium Appetite." Cambridge University Press, Cambridge. Reproduced with permission of the author and Cambridge University Press.

fully for the fluid deficit incurred during a 24-h fast (Rolls *et al.*, 1980a). Yet significant changes in the concentration and volume of plasma do not become apparent until about 10–12 min after the onset of drinking, and predeprivation baselines are attained only after 45–60 min (Ramsay *et al.*, 1977a). The species that incur voluntary dehydration seem less sure of their ability to accurately meter either need or adequacy of the resupply prior to full absorption. They drink more slowly than the first group and pause, before sufficient water is ingested. Full satiety seems to be achieved in these species only after the ingested water has become absorbed and distributed to the various fluid compartments that have undergone dehydration. Orogastric "metering" is nonetheless evident in the early pauses that interrupt the extended period of intermittent drinking typically seen after deprivation in these species.

Humans and the monkey, for instance drink about 75% of the water needed to make up the deficits incurred during 24 h of deprivation within 5–10 min after water is made available. They then continue to take small additional draughts of water for 30–45 min (Rolls *et al.*, 1980a) (Fig. 6.2). In the monkey, the first major pause coincides with the development of significant cellular rehydration, but drinking continues until both cellular and extracellular fluids have returned to predeprivation concentrations (Wood *et al.*, 1980). In humans, drinking slows significantly as much as 10 min before significant changes in plasma sodium concentration and cellular hydration occur (Rolls *et al.*, 1980a). Drinking continues sporadically until plasma concentration and volume have returned to pre-

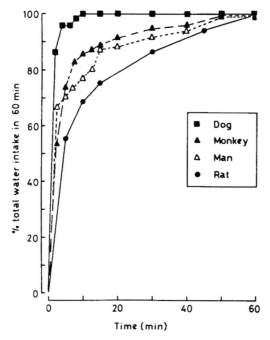

Fig. 6.2. Rate of drinking during the first hour after overnight water deprivation. From: Rolls, B. J., Wood, R. J. and Rolls, E. T. (1980a). Thirst: The initiation, maintenance, and termination of drinking. *In*: "Progress in Psychobiology and Physiological Psychology." Vol. 9 (J. M. Sprague, and A. N. Epstein, eds.) pp. 263–321. Academic Press, New York. Reproduced with permission of the authors and Academic Press.

deprivation baselines about 45–60 min after the onset of drinking (Rolls *et al.*, 1980a).

The rat drinks more slowly than either monkey or humans. Cellular rehydration is all but complete (although plasma volume may remain reduced) at the time drinking terminates (Hatton and Bennet, 1970; Rolls and Wood, 1979; Hall and Blass, 1975; Blass and Hall, 1976).

Preabsorptive Factors

Signals from the mouth and throat do not appear to be essential for the initiation of drinking, as we have seen in Chapter I. However, they do contribute significantly to the maintenance of ingestive behavior, as many experiments on animals with esophageal, gastric, or duodenal fistulae have shown. When animals equipped with esophageal fistulae drink, water wets the mouth and throat but exits from the body before reaching the stomach. Gastric fistulae bypass the mouth and throat and permit the administration of fluids directly into the stomach. Duodenal fistulae go one step further in bypassing the stomach as well.

Esophageal Fistulae

In agreement with Claude Bernard's classic observation, many species (including monkeys, horses, dogs, and rats) "sham drink" far more than the amount required to restore their body's fluid balance (Bellows, 1939; Towbin, 1949; Hall *et al.*, 1976; Maddison *et al.*, 1977).

Modern studies of this phenomenon also show, however, that sham drinking does not continue indefinitely but stops after an amount of water is ingested that is proportional to the animal's physiological need (i.e., the duration of water deprivation). In fact, some species such as sheep, goats, camels, and rabbits are so good at "oral metering" that they sham drink only enough to just about meet the water deficit incurred during deprivation before stopping for a longer rest (Bott *et al.*, 1965; Beilharz *et al.*, 1962; Schmidt-Nielson *et al.*, 1956; Adolph, 1950).

Rats sham drink far more than they ingest normally but do adjust their intake in accordance with the duration of the preceding deprivation period (Blass *et al.*, 1976; Blass and Hall, 1976).

These observations indicate that wetting the mouth and throat provides enough incentive to maintain drinking in all species tested. The fact that drinking does eventually stop and appears to be proportional to water need indicates that many species are capable of estimating the magnitude of their water deficit quite closely and can meter orally ingested water rather precisely.

The mechanisms responsible for this oral metering of water intake are not well understood. Some species have oral receptors that selectively respond to distilled water. Others have receptors that are inhibited by water and, to a lesser extent, by weak saline solutions. The same receptors are activated by hypertonic saline (Liljestrand and Zotterman, 1954; Zotterman, 1956).

It has also been suggested (Andersson and McCann, 1955; Kapatos and Gold, 1972a) that cooling of oral temperature receptors might contribute to satiety. Rats lick a tube from which a puff of cold air emanates whenever the animal touches it. This "air drinking" is seen only in thirsty animals and is proportional to the duration of deprivation. It also reduces subsequent water intake in spite of the fact that the air puffs evaporate saliva (Hendry and Rasche, 1961; Oatley and Dickinson, 1970).

Sensory information from the mouth and throat reaches the brain via the fifth, seventh, ninth, and tenth cranial nerves. Transection of these nerves reduces the amount of water rats ingest ad libitum, but the ability to regulate intake in accordance with need remains essentially intact (Jacquin, 1983; Jacquin and Zeigler, 1983).

Intragastric Infusions

A number of investigators have examined the importance of feedback from oropharyngeal receptors by bypassing them completely.

When water is rapidly intubated into the stomach of water-deprived animals, immediately before water is made available for drinking, water intake is reduced although the magnitude of the effect varies between species. Rats, rabbits, and hamsters reduce their oral intake in direct proportion to the size of the water load and may drink little or nothing when enough water is intubated to fully distend the stomach. These short-term effects are probably due to gastric distension, since similar effects have been observed after the inflation of balloons inserted into the stomach (below) and little or no time is allowed for absorption (Adolph, 1950; Miller et al., 1957; O'Kelly et al., 1954; Fregly et al., 1986).

Other animals, such as the dog, disregard a stomach load of water immediately after the injection but the same amount of intragastric water inhibits drinking when more than 15 min separates the intubation and the first access to oral water (Adolph, 1950).

When water is infused slowly into stomach via a permanent gastric fistula, oral intake is reduced but the compensatory inhibition of oral intake is never complete. When water is infused continuously, at a rate calculated to replace the water normally consumed by mouth, rats have been reported to reduce their oral intake by about 0.4 ml for each 1.0 ml infused into the stomach (Fitzsimons, 1957, 1971c). Even when the volume of the infusion is increased far beyond the normal oral intake (Nicolaidis and Rowland, 1975b), rats consume an additional 10 ml (about 30% of their normal daily intake) by mouth.

It has been pointed out that continuous infusions do not mimic the "periprandial" and diurnal drinking pattern of the rat and might thus not provide enough water during periods of peak need (meals of dry food, eaten at regular intervals, almost exclusively at night). An early test of this hypothesis (Kissileff, 1969b, 1973) did, indeed, show that intragastric infusions of water immediately before and during a meal reduced the oral water intake of rats more successfully (each 1.0 ml of gastric infusion reduced oral intake by 0.9 ml) than the continuous infusions used by earlier investigators (Fig. 6.3).

These results have been replicated (Nicolaidis and Rowland, 1975b) but shown to be influenced by the use of nasopharyngeal catheters, which permit oral metering of the infused fluid. When similar periprandial water injections were administered by means of gastric fistulae that do not traverse the nose, mouth, and esophagus (Holman, 1969; Nicolaidis and Rowland, 1975a; Rowland and Nicolaidis, 1976), the reduction in oral intake was found to be about 0.3 ml per 1.0 ml injected into the stomach, which agrees quite well with the values obtained in the continuous infusion experiments.

Nasopharyngeal gastric fistulae have also been used to demonstrate that rats are capable of regulating their water intake when the act of "drinking" consists of

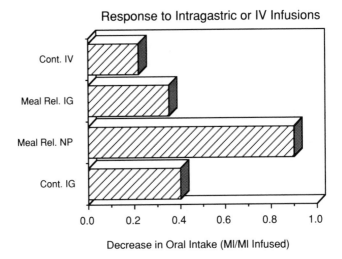

Fig 6.3. Reduction in oral water intake following continuous or meal-related intragastric (IG), nasopharyngeal (NP), or intravenous (IV) infusions of water. Data from: (1) Fitzsimons, J. T. (1971c). The physiology of thirst: A review of the extraneural aspects of the mechanisms of drinking. *In*: "Progress in Physiological Psychology." Vol. 4. (E. Stellar, and J. M. Sprague, eds.) pp. 119–201. Academic Press, New York. (2) Kissileff, H. R. (1969b). Oropharyngeal control of prandial drinking. *J. Comp. Physiol. Psychol.* **67**, 309–319. And (3) Nicolaidis, S., and Rowland, N. (1975b). Systemic versus oral and gastro-intestinal metering of fluid intake. *In*: "Control Mechanisms of Drinking." (G. Peters, J. T. Fitzsimons, and L. Peters-Haefeli eds.) pp. 14–21. Springer Verlag, New York.

a lever press that results in an intragastric injection of water (Epstein, 1960). Much of this regulatory ability appears to be lost when gastric fistulae are used that do not provide oropharyngeal stimulation (Holman, 1969).

Mechanical Distension of the Stomach

When rats are allowed to drink orally and the water is permitted to enter the stomach but its absorption is prevented by a pyloric "noose" that occludes the opening between the stomach and the upper intestine (Hall, 1973; Hall and Blass, 1975, 1977), rats orally ingest far less than they sham drink but do drink a few milliliters more than they would without the noose and appear to be unresponsive to increases in the duration of deprivation. Both effects are probably due to the fact that the amount consumed after even brief periods of deprivation fills and extends the rat's stomach to capacity.

These results prove that gastric distension is a limiting factor under experimental conditions but provide few clues concerning the importance of this mechanism under normal conditions. One must also remember that oral sensations were not excluded in these experiments. At least one experiment (Miller *et al.*, 1957) has shown that water ingested by mouth is more effective in reducing subsequent drinking than an equal amount injected into the stomach.

Earlier reports have noted that an inflated stomach balloon inhibited deprivation-induced drinking as effectively as intragastric injections of water in dogs (Towbin, 1949), rats, and rabbits (Adolph *et al.*, 1954). The drinking response to salt loads is also inhibited by such balloons (Montgomery and Holmes, 1955). The possibility that nausea and discomfort may have contributed to these apparent satiety effects can not be excluded. Miller (1957) has demonstrated that at least in the rat, the inflation of stomach balloons is aversive.

Gastric and Duodenal Cannulae

The information from experiments on gastric infusions and distension has been complemented, more recently, by data from studies that have investigated the effects of draining orally ingested water from the stomach and/or duodenum (Maddison *et al.*, 1980a,b; Wood *et al.*, 1980). This paradigm provides a useful picture of the influence of orogastric mechanisms under more nearly natural conditions.

When gastric cannulae were opened shortly after rhesus monkeys drank to satiation after a 22-h deprivation period, drinking resumed almost immediately and continued without significant pause until a significant portion of the water drained from the stomach was replaced.

When gastric cannulae were opened at the beginning of the 1-h test, drinking continued, essentially without pause throughout the period. The total amount of water consumed averaged five to six times the quantity ingested when the gastric cannula was closed. Similar effects were seen when cannulae implanted in the upper segment of the duodenum were opened at the beginning of the test, although total intake was slightly smaller than when gastric cannulae were opened (Fig. 6.4).

The rapid resumption of drinking after the opening of gastric cannulae in sated monkeys indicates that the presence of water in the stomach is a major factor in preabsorptive satiety in this species. The continued drinking of excessive amounts of water when either gastric or duodenal cannulae were opened before water could accumulate in the stomach shows equally conclusively that oral and esophageal sensations are not a sufficient stimulus for satiety in the monkey.

The satiety value of water in the duodenum was further investigated in a series of experiments that involved the drainage of orally ingested water from stomach cannulae while water or isotonic saline was injected into the duodenum. An

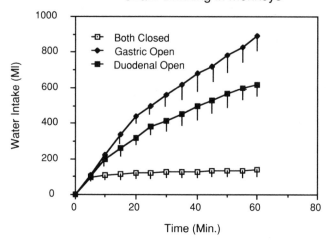

Fig. 6.4. Sham drinking in five monkeys with both gastric and duodenal cannulae after 22.5 h of deprivation. On control tests, both were closed and the monkeys consumed nearly all of their water in the first 10 min of the test. When either the gastric or the duodenal cannula was open, allowing ingested water to drain before being absorbed from the intestine, drinking continued throughout the 60-min test period. After: Maddison, S., Wood, R. J., Rolls, E. T., Rolls, B. J., and Gibbs, J. (1980b). Drinking in the rhesus monkey: peripheral factors. *J. Comp. Physiol. Psychol.* **94**, 365–374. With permission of the authors and the American Psychological Association.

infusion of 100 ml of isotonic saline (a quantity of fluid roughly equivalent to 80% of the amount of water ingested during tests with all cannulae closed) produced no inhibition of sham drinking on these tests. Intraduodenal injections of a comparable quantity of water, on the other hand, reduced sham drinking by about 50%.

These results indicate that the presence of water in the duodenum (which is subject to absorption in the course of the 1-h test period and did, in fact, lower plasma sodium concentration within about 20 min) had significant satiating effects whereas the presence of a comparable quantity of isotonic saline (which did not lower plasma sodium concentration) did not.

What is puzzling about these observations is not the satiating effect of water but the fact that the monkeys continued to ingest orally large amounts of water in spite of the presence of a quantity of water in their intestine that was larger, by far, than that normally transported from the stomach to the duodenum at the time drinking stops after 22 h of deprivation (under the conditions of these experiments only 24 ml of water passed into the duodenum at the time the monkeys ceased drinking).

An extension of these studies to intravenous infusions resulted in some additional riddles. Within 10–15 min after iv infusions of 50 ml of water, plasma sodium concentrations decreased to apparently asymptotic levels that were lower than those produced by an intraduodenal infusion of 100 ml in the test described above. Yet the iv infusion had no effect on sham drinking, in marked contrast to the intraduodenal infusion, which reduced oral ingestion by about 50%. Even an iv infusion of 100 ml of water (which reduced plasma sodium levels even further) reduced oral sham drinking less than the smaller intraduodenal infusions.

It would appear from these results that the absorption of water from the duodenum activates a satiety mechanism that is not sensitive to the general dilution of plasma. It has been suggested that hepatic osmoreceptors may play a role in thirst and related kidney functions (Rogers and Novin, 1983; Adachi *et al.*, 1976), but the available evidence (including the effects of hepatic vagotomy, discussed below) does not provide substantial support for the hypothesis. Most relevant, in the present context, is a report (Kozlowski and Drzewiecki, 1973) of an increase in the osmotic threshold for drinking after hepatic-portal infusions of water in the dog.

It is interesting in this context to note that the oral water intake of 24-h water-deprived rats appears to be inhibited all but completely by intragastric as well as intraperitoneal injections of water. Comparable quantities of isotonic saline are essentially without effect even when the intubation precedes access to oral water by as much as 1 h. Isosmotic solutions of glucose produced a significant reduction in oral intake in these experiments although the effects was smaller than that seen after water (Fregly *et al.*, 1986). The investigators concluded that only solutions that draw solutes from plasma (and thus reduce the osmolality of extracellular as well as cellular fluids) inhibit drinking in the rat.

Vagotomy

It is generally assumed (see Fitzsimons, 1979) that the inhibitory effects of stomach loads and gastric balloons reflect satiety-related feedback from stretch receptors in the walls of the stomach. However, subdiaphragmatic vagotomy, which removes feedback from gastric stretch receptors, produces such complex effects on water intake in the rat that a simple interpretation in terms of a loss of gastric satiety influences seems inadequate.

In the dog, vagotomy affects the pattern of ad libitum drinking (the animals take larger draughts less frequently) (Towbin, 1955) but does not modify the drinking response to salt loads (Holmes and Gregersen, 1950).

In the rat, bilateral abdominal vagotomy has been reported to decrease ad libitum water intake (Kraly, 1978; Kraly *et al.*, 1975) and to attenuate the drinking response to hypertonic saline (Kraly *et al.*, 1975; Smith and Jerome, 1983) as well as to extracellular thirst stimuli such as polyethylene glycol (PG), isoproterenol, and systemic (but not central) angiotensin (Simansky and Smith, 1983; Kraly *et al.*, 1975; Kraly, 1978; Rowland, 1980). It is interesting to note that the significant reduction in cellular dehydration thirst seen in these experiments developed only gradually (Jerome and Smith, 1984).

Bilateral abdominal vagotomy also has been reported to greatly increase the delayed salt appetite after polyethylene glycol (Zimmer *et al.*, 1976). Unilateral abdominal vagotomy apparently has no significant effect on ad libitum drinking in the presence or absence of food or on drinking responses to hypertonic saline in the rat (Vance, 1970).

Attempts to elucidate this complex syndrome by means of selective transections of discrete branches of the subdiaphragmatic vagus nerve have further complicated the picture, as follows.

Gastric vagotomy has been reported to reduce ad libitum water intake in the absence of food (Smith and Jerome, 1983) and to attenuate the drinking response to hypertonic saline (Smith and Jerome, 1983; Jerome and Smith, 1982b) as well as to systemic angiotensin (Jerome and Smith, 1982a).

Celiac vagotomy reduces the drinking response to hypertonic saline (Tordoff and Novin, 1982; Smith and Jerome, 1983) and systemic angiotensin (Jerome and Smith, 1982a) but does not affect ad libitum water intake in the absence of food (Smith and Jerome, 1983) or the dipsogenic effects of polyethylene glycol (Tordoff and Novin, 1982).

Selective hepatic vagotomy has been reported to significantly increase the amount of water drunk after 24 h of deprivation but to have no effects on cellular or extracellular thirst challenges (Smith and Jerome, 1983). The absence of a change in cellular dehydration thirst is particularly noteworthy in view of the fact that vagally innervated osmoreceptor mechanisms have been demonstrated and related to thirst and renal functions (Adachi *et al.*, 1976; Rogers and Novin, 1983).

An interaction between the hepatic and coeliac branch of the vagus is suggested by the observation that the combination of hepatic and celiac vagotomy produced essentially no effect on ad libitum water intake or drinking responses to hypertonic saline in these experiments (Smith and Jerome, 1983).

Unilateral cervical vagotomy, which denervates stretch receptors in the atria of the heart (implicated in the mediation of extracellular thirst stimuli resulting in a decrease in blood volume and/or pressure), has produced inconsistent effects.

Ad libitum water intake in the presence or absence of food appears to be unaffected by either right or left cervical vagotomy (Vance, 1970). The drinking response to hypertonic saline has been reported to be increased after right cervical vagotomy (Moore-Gillon, 1980) and increased (Moore-Gillon, 1980) or decreased (Zimmer *et al.*, 1976) after left cervical vagotomy. Right or left cervical vagotomy has been reported to increase the dipsogenic effects of isoproterenol and polyethylene glycol but to have no effect on drinking after caval ligation (Moore-Gillon, 1980). The facilitatory effect on PG-induced drinking may be mediated by the renin–angiotensin system, since it was not found in nephrectomized rats. Left cervical vagotomy also has been reported to increase the delayed salt appetite seen in rats after polyethylene glycol (Zimmer *et al.*, 1976). This effect was not abolished by nephrectomy.

Although the possibility of complications arising from the transection of motor components of the vagus nerve has not been as systematically ruled out as one would like, the available evidence (deWied, 1966; Blass and Chapman, 1971) suggests that the effects of vagotomy on water intake may reflect a loss of afferent projections to the brain.

Postabsorptive Factors

Intravenous Infusions

In the rat, Nicolaidis and Rowland have systematically investigated the satiety effects of intravenous infusions of water (which bypass gastric as well as oropharyngeal receptors entirely) and compared them to those produced by intragastric water infusions (Nicolaidis and Rowland, 1974, 1975b; Rowland and Nicolaidis, 1974, 1976).

When continuous infusions were used, intragastric infusions were far more effective in reducing oral intake than intravenous infusions. When water was injected only during ad libitum meals, intravenous injections reduced oral intake more effectively than intragastric injections. When the discrete injections were given during the intermeal interval, intravenous and intragastric injections produced comparable effects (which were smaller by far than those of periprandial injections).

None of the intravenous or intragastric injections completely abolished oral intake in any of these experiments. In all cases, the effectiveness of the infusions leveled off at an asymptote equal to about two-thirds of the normal ad libitum oral intake. These observations suggest that ad libitum intake may reflect, in part, a constant oral "thirst" component that cannot be met by systemic infusions. It is interesting that the size of this residual oral water need is almost identical to the reduction observed in animals trained to self-administer water intravenously (see below). It would appear that this 10 ml or so represents water normally consumed in excess of the basic fluid needs of the organism in order to satisfy an oral water appetite.

Nicolaidis and Rowland (1974; Rowland and Nicolaidis, 1974) succeeded in demonstrating water-intake regulation in the rat completely deprived of oral as well as esophageal and gastric cues. When water was not otherwise available, rats leaned to press a lever in order to obtain discrete intravenous injections of about 1.0 ml of water. (The rate of lever pressing, in these experiments, was shown to be a function of the injection volume, within a range extending from

0.25 ml to 2.0 ml per injection.) The total amount of water thus self-administered was lower, by about one-third, than the ad libitum oral intake but appeared to meet the animals' water needs adequately over prolonged periods of testing. Nearly all of the intravenous "drinking" occurred at night just before or during meals, thus closely mimicking the normal meal-associated pattern of water intake. Intravenous drinking was attenuated during periods of food deprivation and increased by the addition of salt to the diet as well as by increases in ambient temperature. Various experimental treatments such as hypertonic salt loads, polyethylene glycol-induced vascular hypovolemia, or intravenous angiotensin did not affect the rate of intravenous water self-administration.

Intravenous infusions have also been made in rhesus monkeys with somewhat different results (Maddison et al., 1980a,b; Wood et al., 1980). The animals were allowed to orally sham drink water which was drained from the stomach before it could be passed on to the duodenum and absorbed. In this paradigm, iv infusions of water, made after 22 h of deprivation at the beginning of a 1-h test, reduced oral intake far less effectively than slow intraduodenal infusions of comparable quantities, even though the iv infusions were more effective in reducing plasma sodium concentrations (see Intragastric Infusions above for detail).

Relative Contribution of Cellular and Extracellular Satiety Signals

If sufficient time for complete absorption of a water preload is allowed, the route of administration becomes a negligible factor in many experimental paradigms. For instance, a 10-ml preload of water, given orally, intragastrically, or intravenously immediately before a 1-h test, has been shown to reduce the water intake of a deprived rat by 64–69% (Ramsay et al., 1977b) (Fig. 6.5).

This figure is a fairly good estimate of the contribution of cellular dehydration to the thirst produced by an overnight period of deprivation since the preload restores plasma sodium concentration to predeprivation levels but has little effect on plasma volume. (Some cellular dehydration may persist in these studies in spite of the return of plasma osmolality because solute is lost during the deprivation period.)

Oral, ig, or iv preloads of isotonic saline, which restore plasma volume without significant changes in osmolality, reduced the 1-h water intake of the same rats by 20–26%, an indication of the magnitude of the contribution of extracellular thirst to the effects of overnight deprivation (Ramsay et al., 1977b).

The comparable figures for dogs are very similar (Ramsay et al., 1977a). In this case, an attempt was made to selectively rehydrate putative central osmoreceptors by infusing water into the lateral carotid artery, which supplies much of the forebrain. This procedure returned the osmolality of the blood supply of the brain (monitored at the jugular vein) to predeprivation levels but

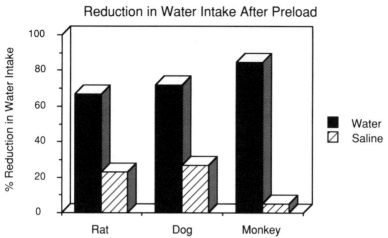

Fig. 6.5. Effects of preloads on water intake after deprivation, expressed as a percentage of the intake on control tests without preloads. Data from: (1) Rolls, B. J., Wood, R. J., and Rolls, E. T. (1980a). Thirst: The initiation, maintenance, and termination of drinking. *In*: "Progress in Psychobiology and Physiological Psychology." Vol. 9 (J. M. Sprague and A. N. Epstein, eds.) pp. 263–321. Academic Press, New York. (2) Wood, R. J., Maddison, S., Rolls, E. T., Rolls, B. J., and Gibbs, J. (1980). Drinking in the rhesus monkey: roles of pre-systemic and systemic factors in drinking control. *J. Comp. Physiol. Pychol.* **94**, 1135–1148. And (3) Ramsay, D. J., Rolls, B. J., and Wood, R. J. (1977a). Thirst following water deprivation in dogs. *J. Physiol.* **232**, 93–100.

had no significant effects on the osmolality of the systemic circulation. The water intake of deprived dogs was reduced by 72%, in spite of the persistence of cellular dehydration throughout most of the body—a convincing demonstration of the influence of brain osmoreceptor mechanisms. Control infusions of isotonic saline into the carotid artery did not affect drinking—an indication that the brain is not equipped with volume receptors as well. When larger iv infusions of isotonic saline were made that restored plasma volume without significant shifts in osmolality, water intake decreased by 27%. When the two procedures were combined, water intake was inhibited all but completely.

The results of a further experiment on rhesus monkeys (Rolls *et al.*, 1980a) indicates that the relative contribution of cellular and extracellular mechanisms may vary considerably between species. In the monkey, iv infusions of water in quantities sufficient to lower plasma sodium and osmolality to predeprivation levels reduced oral intake by 85%. When larger volumes of water were infused, drinking was essentially abolished. Infusions of isotonic saline, which returned plasma volume to baseline levels, reduced drinking only by 5%, and very much larger infusions that resulted in significant hypervolemia produced little additional effects. The monkey, it would seem, relies mainly on feedback from osmoreceptors.

It is well to keep in mind that these are estimates that are undoubtedly affected by the duration of deprivation as well as the conditions of the test itself. In rats (Nicolaidis and Rowland, 1975b; Rowland and Nicolaidis, 1976) as well as monkeys (Maddison *et al.*, 1980a,b; Wood *et al.*, 1980) there is ample evidence (discussed above) of drinking that continues after cellular hydration and extracellular volume have been restored and it is not clear how this "irreducible spontaneous intake by mouth" may affect the data we have just discussed.

Although the precise proportions may be in doubt, it is certain that deprivation-induced thirst is based on extracellular as well as cellular dehydration and that both must eventually be reversed if the body's fluid reserves are to return to predeprivation levels. What is not as certain is the nature of the systemic signal that terminates drinking.

In the case of cellular dehydration, it is well established that a nephrectomized rat, which cannot excrete salt, will drink an amount of water in response to a hypertonic salt load that precisely returns its body fluids to isotonicity (Fitzsimons, 1961a). In so doing, it incurs an ever-growing expansion of the extracellular fluid that seems to have no influence on drinking.

This conclusion is supported by data from normal water-deprived dogs. Intravenous infusions of isotonic saline, in quantities far in excess of the amount needed to restore plasma volume to predeprivation levels (which overexpand the extracellular fluid compartment), have been shown to be no more effective in reducing oral water intake than far smaller infusions that just reverse the volume deficit (Ramsay *et al.*, 1977a).

In the case of extracellular thirst, the obvious signal for satiety is restoration of the vascular fluid volume. This does, indeed, appear to be the salient factor when salt is available in or in addition to water. When only water is available, drinking eventually stops in spite of continuing vascular hypovolemia, presumably because the body fluids become overdiluted and cellular overhydration results. In this case, cellular expansion appears to become a powerful signal for the cessation of drinking.

Many extracellular thirst stimuli result in a delayed and persistent salt appetite, which may be the result of an activation of mechanisms that give rise to a "prophylactic" increase in the intake of sodium. This helps to avoid future occurrences of the dilemma caused by persisting vascular hypovolemia accompanied by cellular overhydration.

Review and Conclusions

When water becomes available after a period of deprivation, many mammals drink just enough within a few minutes to met their physiological need. They stop, apparently on the basis of oral and/or gastric cues, long before cellular or extracellular fluid stores are restored. Others, including humans, stop repeatedly long before their water deficit has been reversed and thus incur voluntary dehydration in the presence of water. Satiety appears to be complete in the species only when the volume and composition of extracellular as well as cellular fluid stores are replenished.

Oral "metering" is apparent in the water intake pattern of all mammals. It has also been demonstrated in numerous experiments that have shown that the "sham-drinking" of esophagostomized animals is proportional to water need. Some species sham drink just enough to reverse their physiological need (if the water were allowed to reach their stomach). Others drink excessively but the total quantity consumed appears to be determined by actual need (i.e., the length of the preceding water deprivation).

The influence of "oral metering" has also been investigated by administering water directly into the stomach. Many of these studies used nasopharyngeal fistulae, which do not completely eliminate oral feedback. These experiments indicated that periprandial injections of water reduced the oral intake of rats by 90%, in contrast to continuous infusions, which achieved only a 40% reduction. However, replications of these studies, using intragastric cannulae that completely eliminate oral feedback, have shown that oral intake is reduced by only 0.3–0.4 ml regardless of the pattern of the gastric infusion.

Experiments on the rhesus monkey have demonstrated the importance of gastric cues in preabsorptive satiety. When water was drained from gastric cannulae shortly after monkeys had completed drinking after a period of deprivation, water intake resumed almost instantly and continued until a significant portion of the lost water was replaced. When the gastric cannulae were opened at the beginning of drinking after deprivation, water intake continued (as it would have in esophagostomized animals) until five to six times the amount of fluid needed to reverse physiological need (had it been allowed to remain in the stomach) was consumed. Oral feedback obviously does not appear to be a predominant satiety factor in this species.

When the orally ingested water that was allowed to drain from gastric cannulae in these experiments was replaced by intraduodenal injections of water, oral intake decreased markedly, indicating that the absorption of water from the duodenum is a major satiety influence. The fact that intraduodenal infusions of isotonic saline had no effect suggests that osmotic pressure is an essential ingredient in duodenal satiety.

Intravenous infusions of quantities of water that reduced plasma osmolality as much as or more than the duodenal infusions had no effect on oral intake, suggesting that duodenal water has access to receptors not shared by the general circulation.

It is widely believed that gastric and perhaps some duodenal influences on satiety are mediated by branches of the vagus nerve. Total abdominal vagotomy as well as transection of the gastric branches of the vagus of the rat decreases ad libitum intake. It also reduces drinking responses to hypertonic saline as well as various extracellular thirst stimuli. Celiac vagotomy has similar effects, although the drinking response to some extracellular thirst stimuli such as PG are spared. Transection of the hepatic branch of the vagus reduces deprivation-induced drinking without significantly lowering the response to hypertonic saline or extracellular thirst stimuli. Unilateral cervical vagotomy, which denervates the stretch receptors of the heart, has produced inconsistent effects in several laboratories.

Postabsorptive influences on satiety have been investigated in the rat and monkey by means of intravenous infusions, which bypass oral and gastric receptors completely. In the rat, periprandial infusions were found to be more effective than continuous infusions. Even large water loads failed, however, to reduce oral intake by more than about two-thirds, indicating an oral water "need" that cannot be met by intravenous or intragastric (above) infusions.

In related experiments, it was shown that rats can be trained to "drink" by pressing a lever that activated a pump such that 0.25–2.0 ml of water is administered iv. The amount of water that is self-administered in this fashion remains at about two-thirds of the normal ad libitum intake. Since the animals appeared to thrive on this amount for prolonged periods of time, it would seem that the normal oral intake occurs, in part, in response to a significant "oral need" that is not related to the cellular and extracellular fluid imbalances that have been the subject of much of our discussion.

Estimates of the relative contribution of cellular and extracellular thirst to deprivation-induced drinking have been obtained in experiments measuring water intake after oral, gastric, or iv preloads of water or isotonic saline.

In the rat and dog, water preloads result in a decrease in oral intake of approximately 70%. Preloads of isotonic saline (which replenish extracellular fluid volume without affecting cellular water) decrease oral intake by 20–30%. Extracellular hypovolemia clearly plays a significant role in thirst in these species although cellular dehydration is the dominant influence.

Rhesus monkeys, on the other hand, reduce their oral intake little if at all after preloads of isotonic saline while responding even more strongly than rats and dogs to preloads of water. Apparently extracellular thirst plays only a minor role in this species, a fact one should take into account when examining the effects of various experimental manipulations on responsiveness to cellular and extracellular thirst stimuli.

Chapter 7

Brain Mechanisms of Thirst: Anatomical Considerations

Historical Perspectives

The physiologists of the eighteenth and nineteenth century generally accepted the conclusion that thirst was a sensation attributable directly to receptors in the mouth and throat. This view did not require the postulation of special brain mechanisms, and few (e.g., Dumas, 1803) bothered to propose any. With the advent of the twentieth century, clinical observations increasingly suggested that central influences might have to be considered. Leschke (1918) proposed that thirst might arise because an increase in the solids of the blood might irritate the cortex. Others (Oehme, 1922; Brunn, 1925) thought some "vegetative center," possibly located in the diencephalon, might translate sensory signals from the mouth and throat into special thirst sensations.

Clinical evidence for an involvement of the diencephalon in thirst became available when diabetes insipidus, which is characterized by excessive urination and continual thirst, was traced to tumor growth or vascular infarct in the region. In the course of related surgery, it was noted that mechanical stimulation of the floor of the third ventricle could elicit thirst sensations.

Experimental study of the brain mechanisms that control thirst and related kidney functions did not get underway until the late 1930s (Bellows and Van Wagenen, 1938, 1939). It was not until the publication of the pioneering work of investigators from the University of Pennsylvania in the 1950s that a picture of hypothalamic "regulation" became apparent that was to dominate the field for decades to come.

Hypothalamus

Electrolytic Lesions

Anand and Brobeck (1951) first reported that rats and cats with lesions in the dorsolateral hypothalamus refused to drink (as well as eat) and would die unless maintained by intragastric intubation. The phenomenon was soon replicated (Teitelbaum and Stellar, 1954; Epstein and Teitelbaum, 1964), and a few cases of apparently "pure" adipsia (normal feeding while intragastrically hydrated) as well as "pure" aphagia (normal drinking but no intake of dry or liquid food) were described (Epstein and Teitelbaum, 1964, Montemurro and Stevenson, 1957; Smith and McCann, 1962).

Teitelbaum and Epstein (1962; Epstein and Teitelbaum, 1964) carefully examined the recovery of ingestive behavior in rats with lateral hypothalamic (LH) lesions. They described a four-stage pattern, which proceeds from an initial acceptance of moist and highly palatable foods while the animal is intragastrically hydrated to a point (often not achieved until after weeks or even months of nursing care) where the animal appears to eat and drink normally although it defends a significantly reduced body weight (Boyle and Keesey, 1975; Powley and Keesey, 1970).

Although the rat that has "recovered" from LH lesions drinks nearly normal quantities of water when both food and water are available ad libitum, its drinking appears to be purely prandial. The animals drink only during meals and stop ingesting water when their food is removed.

When small quantities of water are infused into the mouth of a rat that has recovered voluntary ingestive behavior after LH lesions, drinking is essentially abolished if the water is given during the meal. When the same amount of water is infused directly into the stomach, prandial drinking continues unabated (Teitelbaum and Epstein, 1962; Epstein and Teitelbaum, 1964).

While the normal rat drinks much of its daily ration of water before and after meals, it rarely interrupts a meal to drink. The rat that has "recovered" from LH lesions, on the other hand, is a truly prandial drinker; it eats and drinks concurrently, each meal consisting of alternating bites of food and small draughts of water (Kissileff, 1969a,b, 1971, 1973; Kissileff and Epstein, 1969). Teitelbaum and Epstein (1962) suggested that the "recovered" lateral rat did not drink in response to a loss of body water but only to wet its mouth sufficiently to facilitate the mastication and swallowing of dry food. Although functionally "recovered" it remains truly adipsic in a more general sense.

Subsequent experiments have supported this suggestion. The rat that has "recovered" from LH lesions does not drink after water deprivation unless food is present (Epstein and Teitelbaum, 1964) and drinks little or nothing in response to experimental treatments that produce cellular dehydration (Epstein and Teitelbaum, 1964), vascular hypovolemia (Stricker and Wolf, 1967), or decreased blood pressure (Stricker, 1973, 1976). They also respond poorly or not at all to other experimental treatments that elicit copious drinking in intact rats, including systemic injections of beta-adrenergic drugs (Stricker, 1973, 1976), intracranial angiotensin (Black et al., 1974) or intracranial carbachol (Wolf and Miller, 1964).

These observations unequivocally support the original hypothesis that lateral hypothalamic lesions destroy regulatory mechanisms essential for thirst. A quite different interpretation has, nonetheless, been advanced by investigators (e.g., Marshall et al., 1971, 1974; Marshall and Teitelbaum, 1974; Stricker and Zigmond, 1975, 1976) who paid attention to the often severe sensorimotor disturbances that earlier investigations had ignored. According to this view, the effects of lateral hypothalamic lesions on water intake could be due entirely or in part to an impairment of nonspecific arousal or "activation" rather than an interference with mechanisms specifically related to thirst.

The principal data base that suggests such an interpretation is as follows:

1. Large lesions in the dorso-lateral hypothalamus produce sensorimotor and arousal dysfunctions that are often severe during the initial post-operative period when the animals are adipsic (as well as aphagic) and tend to recover as voluntary ingestive behavior recovers (Balagura et al., 1969; Marshall et al., 1971; Marshall and Teitelbaum, 1974; Levitt and Teitelbaum, 1975).
2. Lesions in relay stations of the extrapyramidal motor system such as the globus pallidus (Morgane, 1961) and substantia nigra (Ungerstedt, 1971) that project through the far-lateral hypothalamus and adjacent portions of the internal capsule, or knife cuts that interrupt some of these projections without direct damage to hypothalamic tissue (McDermott et al., 1977a,b; Alheid et al., 1977a,b; Gold, 1967), produce effects on ingestive behavior, arousal, and sensorimotor competence that are similar in many respects to those seen after the classic LH lesions.
3. Intraventricular or intraparenchymal injections of neurotoxins which destroy brain catecholaminergic neurons, including the dopaminergic nigrostriatal bundle that passes through the lateral hypothalamus, also reproduce the acute effects of LH lesions although the long-term consequences tend to be less severe (Ungerstedt, 1971; Zigmond and Stricker, 1973).

Teitelbaum and associates (see Teitelbaum et al., 1980, 1983; Fibiger et al., 1973a,b; Stricker and Zigmond, 1974, for review) have analyzed the sensorimotor dysfunctions of the rat and cat with lateral hypothalamic lesions in detail. They describe an initial syndrome that has been likened to a functional decerebration and includes somnolence, akinesia (a general lack of movement), and catalepsy (the prolonged maintenance of unusual and presumably uncomfortable postures). Teitelbaum points out that similar states can be induced by many drugs that directly or indirectly interfere with brain catecholaminergic systems.

Unlike the true decerebrate animal, the rat and cat with LH lesions show progressive recovery, which is reflected in the gradual reappearance of increasingly complex behaviors such as orienting, walking, eating, etc.

Teitelbaum argues that these units of behavior are not lost during the initial phases of the LH lesion syndrome but are merely unresponsive to the stimuli that normally elicit them. This interpretation is based, in part, on observations that indicate that complex behaviors can be elicited during the initial stages of unresponsiveness by unusually strong stimulation. Painful tail-pinch, for instance, can arouse an apparently cataleptic cat or rat sufficiently to instigate active climbing, jumping, or even feeding, all behaviors not otherwise observed at this stage (Teitelbaum and Wolgin, 1975; Marshall *et al.*, 1974, 1976; Antelman *et al.*, 1976). Amphetamine-induced arousal elicits feeding in rats at this stage even though the same dose of the drug inhibits feeding in normal rats as well as "recovered" rats with LH lesions (Wolgin *et al.*, 1976). Similarly, behavior that has recovered can be suppressed at a later stage of recovery by stimuli that reduce general activation. An example of this is the sleeplike immobility seen after stomach loads of a liquid diet in rats that have recovered spontaneous mobility and voluntary ingestive behavior after LH damage (Levitt and Teitelbaum, 1975).

An interesting perspective of the role of dopaminergic pathways in the mediation of activational responses to natural thirst stimuli and experimentally induced cellular and extracellular hypovolemia has been presented by Bruno and colleagues. Neonatal rats given brain lesions which all but completely depleted brain dopamine displayed none of the dysfunctions seen in animals given similar lesions in adulthood (Bruno *et al.*, 1984) but displayed impaired drinking responses to a fairly high dose (5 ml of a 30% solution, sc) of PG when tested as adults. A delayed response to PG was reinstated by the administration of caffeine 24 h after the PG treatment (Bruno *et al.*, 1986).

Although the severe cataleptic-akinesia syndrome is seen only in animals with very large lateral hypothalamic lesions, there is little doubt that sensorimotor and arousal dysfunctions contribute to and possibly account for the initial period of aphagia and adipsia seen after LH lesions. Teitelbaum's exquisite and detailed analysis suggests that even in the superficially recovered animal, "subclinical" behavioral impairments (such as an inability to walk backward) persist and become apparent only upon careful scrutiny.

The critical question in the context of the present discussion is whether the apparently permanent adipsia in the absence of food, and the persisting impairments in the responses to cellular as well as extracellular thirst stimuli that are consistently seen after large LH lesions can be explained in terms of similar "subclinical" reductions in general arousal or, perhaps more specifically, reactivity to internal stimuli as Stricker and Zigmond (1976) have suggested.

Stricker (1976) has reported that rats that recovered voluntary food and water intake after relatively brief periods of aphagia and adipsia did not drink in the first hours after cellular (hypertonic NaCl) or extracellular (polyethylene glycol) dehydration, caval ligation, or isoproterenol but appeared capable of increasing their 24-h intake, albeit only slightly, following some of these experimental treatments.

Stricker suggested that the recovered lateral animals may be incapable of responding to experimental thirst stimuli during short-term tests (when normal animals do most, if not all of their drinking) because the stress inherent in these procedures overloads the capability of arousal or activation mechanisms that have only partially recovered from the lesion. He argues, further, that the delayed drinking seen in some of the tests may be very much smaller than that seen in normal controls because the experimentally induced deficits in body fluid composition or distribution may be compensated by a combination of renal conservation (which tends to be intact after LH lesions) and the small amount of water that is ingested.

It seems only fair to point out that the traditional alternative interpretation of the relatively small and delayed responses to the recovered LH-lesioned rat, in terms of partial recovery of incompletely damaged mechanisms specifically related to thirst, would seem to arrive at much the same predictions. Indeed, the rats with LH lesion that were tested in Stricker's experiments recovered voluntary intake after only a few days or, at most, weeks of adipsia and appear to drink, albeit less than controls, during periods of food deprivation. This suggests that these lesions may not have destroyed thirst-related functions as completely as was the case in the exhaustive studies of Epstein and Teitelbaum, who reported periods of aphagia and adipsia that lasted for many weeks and even months (Teitelbaum and Epstein, 1962; Epstein and Teitelbaum, 1964).

The fact that Stricker's rats responded quite differently to various cellular and extracellular thirst stimuli (see also Rowland, 1976c) would seem to be more compatible with lesion effects that are related to specific damage to thirst-related neural mechanisms than a nonspecific deficit in general arousal or activation.

This does not in any way detract from the salient point that Stricker as well as Teitelbaum (and, indeed, many experimental psychologists before them) have made: any behavior requires a certain level of general activation and arousal in addition to the specific motivation that leads to the selection of specific behaviors. Lateral hypothalamic lesions undoubtedly interfere with this nonspecific component of motivation, and this must be taken into account when one tries to interpret the consequence of the lesion on drinking and related behaviors.

The fact that the rat that has "recovered" from large LH lesions does drink during a meal indicates that it can perform the behavior and is capable of being motivated to execute it (presumably entirely by the requirements of ingestion and digestion of dry food).

The fact that it drinks more when additional salt is put into its food (Rowland, 1977) may not say anything about its ability to respond to cellular dehydration but may merely emphasize the importance of sensory feedback from the mouth and throat. The recovered LH-lesioned rat has been shown to refuse water but readily accept milk shortly after the administration of a salt load (Williams and Teitelbaum, 1959), a clear indication that it is sufficiently aroused to drink a preferred fluid but seemingly lacking the motivation to consume plain water.

The existence of lateral hypothalamic mechanisms that appear to be concerned specifically with thirst and, indeed, specific types of thirst is also indicated by the results of experiments that have shown that lesions in medial portions of the LH attenuate drinking responses to intracranial angiotensin or systemic injections of renin or isoproterenol without reducing drinking responses to hypertonic saline. Lesions in lateral portions of the LH produced an opposite pattern of effects, cellular dehydration thirst being selectively impaired or abolished (Kucharczyk and Mogenson, 1975; Sclafani *et al.*, 1973).

It is interesting to note that a similar dissociation of lesion effects on cellular and extracellular thirst has been reported by damage to the anterolateral hypothalamus and preoptic area (Blass and Epstein, 1971) as well as portions of the zona incerta immediately rostral to the LH (Walsh and Grossman, 1976, 1978) (see below).

Kainic Acid Lesions

Reports from several laboratories have indicated that the lateral hypothalamus contains nerve cell bodies that appear to be involved in thirst. Microinjections of the neurotoxin kainic acid (which destroyed nerve cell bodies but not fibers of passage) into the LH of rats have been reported to produce transient adipsia (and aphagia) followed by hypodipsia. Kainic acid also attenuated the drinking response to hypertonic saline. The animals showed no evidence of somnolence, catalepsy, or akinesia and tended to be hyperactive and hyperreactive to sudden and intense stimuli (Grossman *et al.*, 1978; Stricker *et al.*, 1978; Wayner *et al.*, 1981).

Kainic acid tended to spread to the rostrally adjacent aspects of the zona incerta in these experiments, and the possibility cannot be excluded that this may have contributed to the behavioral results (see below). Attempts to minimize diffusion by iontophoretic application of kainic acid to the lateral hypothalamus (Grossman and Grossman, 1982) produced much less local destruction of nerve cells in the LH, no detectable spread to the zona incerta, and statistically significant but smaller inhibitory effects on ad libitum intake as well as drinking responses to hypertonic saline.

Knife Cuts

The possible significance of damage to fibers of passage in the etiology of the complex lateral hypothalamic lesion syndrome has also been investigated by means of surgical knife cuts that transect nerve fibers running across the plane of travel of a wire knife without producing significant direct damage to cellular components of the region. The instrument used in these experiments consists essentially of a thin stainless-steel guide tube that is stereotaxically lowered into the brain before a fine steel wire is extended at roughly right angles to its tip. The entire assembly is then raised, lowered, or rotated to produce cuts in the coronal, parasagittal, or horizontal plane.

When semicircular cuts were made along the rostrolateral border of the hypothalamus (separating it from the adjacent zona incerta), a pattern of effects on water and saline intake was seen that was similar to that seen after electrolytic lesions in the zona incerta itself (below). After a few days of hypodipsia, ad libitum water intake in the presence of dry food returned to normal levels. However, during 24 h of food deprivation the animals drank essentially no water (1.2 ml) or 0.5 M saline (0.3 ml). After sc injections of formalin, water as well as saline intake increased slightly but far less than in control animals.

Similar cuts made between the zona incerta and ventral thalamus produced comparable inhibitory effects on ad libitum as well as formalin-induced sodium intake but had no significant effects on water intake (Walsh and Grossman, 1977).

It is significant in the context of our discussion of the potential influences of nonspecific arousal and activation deficits in the LH lesion syndrome that neither of these cuts produced any evidence of somnolence, akinesia, or other detectable sensorimotor deficits that might have interfered with drinking. Indeed, the fact that ad libitum food and water intake was only mildly depressed in the immediate postoperative period and returned to normal levels within a few days afterward attests to the fact that the animals' ability to drink was not compromised.

Knife cuts in the parasagittal plane, along the lateral border of the LH, which effectively transected all laterally coursing fibers entering or leaving the hypothalamus laterally, reproduced, in every detail, the effects of large LH electrolytic lesions even though cellular components of the region were not directly damaged by the knife cuts (Grossman and Grossman, 1971, 1973). The rats were adipsic (and aphagic) for weeks and sometimes months, did not drink during periods of food deprivation long after ad libitum intake had returned to baseline levels, and did not drink after hypertonic saline or polyethylene glycol. The animals also displayed the sensorimotor and arousal dysfunctions typical of the rat with LH lesions (Fig. 7.1).

Smaller parasagittal cuts along the rostrolateral border of the hypothalamus produced more transient effects on ad libitum water intake (on the average, the animals were adipsic for 5.5 days) but sharply reduced water intake during 24 h of food deprivation and significantly attenuated drinking responses to hypertonic saline or polyethylene glycol when tested long after ad libitum water intake had returned to normal levels (McDermott et al., 1977a,b; Alheid et al., 1977a,b).

In all of these experiments, severe striatal dopamine (DA) depletions were observed, indicating that nigrostriatal projections had been interrupted. Yet many of the cuts produced only relatively minor and transient sensorimotor and

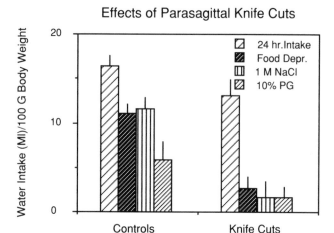

Fig. 7.1. Daily water intake, with and without food available, in 12 rats that recovered voluntary ingestive behavior 20–60 days after parasagittal knife cuts along the lateral border of the hypothalamus. (Seven additional animals did not recover within 90 days.) When tested 34–42 days after recovery of voluntary drinking, there was no evidence of responsiveness to either 1 *M* NaCl or 5 ml of a 10% PG solution, which elicited drinking reliably in controls. Data from: Grossman, S. P., and Grossman, L. (1973). Persisting deficits in rats "recovered" from transections of the fibers which enter or leave the hypothalamus laterally. *J. Comp. Physiol. Psychol.* **85**, 515–527.

arousal dysfunctions. The severity or persistence of the observed deficits in water-intake regulation was not correlated with the magnitude of the striatal DA depletions.

Knife cuts in the coronal plane, across lateral components of the medial forebrain bundle, produced severe and persistent adipsia (and aphagia) even though striatal DA depletions were relatively small. Those animals that could be nursed until voluntary ingestive behavior returned drank less than controls during 24 h of food deprivation and during a 6-h test following hypertonic saline, but the impairments were not as large as those seen after parasagittal cuts (or electrolytic lesions of the LH) (McDermott *et al.*, 1977a,b).

Hyperdipsia (Smith and McCann, 1962, 1964) as well as increased drinking responses to hypertonic saline (King and Grossman, 1977) have been reported after electrolytic lesions in the posteromedial hypothalamus, and it has been suggested that this may be a response to local tissue irritation (Rolls, 1970). Since the hyperdipsia persisted after nephrectomy, it would appear likely that it was not entirely secondary to a disturbance of antidiuretic hormone secretion and the resulting polyuria (Smith and McCann, 1962, 1964).

Transections of the caudal connections of the medial hypothalamus produce similar effects in the female rat (Hennessy and Grossman, 1976; Grossman and Hennessy, 1976; Grossman, 1971). Some of these cuts produced marked hyperdipsia without concurrent hyperphagia, indicating that increased prandial water requirements are not the cause of the excessive water intake (Fig. 7.2).

Further study of the phenomenon demonstrated that very large doses of vasopressin reduced but did not eliminate the increased water intake, indicating that an interruption of pathways necessary for the control of vasopressin release may be only partly responsible for the hyperdipsia.

That other factors may also be involved is further indicated by the fact that the hyperdipsic animals concentrated urine fairly well and continued to drink 300% above control level during the oliguric phase when rats with experimentally induced diabetes insipidus show only a very small elevation of intake (Hennessy et al., 1977).

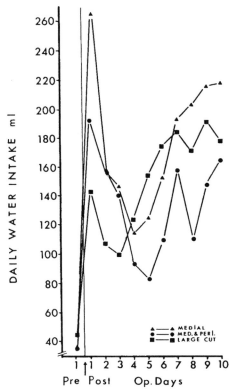

Fig. 7.2. Daily water intake of rats before and 10 days after knife cuts in the coronal plane that interrupted the posterior connections of the hypothalamus. "Medial" cuts (which were most effective) were restricted to the area immediately behind the ventromedial nucleus. "Medial & Perifornical" cuts extended lateral to the region of the fornix, and those identified as "Large" involved portions of the lateral hypothalamus as well. From: Hennessy, J. W., Grossman, S. P., and Kanner, M. A (1977). A study of the etiology of the hyperdipsia produced by coronal knife cuts in the posterior hypothalamus. *Physiol. Behav.* **18**, 73–80. Reproduced with permission of the authors and Pergamon Press.

Hyperdipsia has also been reported after electrolytic lesions (Coscina *et al.*, 1972; Lorens *et al.*, 1971; Osumi *et al.*, 1975) or coronal knife cuts (Grossman and Grossman, 1977; Grossman *et al.*, 1977) in the lower midbrain that deplete hypothalamic and forebrain serotonin and norepinephrine. The effect is often quite large but generally transient, water intake typically returning to baseline levels within 1–2 weeks.

Electrical Stimulation

The prominent role traditionally accorded to the lateral hypothalamus in many models of thirst-related brain mechanisms is supported by the observation that electrical stimulation of the dorsolateral hypothalamus elicits copious drinking in the rat (Greer, 1955; Mogenson and Stevenson, 1966, 1967; Mogenson *et al.*, 1971; Miller, 1960) and goat (Andersson, 1955; Andersson and McCann, 1955).

The stimulation-elicited drinking has been described as "compulsive" by some investigators (Valenstein *et al.*, 1968; Mogenson and Stevenson, 1967; Andersson, 1955) and may result in the ingestion of very large quantities of water (Andersson and McCann, 1955; Mogenson and Stevenson, 1966, 1967) or even highly aversive fluids such as concentrated salt solutions or urine (Andersson, 1955). At some electrode sites in the goat, drinking is accompanied by a pronounced reduction in urine flow indicating a concurrent stimulation of antidiuretic hormone release (Andersson, 1955).

That these effects of hypothalamic stimulation may indeed reflect an activation of neural mechanisms specifically related to thirst is suggested by several observations. Preloads of water that reduce deprivation-induced drinking have been shown to increase the threshold for stimulation-elicited drinking in the rat (Mendelson, 1970). Goats perform water-rewarded instrumental responses learned while water-deprived when hypothalamic stimulation is applied (Andersson and Wyrwicka, 1957).

In spite of the consistent results of these experiments, doubts about their interpretation have been raised because electrical stimulation of the lateral hypothalamus, particularly as practiced by many of the pioneers in this field, elicits not only drinking but other behaviors, notably other *ingestive* behaviors as well (Miller, 1960; Wise, 1968, 1969; Cox and Valenstein, 1969a,b; Mogenson, 1971).

Moreover, there are numerous reports of animals that initially drank when stimulated but subsequently switched to eating (or vice versa) when water was removed from the environment or the stimulation parameters were changed (Valenstein *et al.*, 1968; Wise, 1968; White *et al.*, 1970; Mogenson, 1971; Mogenson and Morgan, 1967; Milgram *et al.*, 1971; Wayner, 1970) (Fig. 7.3).

These observations are open to several interpretations. Perhaps the simplest derives from the undeniable fact that electrical stimulation, consisting of rather arbitrarily selected patterns of sine or square waves, which most assuredly never

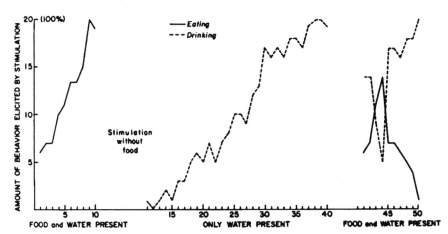

Fig. 7.3. Effects of electrical stimulation of the hypothalamus of a rat. Initially, where food and water were both present, stimulation evoked feeding and did so, after 10 test sessions, 100% of the time. Following a prolonged period of intermittent stimulation with only water present, the animal began to drink in response to stimulation and came to do so 100% of the time after 40 test sessions. When food was then reintroduced, both feeding and drinking occurred but drinking became the dominant response within 10 additional test sessions (each consistent of twenty 20-sec stimulation periods). From: Valenstein, E. S. (1973). Invited comment: Electrical stimulation and hypothalamic function: historical perspective. *In*: "The Neuropsychology of Thirst." (A. N. Epstein, H. R. Kissileff, and E. Stellar, eds.) pp. 155–161. V. H. Winston & Sons, Washington D.C. Reproduced with permission of the author and V. H. Winston & Sons.

duplicate or even approximate normal neural activity, almost certainly cannot selectively activate any functionally defined neural system. It indeed seems miraculous that any complex behavior, such as drinking, can be elicited at all with any regularity. This would seem to be particularly true in areas such as the hypothalamus that appear to be traversed by numerous neural systems known to be related to a wide variety of behavioral functions. Electrical stimulation of such a region can, at best, concurrently activate, albeit in a most unnatural way, a number of functionally unrelated neural systems. The end result cannot conceivably duplicate the unambiguous sensations experienced as a result of water deprivation. It should not come as a surprise that an animal may be willing to perform a number of different related behaviors such as eating, drinking, gnawing, etc. (the most commonly seen behaviors after stimulation of the lateral hypothalamus).

In one form or another, this explanation is accepted by many investigators in the field, but Valenstein (1969, 1970, 1973; 1976) has proposed an alternative that is compatible with the hypothesis that some, if not all, of the effects of LH lesions on water intake may be due to an impairment in nonspecific arousal. He suggests, in essence, that feeding or drinking may be elicited by hypothalamic stimulation, not because motivational states similar to hunger or thirst are evoked but because an increase in general arousal or activation results in the appearance of "prepotent" responses to significant aspects of the environment (food or water usually being the only objects available in a rat's cage during most tests). Valenstein agrees that stimulation at different sites may well predispose the resulting activation to be "channeled" preferentially so that certain behaviors may be more likely to be elicited than others. However, he believes that the consequences of electrical brain stimulation at different sites "are not sufficiently designated to preclude response substitution or to justify the application of terms that imply specific drive states" (Valenstein, 1969, p. 313).

Valenstein's interpretation complements Stricker's interpretation of LH lesion effects (above) and both have attracted a good deal of attention and controversy. Valenstein's hypothesis is opposed by investigators who have observed:

1. Only drinking at some electrode sites and only feeding at others (Mogenson, 1971), especially when very small electrodes are used (Olds *et al.*, 1971; Huang and Mogenson, 1972).
2. Consistently different thresholds for the elicitation of drinking or feeding (Wise, 1968, 1969; Milgram *et al.*, 1971).
3. Different behaviors in response to low- and high-frequency stimulation of the same region (Mogenson et al., 1971).
4. Specific effects of prestimulation food or water ingestion on the thresholds for stimulation-elicited feeding or drinking (Devor *et al.*, 1970).

Proponents of Valenstein's view have taken comfort from the observation that a mild tail-pinch can elicit some of the behaviors commonly seen after hypothalamic stimulation (although drinking appears to be a conspicuous exception in most experiments) (Antelman *et al.*, 1977).

The issue of specificity has been debated in a number of scholarly reviews (e.g., Mogenson, 1973; Teitelbaum, 1973; Valenstein, 1973; Caggiula, 1969; Roberts, 1969) and obviously transcends the problems of stimulation-elicited thirst. Yet it is in this context that it has raised major questions that have led some investigators in the field to dismiss the lateral hypothalamus entirely. I do not favor this view because the confluence of data from experiments employing such different techniques as lesions, electrical stimulation, electrophysiological recordings, and chemical "stimulation" (below) presents too consistent a picture to justify dismissal of such a large body of information.

Microinjections

Much of the initial impetus for investigations of the hypothalamus as a regulatory mechanism for thirst came from the pioneering work of Andersson (1953), who reported that microinjections of hypertonic saline into the anterior hypothalamus of goats induced copious drinking. This seemed to provide a direct parallel to the brain osmoreceptors that Verney (1947) had earlier demonstrated to be active in the regulation of antidiuretic hormone (ADH) release from the pituitary.

Andersson's findings have been replicated in other species such as the rat (Blass and Epstein, 1971) and rabbit (Peck and Novin, 1971). These studies, as well as more recent research from Andersson's own laboratory, have given rise to some controversy. The problem arises from the fact that at many hypothalamic (or ventricular) injection sites drinking can, indeed, be elicited by hypertonic saline but not, in most cases, by isosmotic solutions of other osmotically active solutions such as sucrose.

Andersson (1978; Andersson et al., 1982) has interpreted this to indicate that thirst is regulated not by central osmoreceptors but by receptors specifically sensitive to sodium, the principal osmotic stimulus that requires a response by the intact organism under normal circumstances (see our discussion of cellular thirst for further detail).

Others have taken the position that the relatively few sites that have been discovered in the lateral preoptic region of the rat and rabbit that do appear to respond to hypertonic sucrose as well as saline provide evidence that brainstem osmoreceptors are, in fact, active in the control of cellular dehydration thirst. According to this view (e.g., Epstein, 1983), brain sites responsive to hypertonic saline but not sucrose should be dismissed because the response reflects non-specific activation rather than the reaction of osmoreceptors. I agree with that conclusion, although the goat and possibly sheep may rely on sodium receptors. I do, however, believe that the pattern of injection sites where hypertonic saline specifically elicits drinking would seem to be of interest since it almost certainly identifies thirst-related neurons. A brief review of some of these data may be useful, as follows.

Peck and Novin (1971) explored more than 600 injections sites in the hypothalamus of the rabbit and identified a band of tissue extending throughout the rostrolateral hypothalamus from which hypertonic saline (but not sucrose) elicited drinking. As in the case of electrical stimulation, feeding and gnawing were also sometimes evoked. In the rat, Blass and colleagues (Blass and Epstein, 1971; Blass, 1974; Peck and Blass, 1975) have attempted a similar survey but used far fewer injection sites, which were concentrated in the lateral preoptic region (discussed below). In these experiments, a surprisingly small percentage of injection sites responded to sucrose as well as to hypertonic saline, and only a few were found in the lateral hypothalamus itself.

Electrophysiology

A number of investigators have identified single cells in the lateral hypothalamus of rats (Nicolaidis, 1968; Blank and Wayner, 1975; Weiss and Almli, 1975b), cats (Emmers, 1973), and monkeys (Vincent et al., 1972) that respond, apparently specifically, to systemically administered hypertonic saline. Sucrose or other osmotically active substances were not tested in these studies. Some hypothalamic cells also respond to salt on the tongue (Nicolaidis, 1968) or direct iontophoretic application of sodium (Oomura et al., 1969).

Zona Incerta

The zona incerta is an often poorly defined and odd-shaped tissue that is contiguous with the dorsolateral hypothalamus. In the rat, it extends from the rostral pole of the substantia nigra and ventral nucleus of Tsai where it takes up a lateral and ventral position all the way up to the anterior hypothalamus where it is located dorsomedially.

Electrical stimulation of the zona incerta has been reported to specifically and uniquely elicit drinking (Huang and Mogenson, 1972; Olds et al., 1971), in experiments that demonstrated only feeding responses from electrodes in the lateral hypothalamus proper.

Lesions of the rostromedial zona incerta, just dorsal and medial to the portion of the dorsolateral hypothalamus where lesions have the most dramatic and persistent effects on water (as well as food) intake, result in a complex pattern of effects on drinking, which indicates that this region may integrate information from many thirst-related channels.

Rats with rostromedial zona incerta lesions are hypodipsic immediately after surgery and recover normal or nearly normal ad libitum intake within about 8–10 days. During the first few days after the lesion, the animals are also mildly hypophagic and lose 10–15% of body weight, which is not subsequently recovered. The subsequent water intake is appropriate to this reduced body weight though slightly below preoperative baselines (Grossman and Grossman, 1978; McDermott and Grossman, 1979, 1980a,b; Walsh and Grossman, 1973, 1975, 1977, 1978).

The lesioned animals drink nearly all of their daily water at night (McDermott and Grossman, 1980a), displaying an exaggerated circadian rhythm also typical of the recovered lateral rat (Kakolewski et al., 1971; Kissileff and Epstein, 1969; Rowland, 1976a,b).

During periods of food deprivation, it becomes apparent that the rat with rostromedial zona incerta lesions drinks only to facilitate the ingestion and digestion of dry food. Water intake stops as soon as food is removed and remains at nearly zero levels for periods a long as 3 days (the longest period tested) (Walsh and Grossman, 1973) (Fig. 7.4). No recovery of this primary adipsia has been observed in tests performed as long as 6 months after surgery (Grossman and Grossman, 1978; Rowland et al., 1969; Walsh and Grossman, 1976, 1978).

Like the rat that has "recovered" from LH lesions (Teitelbaum and Epstein,

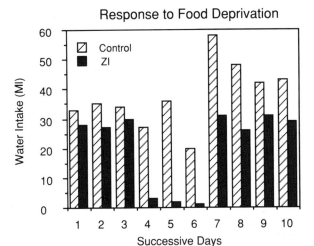

Fig. 7.4. Daily water intake of rats with rostromedial zona incerta (ZI) lesions during 3 days of ad libitum access to food, followed by 3 days of food deprivation and 4 additional days of ad libitum access to food. Note that rats with ZI lesions did not increase their water intake after 3 days of nearly complete abstinence from water. Data from: Walsh, L. L., and Grossman, S. P. (1973). Zona incerta lesions: Disruption of regulatory water intake. *Physiol. Behav.* **11**, 885–887.

1962; Epstein and Teitelbaum, 1964), the rat with zona incerta (ZI) lesions remains a purely prandial drinker. When maintained on a liquid diet, rats with ZI lesions are fully adipsic (Evered and Mogenson, 1976).

When food is returned to the rat with ZI lesions after 24 h of deprivation it will drink little or nothing until it has consumed a significant amount of food. If food and water are available ad libitum during the ensuing 24 h, the rat with ZI lesions makes little or no effort to make up for the self-imposed water restriction during the period of food deprivation. Controls, on the other hand, overdrink and more than compensate for the relatively small water deficit incurred during food deprivation (Walsh and Grossman, 1973).

When rats with ZI lesions are water (but not food) deprived for 24 h, they drink more than twice as much during the first hour of ad libitum access to water than they had during a 24-h period of food deprivation (Walsh and Grossman, 1978; Evered and Mogenson, 1976).

The deprivation-induced drinking of the rat with ZI lesions is smaller than that of controls, and it is not clear whether accumulated prandial and digestive needs (such as oral dryness and gastric discomfort) provide the principal stimulus for it. The "recovered" lateral rat has been reported (Epstein and Teitelbaum, 1964) to drink little or nothing after an overnight period of water deprivation even when food is available during the deprivation period. It is unfortunately not clear whether this reflects a more severe impairment or merely a shorter deprivation period.

Rats with rostromedial ZI lesions drink little or nothing in response to sc, ip, or iv injections of a wide range of doses of hypertonic saline (Grossman and Grossman, 1978; McDermott and Grossman, 1980a; Rowland *et al.*, 1979; Walsh and Grossman, 1976, 1978; Walsh *et al.*, 1977) (Fig. 7.5). The effect appears to be permanent, although some recovery of osmotic thirst has been observed 6 months after surgery (McDermott and Grossman, 1980a).

Impairments in drinking after hypertonic saline have also been observed in rats with LH lesions (Epstein and Teitelbaum, 1964) as well as in rats with lesions in the lateral preoptic area (Blass and Epstein, 1971) or damage to anteromedial aspects of the preoptic region (Buggy and Johnson, 1977b; Johnson and Buggy, 1978). It has generally been assumed that these deficits reflect a loss or severe impairment in the animal's response to cellular dehydration. In recent years, this assumption has been questioned on the basis of reports of delayed drinking responses to hypertonic saline in rats with LPO or LH lesions that did not drink on short-term tests, especially when the tests were administered during the dark, active phase of the rat's diurnal cycle (Coburn and Stricker, 1978; Stricker, 1976; Rowland, 1976a,b).

Grossman and Grossman (1978) observed that some animals with ZI lesions that did not drink 1 or 6 h after any of a wide range of doses of hypertonic saline did drink modest amounts of water when the test was extended to 24 h. However, a significant number of rats with ZI lesions failed to increase their intake even

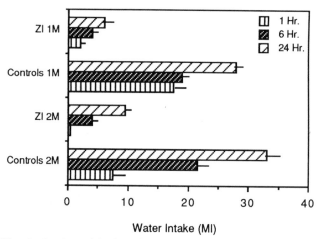

Fig. 7.5. Water intake after sc injections of 5 ml of 1 *M* or 2 *M* NaCl in sterile water by rats with bilateral rostromedial zona incerta (ZI) lesions and by sham-operated controls. Data from: Grossman, S. P., and Grossman, L. (1978). Parametric study of the regulatory capabilities of rats with rostromedial zona incerta lesions: Responsiveness to hypertonic saline and polyethylene glycol. *Physiol. Behav.* **21**, 432–440.

during this extended test, suggesting that the improvements seen in some animals may reflect incomplete destruction of the incertal mechanisms involved in drinking responses to cellular dehydration signals. Rowland *et al.* (1979) pursued this issue by showing that rats with ZI lesions that did not drink during the first 6 h after ip injections of hypertonic saline did excrete a significant portion of the salt load in urine. These same animals did not, however, increase their water intake after iv loads of hypertonic saline, even after they had been nephrectomized to prevent the excretion of sodium during the test. These animals did increase their ad libitum water intake when salt was added to their already quite salty diet. Since they failed to respond to sodium administered by any other route, the increased drinking response to salt in the food probably reflects oropharyngeal and possibly gastric factors rather than a true response to cellular dehydration.

McDermott and Grossman (1980a) investigated the possibility that tests administered during the dark, active phase of the rat's diurnal cycle might be more effective than the more common daytime tests. As in the case of the delayed testing described above, administering the hypertonic saline 6 h before the onset of darkness (so that 12 h of darkness were part of the ensuing 18-h test) resulted in significant drinking (though impaired when compared to controls) in some rats with ZI lesions that had not drunk on short-term tests administered during the day. However, a significant number of ZI rats failed to drink even on this extended test.

Brown and Grossman (1980) have reported results indicating that the loss of drinking to hypertonic saline after ZI lesions is due to the destruction of nerve cell bodies indigenous to the area rather than an interruption of fibers of passage. In their experiments, iontophoretic applications of the neurotoxin kainic acid severely depleted the zona incerta of neurons and produced transient hypodipsia as well as a persisting impairment in responding to sc hypertonic saline.

Rats with rostromedial zona incerta lesions do not respond to cellular dehydration but seem to drink water normally (Walsh and Grossman, 1976) or nearly so (Grossman and Grossman, 1978; Walsh and Grossman, 1977, 1978) in response to high sc polyethylene glycol or formalin treatments, which result in vascular hypovolemia (although the specific salt appetite seen in normal rats after these treatments is severely attenuated). The drinking response to low doses of PG is reduced (Walsh and Grossman, 1977; Grossman and Grossman, 1978) (Fig. 7.6). Rats with rostromedial ZI lesions do not drink in response to sc isoproterenol or iv or icv angiotensin (Walsh and Grossman, 1978; Rowland *et al.*, 1979) (Fig. 7.7).

On balance, the rat with ZI lesions responds very much like rats with lesions in the anteromedial preoptic region (discussed below) where a loss of drinking in response to hypertonic saline (Buggy and Johnson, 1977a), angiotensin (Buggy and Johnson, 1977a), caval ligation (Johnson, 1979), and isoproterenol (Lind and Johnson, 1981) often coexists with normal or nearly normal drinking in

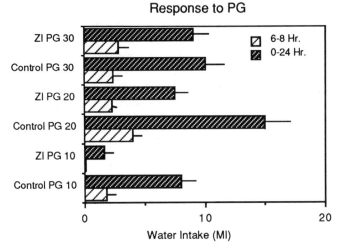

Fig. 7.6. Water intake after sc injections of 5 ml of a solution containing 10, 20, or 30% poly-ethylene glycol (PG). Intake was measured for 2 h beginning 6 h after the administration of PG and again 24 h after the injection. Data from: Grossman, S. P., and Grossman, L. (1978). Parametric study of the regulatory capabilities of rats with rostromedial zona incerta lesions: Responsiveness to hypertonic saline and polyethylene glycol. *Physiol. Behav.* **21**, 432–440.

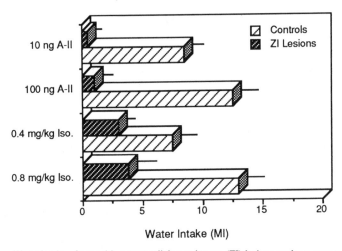

Fig. 7.7. Water intake of rats with rostromedial zona incerta (ZI) lesions or sham-operated controls during 30 min after intracerebroventricular injections of 10 ng or 100 ng of angiotensin II and 3 h after ip injections of 0.04 or 0.8 mg/kg isoproterenol. Data from: Walsh, L. L., and Grossman, S. P. (1978). Dissociation of responses to extracellular thirst stimuli following zona incerta lesions. *Pharm. Biochem. Behav.* **8**, 409–416. And S. P. Grossman, unpublished observation.

response to polyethylene glycol (Buggy and Johnson, 1977a; Johnson and Buggy, 1978). In both cases, food intake appears to be normal and there is no evidence of overt sensorimotor dysfunctions which might be responsible for the observed impairments in water intake regulation.

It should be noted that lesions in more posterior aspects of the zona incerta have been reported to produce a different pattern of effects, which is characterized by persisting hypodipsia presumably related to sensorimotor dysfunctions that decrease the amount of water ingested per tongue movement (Evered and Mogenson, 1976, 1977). I have observed similar effects of such lesions, as well as more severe sensorimotor dysfunctions that make it extremely difficult for a rat to ingest water or dry food.

Lateral Preoptic Area

The lateral preoptic region (LPO) has attracted attention because of experimental observations indicating that it contains central osmoreceptor mechanisms that monitor cellular hydration. The complex problems surrounding the attempts to define, locate, and study central osmoreceptors have been discussed in some detail in Chapter III on cellular dehydration thirst. Here, only the data relevant to their possible location in the LPO will be presented.

Lesions

Electrolytic or surgical lesions in the LPO of dogs (Andersson and Larsson, 1956), rats (Blass and Epstein, 1971; Teicher and Blass, 1976; Coburn and Stricker, 1978), and rabbits (Peck and Novin, 1971) have been reported to severely attenuate the normal drinking response to systemic hypertonic saline without, in some cases, affecting ad libitum drinking or the response to water deprivation (Fig.7.8).

Rats with LPO lesions do not appear to be entirely without defense against cellular dehydration. Although they drink little or nothing during the first few hours after an ip salt load, their ability to excrete salt via the kidney appears to be intact. This, in combination with some delayed drinking, eventually restores plasma osmolality (Coburn and Stricker, 1978).

Rats with LPO lesions also drink essentially normally in response to intravenous infusions of hypertonic saline as well as salt added to their diet (the latter could reflect a response to oral irritation rather than changes in the osmolality of body fluids) (Coburn and Stricker, 1978) (Fig. 7.9). Rats with LPO lesions also increase their water intake when hypertonic saline is administered after water deprivation (Teicher and Blass, 1976).

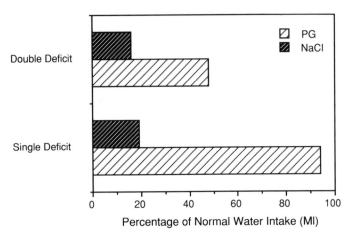

Fig. 7.8. Water intake after ip injections of 2 ml of 2 *M* NaCl or 2 ml of a 40% polyethylene glycol solution in rats with lesions in the lateral preoptic area (LPO). Some animals displayed an apparently selective loss of drinking after salt loads; others were also impaired in their response to vascular hypovolemia. After: Blass, E. M., and Epstein, A. N. (1971). A lateral preoptic osmosensitive zone for thirst in the rat. *J. Comp. Physiol. Psychol.* **76**, 378–394. With permission of the authors and the American Psychological Association.

The effects of LPO lesions on drinking responses to extracellular thirst stimuli have been the subject of some controversy. Both Blass and Epstein (1971) and Coburn and Stricker (1978) have reported that some LPO lesions impair acute drinking in response to ip salt loads without affecting the response to poly-

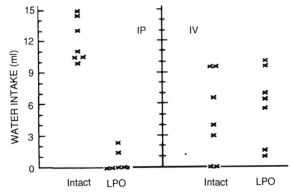

Fig. 7.9. Water intake of rats with lesions in the lateral preoptic area (LPO) during a 4-h test following the administration of 2 ml of a 2 *M* NaCl solution ip (left) or 4 ml of a 1 *M* NaCl solution iv (right). The same animals were used in both tests. After: Coburn, P. C., and Stricker, E. M. (1978). Osmoregulatory thirst in rats after lateral preoptic lesions. *J. Comp. Physiol. Psychol.* **92**, 350–361. With permission of the authors and the American Psychological Association.

ethylene glycol (PG). However, both examined the drinking response to a single high dose of NaCl and to a single low dose of PG. Blass and Epstein (1971) reported only marginal drinking responses to PG even in their controls. Coburn and Stricker (1978) observed more significant drinking after PG but found only small impairments in the long-term response to ip salt loads and essentially no impairment in the response to iv infusions of hypertonic saline or to increases in dietary salt.

Almli and Weiss (1974) have reported that lesions restricted to the LPO significantly increased the latency of drinking responses to PG without affecting the amount of water consumed. Larger lesions also reduced PG-induced water intake. Blass and Epstein (1971) also reported such "double deficits" after large lesions in the region of the LPO and suggested that incidental damage to the lateral hypothalamus might be responsible. However, Coburn and Stricker (1978) have reported normal drinking responses to low doses of PG in rats with large lesions in the posterior LPO that extended bilaterally into the anterolateral hypothalamus. To confound matters further, there is a report (Peck, 1973) that some LPO lesions attenuate drinking responses to systemic angiotensin and isoproterenol while leaving intact the drinking response to hypertonic saline. There has as yet been no replication of this unusual finding.

McGowan et al. (1988b) depleted a subpopulaion of nerve cells from the LPO of rats by applying the neurotoxin kainic acid (KA) to the LPO iontophoretically. When tested several weeks later, the KA-treated animals drank normally, or nearly so, in response to small salt loads (5 ml of a 0.5 M solution) as well as low concentrations of polyethylene glycol (5 ml of a 10% or 20% solution). Yet these animals consistently displayed significant impairments in their response to more intense challenges (5 ml of a 1.0 M NaCl solution or 5 ml of a 30% PG solution).Their drinking response to 1.5 mg/kg of angiotensin II was delayed (Fig. 7.10).

The observation that iontophoretic application of kainic acid to the LPO reduced the drinking response to polyethylene glycol administered in high concentration indicates that a reevaluation of the region's contribution to water intake regulation may be fruitful. The impaired response to vascular hypovolemia and angiotensin is not in conflict with the hypothesis that the region may act as an osmoreceptor mechanism related to cellular dehydration thirst. It does suggest that the LPO may also be a source of more general influences on thirst.

The essentially intact drinking response to a small salt load in animals with KA-induced LPO damage may be due to the survival of some LPO neurons, which participate in the organization of drinking responses to cellular dehydration. However, it is plausible that other areas of the brain may also be able to organize drinking responses to cellular dehydration under some conditions. This interpretation is supported by Coburn and Stricker's (1978) report that rats with large electrolytic lesions in the LPO are capable of (a) delayed drinking after

KA-Induced Neuron Depletion in LPO

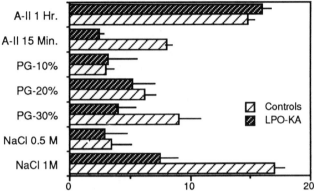

Fig. 7.10. Water intake of rats with kainic acid-induced neuron depletions in the LPO in response to sc injections of 1.5 mg/kg of A-II; high (5 ml of 1 *M* sc) and low (5 ml of 0.5 *M* sc) doses of NaCl; and high (5 ml of 30% sc) and low (5 ml of 10% or 20% sc) doses of polyethylene glycol (PG). Data from: McGowan, M. K., Brown, B., and Grossman, S. P. (1988b). Depletion of neurons from lateral preoptic area impairs drinking to various dipsogens. *Physiol. Behav.* **43**, 815–822.

larger ip salt loads, and (b) essentially intact drinking after IV infusions of hypertonic NaCl solutions or increased dietary salt. The hypothesis is also consistent with the fact that lesions in several upper brainstem and forebrain regions, such as the lateral hypothalamus (Epstein and Teitelbaum, 1964), zona incerta (Walsh and Grossman, 1976, 1978; Grossman and Grossman, 1978), antero-ventral third ventricle (Johnson and Buggy, 1977, 1978), organum vasculosum of the lamina terminalis (Thrasher *et al.*, 1982b), and nucleus medianus (Gardiner and Stricker, 1985a,b), have been shown to impair or abolish drinking responses to cellular dehydration. The fact that rats with LPO lesions recover normal ad libitum water intake as well as drinking after deprivation even when preloads of isotonic saline remove the hypovolemic component of deprivation thirst also supports such an interpretation (Blass and Epstein, 1971; Teicher and Blass, 1976; Coburn and Stricker, 1978).

Coburn and Stricker (1978) interpreted the residual capabilities of rats with LPO lesions in the framework of Stricker's earlier analysis of the arousal deficits seen in rats with lateral hypothalamic lesions. More specifically, Coburn and Stricker argued that LPO lesions (as well as lesions in the caudally adjacent lateral hypothalamus) interrupt catecholaminergic fibers of passage essential for "nonspecific activational components of behavior." The behavioral impairments seen in rats that are thus "centrally sympathectomized" are due, according to this view, to the animals' inability to "tolerate the stress that accompanies acute homeostatic imbalances."

The observation by McGowan *et al.* (1988b) that rats with KA-induced damage to the LPO respond essentially normally to low salt loads and concentrations of polyethylene glycol but display deficits when higher doses are used could be interpreted to support Coburn and Stricker's hypothesis. However, the fact that these effects were seen after iontophoretic KA injections that do not affect fibers of passage clearly implicates neurons indigenous to the LPO.

Electrophysiology

That the lateral preoptic area may, indeed, contain thirst-related osmoreceptors is indicated by the fact that systemic injections of hypertonic solutions modulate the firing rate of cells in the preoptic region (Von Euler, 1953; Cross and Green, 1959; Novin and Durham, 1969). Most of these cells are in the region of the supraoptic nuclei, and there is good evidence that these are the neurosecretory cells that produce antidiuretic hormone and control its release by the pituitary. However, cells that respond apparently specifically to systemic salt loads have also been found in the lateral preoptic region itself (Weiss and Almli, 1975b; Blank and Wayner, 1975; Malmo and Mundl, 1975; Emmers, 1973; Malmo and Malmo, 1979, 1981).

Microinjections

A number of studies have demonstrated drinking in sated rats (Blass and Epstein, 1971; Blass, 1974; Peck and Blass, 1975) and rabbits (Peck and Novin, 1971) following microinjections of hypertonic saline or hypertonic sucrose (but not hypertonic urea) into the LPO. Microinjections of water into these sites have been reported to reduce the drinking response to systemic hypertonic saline in the rat (Blass and Epstein, 1971). Rabbits given a choice between a normally preferred dilute saline solution and water drank mainly water (Peck and Novin, 1971), a behavior seen also after systemic injections of hypertonic saline in the rat (Stellar *et al.*, 1954).

Although these observations complement the results of experiments relying on electrophysiological and lesion procedures (discussed above), they have engendered a good deal of controversy (Andersson, 1973; Peck, 1973; Peck and Blass, 1975). One issue that has not yet been entirely resolved is the apparent scarcity of the osmosensitive sites. Even though large volumes of saline or sucrose solutions at concentrations beyond the normal physiological range were injected, Peck and Novin's (1971) extensive survey of 600 injection sites turned up only six that were positive for both sodium and sucrose. Blass and Epstein's (1971) contemporary study in the rat attempted far fewer placements but also found only five that responded to both saline and sucrose, and it is not entirely clear whether all five of these were definitively in the LPO. Subsequent studies by Blass and associates (Blass, 1974; Peck and Blass, 1975) provided a somewhat larger sample of positive placements and reduced the osmolality of their injections so that they approached the upper end of the normal physiological range but, in turn, used very large injection volumes of a saline–sucrose mixture. It is not clear why the ratio of positive placements (19 of 86 placements resulted in specific drinking responses in the most recent study) should have been so low, in spite of injection volumes of 2.0 μl, which should have been able to flood all of the LPO as well as adjacent tissue.

Anteroventral Third Ventricle (AV3V)

The tissues surrounding the anteroventral aspects of the third ventricle (AV3V), the medial preoptic area, the organum vasculosum of the lamina terminalis (OVLT), and the nucleus medianus have all been implicated in the regulation of the organism's fluid balance and thirst (Fig. 7.11). Because the investigators who discovered the importance of this region in the regulation of thirst were not aware of the possibility that each subfield may contribute in unique ways to the regulation of the organism's fluid and sodium balance, their lesions and other experimental procedures were aimed at the AV3V without concern for invasion of rostrally or laterally adjacent regions. An attempt will be made to sort this literature into groupings according to the principal structure investigated. How-

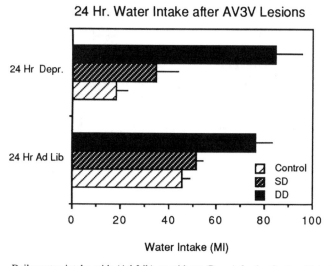

Fig. 7.11.   Daily water intake with (Ad Lib) or without (Depr.) food, of rats with lesions in the tissues surrounding the AV3V. Tests were performed after the animals had recovered from the adipsia observed in the immediate post-operative period. SD = rats which drank in response to A-ll but not hypertonic saline; DD = rats which did not drink to either of the two treatments (See Fig. 7.12). Data from Buggy and Johnson (1797b).

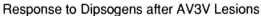

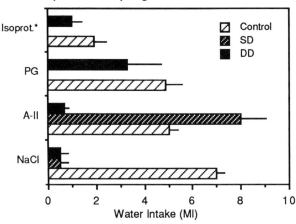

Fig. 7.12. Response to various dipsogenic stimuli in rats with AV3V lesions. Smaller lesions tended to impair drinking response to hypertonic saline (sc injections of 0.4 ml of 12%/100 g body weight or 1 ml of 10%) without reducing the response to angiotensin II (1.56 mg/kg or 500 μg/rat, sc) labelled SD (single deficit). Larger lesions in the same region reduced drinking to both dipsogens (double deficit or DD) but failed to reliably impair the drinking response to polyethylene glycol (1 ml of 20% PG/kg body weight, sc). Data from: Buggy, J., and Johnson, A. K. (1977b). Preoptic-hypothalamic periventricular lesions: thirst deficits and hypernatremia. *Am. J. Physiol.* **233**, R44–52. In a separate experiment, similar lesions were shown to reduce the drinking response to several doses of isoproterenol (only the response to 2.0 μg/kg, which produced the largest response is shown here). Data from: Lind, R. W., and Johnson, A. K. (1981). Periventricular peptic-hypothalamic lesions: Effects on isoproterenol-induced thirst. *Pharm. Biochem. Behav.* **15**, 563–565.

ever, one should keep in mind that the results of many investigations may well be influenced significantly by incidental involvement of adjacent structures.

Rats (Johnson and Buggy, 1977, 1978), goats (Andersson *et al.*, 1975), and sheep (McKinley *et al.*, 1982, 1986) with large lesions involving the tissues surrounding the anterior aspects of the third ventricle (AV3V) are adipsic but not aphagic if hydrated properly (Andersson *et al.*, 1975; Johnson and Buggy, 1977, 1978; McKinley *et al.*, 1986).

The animals fail to initiate appropriate antidiuretic responses and become exceedingly hypernatremic, indicating that vasopressin release is inhibited by the lesion (McKinley *et al.*, 1983, 1986; Brody and Johnson, 1980; Brody *et al.*, 1980; Buggy and Johnson, 1977a,b). As many as 50% of these animals do not regain voluntary drinking and die within about a week of the consequences of hypernatremia, pulmonary edema, and/or hyperthermia (Buggy and Johnson, 1977a; Johnson and Buggy, 1978; Nagel and Satinoff, 1980; Satinoff *et al.*, 1982; McKinley *et al.*, 1986). Others regain voluntary ingestive behaviors after a few days, particularly when survival is promoted by gavage or the availability of highly palatable fluids. These animals return to ad libitum drinking, which results in normal or even supranormal daily intakes (Buggy and Johnson, 1977a,b; McKinley *et al.*, 1986) (Fig. 7.11).

The recovered survivors drink little or nothing in response to water deprivation (Buggy and Johnson, 1977a,b; McKinley *et al.*, 1986), hypertonic saline (Johnson and Buggy, 1978; Buggy and Johnson, 1977a,b; McKinley *et al.*, 1986), isoproterenol (Lind and Johnson, 1981), and peripheral or central angiotensin (Buggy and Johnson, 1977b, 1978; Johnson and Buggy, 1977). The peripheral pressor responses to iv or icv angiotensin are also attenuated (Johnson *et al.*, 1978; Brody and Johnson, 1980; Buggy *et al.*, 1977). The drinking response to polyethylene glycol-induced vascular hypovolemia does not appear to be signficantly reduced by the lesion (Buggy and Johnson, 1977b; Johnson and Buggy, 1978) (Fig. 7.12).

Rats with AV3V lesions also display a reduced sodium preference when maintained on a low-sodium diet but increase their intake of hypertonic saline after an acute formalin challenge (Bealer and Johnson, 1979).

Microinjections of angiotensin or hypertonic saline or sucrose into the AV3V have been reported to elicit drinking as well as short-latency pressor and antidiuretic responses in the rat (Buggy, 1977; Buggy *et al.*, 1979). Combined injections of angiotensin and hypertonic saline did not result in greater drinking than the sum of the two injections given alone. Injections of hypertonic solutions into the AV3V were more effective than comparable injections into the LPO. Injections of angiotensin were equally effective at both sites.

In the goat (Andersson and Eriksson, 1971), the combination of angiotensin and hypertonic saline produces greater drinking than the sum of the effects of the two injections given separately.

Medial Preoptic Area

Lesions in the medial preoptic area (MPO) in rats have been reported to result in persisting impairments in body fluid and salt regulation in rats. Following an acute postoperative malaise, characterized by aphagia and adipsia, ad libitum food and water intake returns to normal levels. However the animals remain chronically hypernatremic and fail to respond to systemic salt loads. Their drinking response to polyethylene glycol-induced hypovolemia, on the other hand, appears to be unaffected (Black, 1976).

Rats with similar MPO lesions also emit fewer water-rewarded operant responses than controls. This decrease is not the result of an interference with sensorimotor abilities, or of an overall decrease in motivated behavior, since operant responding for food reward remains within the range of control levels.

When only quinine-adulterated water is made available ad libitum, animals with MPO lesions drink significantly less than controls (Carey and Procopia, 1974).

It is not clear whether the reported effects of MPO lesions are attributable to the destruction of AV3V tissue or, for that matter, whether some or all of the effects of AV3V lesions are due to the destruction of medial portions of the MPO.

McGowan *et al.* (1988a) have attempted to address this question. Rats with electrolytic lesions that were strictly confined to the tissue immediately surrounding the wall of the anteroventral portion of the third ventricle (AV3V), without invading the MPO, displayed normal ad libitum water intake and plasma osmolality as well as drinking responses to deprivation, hypertonic saline (0.5 or 1.0 *M*), angiotensin II (1.5 mg/kg), and isoproterenol (30 μg/kg). Electrolytic lesions in the medial preoptic region itself had no significant effects on ad libitum food and water intake, but impaired the drinking response to 1 *M* NaCl and resulted in a persistent increase in plasma osmolality (Fig. 7.13). These observations suggest that damage to the ependymal lining of the anterior third ventricle and immediately adjacent cells is not, by itself, sufficient to impair cellular or extracellular thirsts.

McGowan *et al.* (1988a) also addressed a second issue that is raised by the proliferation of upper brainstem and forebrain tissues, which appear to exert

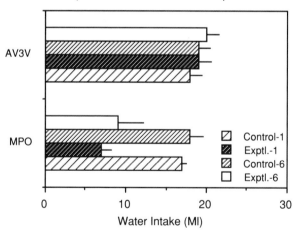

Fig. 7.13. Water intake, 1 and 6 h after systemic injections of 5 ml of a 1 *M* NaCl solution in rats that had electrolytic lesions confined to the immediate vicinity of the anterior third ventricle (AV3V) or in the medial preoptic region, sparing the immediate vicinity of the AV3V. Data from: McGowan, M. K., Brown, B., and Grossman, S. P. (1988a). Lesions of the MPO or AV3V: Influences on fluid intake. *Physiol. Behav.* **42**, 331–342.

similar influences on thirst. In view of the strategic central location of the MPO in this network, it appears plausible that the effects of MPO and/or large AV3V lesions might be due to an interruption of fibers of passage. To test this hypothesis, McGowan *et al.* (1988a) depleted neurons from the MPO of rats by iontophoretic application of the neurotoxin kainic acid (KA), which destroys nerve cell bodies without damage to fibers of passage. The KA-induced neuron depletion in the MPO of rats reduced the drinking response to 1.0 *M* saline, to 30% PG, and to 30 μg/kg isoproterenol. Ad libitum water intake and drinking responses to deprivation, or to low concentrations (0.5 *M*) of hypertonic saline, low concentrations (10 or 20%) of PG, and to systemic administration of 1.5 mg/kg angiotensin II were within the normal range (Fig. 7.14).

OVLT and Nucleus Medianus

In recent years, the tissue just anterior to the third ventricle has been divided into an anteroventral region [containing the organum vasculosum of the lamina terminalis (OVLT), the ventral, subcommissural, portion of the nucleus medianus, and periventricular tissue] and an anterodorsal region (containing the subfornical

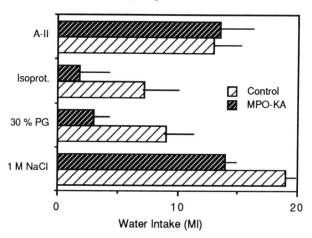

Fig. 7.14. Water intake after various dipsogens in rats that sustained significant depletions of neurons from the medial preoptic (MPO) area as a result of iontophoretic injections of kainic acid (KA). The data shown represent, from bottom to top, 2-h intake after sc injections of 5 ml of 1 *M* NaCl; 8-h intake after ip injections of 5 ml of a 30% solution of polyethylene glycol (PG); 2-h intake after sc injections of 30 μg/kg of isoproterenol; and 1-h intake after sc injections of 1.5 mg/kg of angiotensin II. Data from: McGowan, M. K., Brown, B., and Grossman, S. P. (1988a). Lesions of the MPO or AV3V: Influences on fluid intake. *Physiol. Behav.* **42**, 331–342.

organ, dorsal nucleus medianus, and ventromedial septum) (McKinley *et al.*, 1982, 1983, 1986; Gardiner and Stricker, 1985a,b; Gardiner *et al.*, 1986).

In sheep, lesions of the AV3V have been reported to have only minor, transient effects on water intake regulation. However, larger lesions that involved the tissue rostral to the anterior wall of the third ventricle, including the organum vasculosum of the lamina terminalis reproduced the effects seen in rats after large AV3V lesions. The animals were adipsic (some never recovered voluntary drinking) and extremely hypernatremic. The animals did not drink in response to injections of hypertonic saline or A-II, even after recovery of normal ad libitum intake. Although systemic injections of hypertonic saline did not elicit drinking, they did reduce the intake of hypertonic saline (McKinley *et al.*, 1982, 1983). Studies in the goat have produced similar results: destruction of the tissue rostral to the anterior wall of the third ventricle resulted in adipsia as well as a significant decrease in antidiuretic hormone (ADH) release (Andersson *et al.*, 1975).

In the dog, attempts have been made to destroy the organum vasculosum of the laminae terminalis selectively (Thrasher *et al.*, 1982b; Thrasher and Ramsay, 1986). Such lesions had little or no effect on ad libitum water intake but attenuated the drinking response to iv hypertonic saline and also increased the osmotic threshold for vasopressin release. Dogs with OVLT lesions also drank little or nothing in response to iv infusions of angiotensin and did not increase vas-

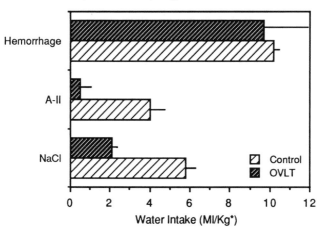

Fig. 7.15. Water intake after several dipsogens in dogs with OVLT lesions. The lesions impaired drinking to a salt load (14.6 m*M*/kg body weight) and systemic A-II (iv infusions of 20 pmol/kg/min for 30 min) but had no effect on drinking after hemorrhage (20 ml/kg). To avoid distortions of scale, the data from the NaCl test are expressed as ml/100 g body weight. Data from: Thrasher, T. N., and Ramsay, D. J. (1986). The organum vasculosum laminae terminalis. *In*: "The Physiology of Thirst and Sodium Appetite." (G. deCaro, A. N. Epstein, and M. Massi, eds.) pp. 327–332. Plenum Press, New York.

opressin release. The lesion did not reduce the drinking or vasopressin response to hemorrhage (Fig. 7.15). This indicates that hypovolemic thirst stimuli are not affected by OVLT lesions, a conclusion congruent with the fact that large AV3V lesions do not impair drinking in response to polyethylene glycol-induced hypovolemia in the rat (Buggy and Johnson, 1977b; Johnson and Buggy, 1977, 1978).

In the rat, lesions in the region immediately rostral to the third ventricle, which destroyed most or all of the ventral nucleus medianus and, in most cases, adjacent tissues of the OVLT, periventricular lining, and medioventral septum have been reported (Gardiner and Stricker, 1985a,b) to produce transient adipsia in a significant number of the animals tested. Others were normodipsic but polyuric (and hence in negative water balance) in the immediate postoperative period. About one-third of the animals became hyperdipsic within a few days or weeks after the lesions. This group included a significant number of animals that had been adipsic in the immediate postoperative period as well as others that had been normodipsic prior to the delayed onset of hyperdipsia. In most animals, the hyperdipsia was manifest primarily or exclusively at night, daytime intakes being within the normal range for most but not all animals. The water intake of the experimental animals was not reduced during periods of sodium or food restriction when they would generally consume less.

Some of the experimental and control (sham-operated) animals from the preceding study were further tested for their responsiveness to experimental treatments that result in cellular dehydration (sc hypertonic saline) or vascular hypovolemia (sc polyethylene glycol) (Gardiner and Stricker, 1985a,b). The brain-damaged rats responded poorly if at all to both hypertonic saline and PG when tested during the day but displayed essentially normal responses when tested at night or after pretreatment with caffeine. This pattern of results suggests that the region rostral to the anterior third ventricle may be the source of activational influences that play a significant role in the organization of drinking.

Subfornical Organ

The subfornical organ (SFO) protrudes into the dorsal aspects of the anterior third ventricle. It has been implicated in angiotensin-mediated thirst (see Chapter VIII on the central mechanism of angiotensin thirst) and in carbachol-elicited thirst.

The SFO is arguably the most sensitive brain site for both angiotensin and carbachol (Simpson and Routtenberg, 1972, 1973; Simpson et al., 1978a). Its role as a likely target for plasma angiotensin is discussed at length in Chapter VIII. The role of cholinergic brain pathways in thirst is discussed in detail in Chapter IX.

Lesions of the SFO have been reported to abolish or severely attenuate drinking responses to systemic angiotensin in rats (Simpson *et al.*, 1978a,b), dogs (Thrasher *et al.*, 1982a), and opossums (Elfont *et al.*, 1980). In rats, SFO lesions also attenuate the drinking response to intracranial carbachol (Simpson and Routtenberg, 1972), to polyethylene glycol-induced vascular hypovolemia, and to systemic isoproterenol (Simpson *et al.*, 1978a,b).

Several observations suggest that while the SFO may influence drinking responses to various extracellular thirst stimuli, it is not essential for their elaboration. Lesions in the SFO have been reported to significantly attenuate drinking after SC injections of a moderate dose (5 ml of a 20% solution) of PG but had little or no effect on drinking after 5 ml of a 30% solution. The rats with SFO lesions did drink, apparently normally, when the lower dose of PG was preceded by an injection of caffeine or hypertonic saline (Hosutt *et al.*, 1981). It is interesting to contrast this pattern of impairments in responding to low but not high doses of PG with a similar pattern seen after zona incerta lesions (Grossman and Grossman, 1978) and an opposite pattern seen after LPO or MPO neurotoxin lesions, which impair the rats' ability to respond to high doses of both hypertonic saline and PG without significantly impairing responses to low doses (McGowan *et al.*, 1988a,b).

Septal Area

Some, but not all, septal lesions produce hyperdipsia in rats (Harvey and Hunt, 1965; Lubar *et al.*, 1968; Black and Mogenson, 1973). It has been suggested (Besch and van Dyne, 1969) that damage to ventral aspects to the septum or, perhaps, ventral fiber connections (Tondat and Almli, 1975) might produce the most consistent effects. Others (e.g., Lubar *et al.*, 1968, 1969) have obtained best results from posterior lesions, and many other investigators have been unable to detect support for either suggestion in their data (Sorenson and Harvey, 1971; Carey, 1969).

A recent analysis of the problem (Iovino and Steardo, 1986) came to the conclusion that medioventral lesions that extended significantly below the level of the anterior commissure were more effective (60% of the rats became hyperdipsic) than lesions confined to the lateral septum (35%) or very large lesions that destroyed the entire septum (25%).

The hyperdipsia seen after some septal lesions does not appear to be secondary to polyuria (Lubar *et al.*, 1969; Blass and Hanson, 1970; Black and Mogenson, 1973), although some earlier reports suggested inhibitory effects on antidiuretic hormone secretion (Lubar *et al.*, 1968; Besch and van Dyne, 1969). Recent studies (Iovino *et al.*, 1983; Iovino and Steardo, 1986) have indicated that septal lesions have no effect on antidiuretic hormone release in response to polyethylene glycol but do significantly reduce plasma levels after hypertonic saline.

The increased water intake, on the other hand, appears to be due specifically to a facilitatory effect on drinking responses to extracellular thirst stimuli. Rats made hyperdipsic by septal lesions also drink significantly more in response to polyethylene glycol, caval ligation, ip renin, iv angiotensin, or sc isoproterenol. Water intake in response to gastric, ip, or iv loads of hypertonic saline are unaffected (Blass and Hanson, 1970; Blass *et al.*, 1974) (Fig. 7.16).

The effects of septal lesions on polyethylene glycol-induced drinking have been the subject of some controversy. Although rats with septal lesions consistently drink more than controls in response to ip injections of PG (Blass and Hanson, 1970; Blass *et al.*, 1974), there are several reports of normal drinking responses to sc injections that are equally effective in controls (Blass *et al.*, 1974; Black and Mogenson, 1973).

Stricker has reported that septal lesions do, in fact, result in exaggerated responses to PG given via either route of administration. However, the enhanced response to sc injections is delayed beyond the time (8–10 h) when the effect of PG is normally measured (Stricker, 1978b) and is significant only when higher concentrations of PG are used (Stricker, 1984). These observations help us to understand the immediate cause of an apparent contradiction in the literature but leave us with a far more difficult question: Stricker argues that the delayed response to sc PG must be due to very high plasma angiotensin levels to which

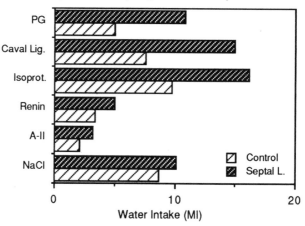

Fig. 7.16. Response to various dipsogens in rats with septal lesions. Polyethylene glycol was administered ip (2 ml of a 40% solution) and water intake was recorded 6–8.5 h after the injection. The value shown for caval ligation is the cumulative intake for 24 h after ligation of the inferior vena cava. Isoproterenol was administered sc (330 μg/kg) and water intake was collected for 2 h after the injection. Hog renin (2 U/100 g body weight) was administered ip and water intake was recorded for 3 h. Angiotensin II was infused iv (80 μg/kg in a concentration of 0.05 μg/μl). The salt load was administered iv for an unspecified time. Data from: Blass, E. M., Nussbaum, A. I., and Hanson, D. G. (1974). Septal hyperdipsia: Specific enhancement of drinking to angiotensin in rats. *J. Comp. Physiol. Psychol.* **87**, 422–439.

the rat with septal lesions appears to be particularly sensitive. Yet ip injections of PG produce far smaller volume deficits and, presumably, lower angiotensin levels by the time they become effective in stimulating excessive drinking in the rat with septal lesions. If the response to sc PG is the result of hyperreactivity to very high levels of angiotensin, why does the septal animal overdrink in response to ip PG?

Blass and colleagues (1974) suggested that the apparently general facilitatory effects of septal lesions on drinking responses to all extracellular stimuli might be due to the fact that they are all mediated by the renin–angiotensin system. As we have seen in our earlier discussion of systemic angiotensin, it is probably not the principal route used to signal hypovolemic conditions to the brain. Stricker's demonstration of very large temporal differences in the effectiveness of sc and ip polyethylene glycol suggests that an exaggerated response to angiotensin is almost certainly not responsible for the hyperdipsic effects of septal lesions.

It should be pointed out, in this connection, that single neurons in the medial septum have been shown to change their firing rate in response to osmotic as well as volemic thirst stimuli (Bridge and Hatton, 1973).

Electrical stimulation of the septal area inhibits drinking responses to cellular as well as extracellular thirst stimuli (Moran and Blass, 1976), water deprivation (Wishart and Mogenson, 1970), or lateral hypothalamic electrical stimulation (Sibole et al., 1971).

Although no clear picture has as yet emerged from the experimental literature on the septum, it appears likely that it is the source of inhibitory (satiety?) signals that affect water intake under most natural circumstances. What remains puzzling is the fact that septal lesions, even quite large ones, have such variable effects on water intake. One is tempted to think of a secondary, irritative or ischemic reaction in neighboring tissues (which might be differentially affected by lesions in different animals, depending perhaps on the exact course of blood vessels or other conductive tissue). The notable failure of several investigators to consistently find segments of the area where lesions might be especially effective unfortunately does not offer much support for such a conclusion.

Review and Conclusions

Traditionally, investigators in search of brain mechanisms regulating thirst and related renal functions have looked to the hypothalamus because the early clinical literature implicated the area in the excessive thirst and diuresis of diabetes insipidus. The development of stereotaxic surgery in the 1930s made it possible to explore subcortical structures and it was not long after the end of World War II that researchers from the University of Pennsylvania reported adipsia in rats and cats after damage to the lateral hypothalamic area.

Intensive study of the phenomenon demonstrated gradual recovery of food-associated drinking but little or no return of drinking responses to experimental procedures that result in cellular or extracellular dehydration. Rats that "recovered" from the acute effects of LH lesions also returned to a state of adipsia during periods of food deprivation. The animals appeared to be capable of drinking but devoid of systemic cues to do so except when the oral (and perhaps digestive) requirements of food ingestion indicated a specific and apparently local "need." As a consequence of this research, it was widely accepted in the 1950s and 1960s that the lateral hypothalamus contained neural mechanisms essential for the elaboration of thirst.

A different interpretation of the by now classic "lateral hypothalamic syndrome" was proposed in the 1970s when it became clear that lateral hypothalamic lesions produced not only adipsia (usually accompanied by aphagia) but also severe sensorimotor and arousal dysfunctions that appeared to recover in parallel with ingestive behavior. This aspect of the lesion syndrome was shown to be due, at least in part, to an interruption of ascending catecholaminergic components of the medial forebrain bundle that course though the LH and adjacent portions of the internal capsule.

Intracerebroventricular or intradiencephalic injections of the neurotoxin 6-hydroxydopamine were particularly effective in producing the LH lesion syndrome when administered in conjunction with drugs that promote the preferential destruction of dopaminergic neurons. The nigrostriatal projections that rely exclusively on DA neurons thus became the primary candidate for a neural substrate for activational responses to internal stimuli related to thirst and hunger.

Today there is little doubt that the sensorimotor and arousal dysfunctions seen in the acute recovery phases of LH lesions contribute significantly to the acute impairments in ingestive behavior. The principal unresolved issue is whether the persisting adipsia during periods of food deprivation and often severe unresponsiveness to cellular as well as extracellular thirst stimuli seen in rats with LH lesions should be interpreted entirely or even in part in terms of persisting "subclinical" arousal dysfunctions as a number of investigators have proposed.

Stricker, for instance, has shown that rats with LH lesions can excrete salt loads in concentrated urine and display delayed and relatively small drinking responses to hypertonic saline as well as to several extracellular thirst stimuli. He suggests that the normal drinking response to these dipsogens is absent because the animal's damaged arousal system cannot deal with the stress imposed by experimental procedures. The logic of this argument is sound, but it seems only fair to note that exactly the same pattern of drinking would be expected if a neural mechanism specifically related to thirst were partially damaged and thus unable to deal with what amounts to unphysiological emergencies. It is not clear, in any case, why a "recovered" animal with LH lesions should be adipsic during periods of food deprivation.

There have been numerous attempts to address the issue experimentally. Intra-hypothalamic injections of the neurotoxin kainic acid, which destroys some nerve cell bodies but has no effect on fibers of passage, have been shown to produce transient adipsia, hypodipsia, and reduced responsiveness to systemic hypertonic saline. These injections do not produce dopamine depletions or somnolence, akinesia, or reduced reactivity to sensory input (they do, in fact, elicit hyperactivity). Their effects on drinking have been significant but not as severe and persistent as those of electrolytic lesions.

Surgical knife cuts dorsal, caudal, rostral, or lateral to the critical region of the dorso-lateral hypothalamus have been shown to have a wide variety of effects on ad libitum water intake and drinking in response to cellular or extracellular dipsogens. These cuts also produce effects on striatal dopamine and sensorimotor and arousal functions, which vary from the very severe and persistent to the negligible. Attempts to correlate the severity of the thirst deficits with the magnitude and persistence of the sensorimotor dysfunctions or dopamine depletions have been unsuccessful. These studies demonstrate the importance of various afferent and efferent connections to and from the lateral hypothalamus in thirst. They do not, on balance, support the notion of a stress-induced nonspecific dysfunction at the heart of the LH lesion syndrome, but also do not completely rule out the more restrictive hypothesis that arousal dysfunctions may well play a role in its acute phase.

Electrical stimulation of many lateral hypothalamus sites elicits drinking. Although this seems to provide strong support for the hypothesis that neural mechanisms specifically related to thirst and drinking are represented here, Valenstein has offered an alternative interpretation. He noted that electrical stimulation at some hypothalamic sites elicits behaviors (such as eating, food-carrying, etc.) other than drinking when water is not available and that some animals would switch between different behaviors depending on situational variables. Valenstein proposed therefore that stimulation of the LH might activate "prepotent" responses to prominent features of the environment due to an increase in general activation rather than a specific behavior such as drinking or a related motivational state such as thirst. Numerous investigators have attempted to demonstrate the specificity of the stimulation effect. The weight of the evidence here, as in the case of LH lesions, favors the hypothesis that thirst-related mechanisms are present in this region. Unfortunately, the weight is not sufficient to allow one to disregard Valenstein's version of the nonspecific arousal hypothesis.

It may be useful to emphasize that the lateral hypothalamus is indeed traversed by fibers of passage known to participate in arousal. Lesions and stimulation in the area should, consequently, affect reactivity to environmental as well as internal stimuli. The question at issue here is whether the area also contains neurons specifically concerned with thirst and the regulation of body fluids.

At least partially in response to the uncertainties that have surrounded the interpretation of the effects of hypothalamic lesions and stimulation, investigators have turned their attention to other regions of the brain. The tissues immediately dorsal or rostral to the hypothalamus have been the subject of most contemporary interest.

Rats with lesions confined to the rostromedial zona incerta are not afflicted with disabling sensorimotor or arousal dysfunctions but display a pattern of drinking that is all but identical to that seen in rats that have "recovered" from the acute effects of LH lesions. After a brief postoperative interlude of hypodipsia, ad libitum water intake is normal. However, the animals become adipsic when food deprived and remain so for several days. They drink little if at all in response to systemic salt loads as well as isoproterenol or iv or icv angiotensin. To complete a pattern that appears to be typical of damage to more rostral regions, rats with ZI lesions drink normally or nearly so in response to high doses of polyethylene glycol or formalin, whereas the response to low doses is generally impaired.

The effects of ZI lesions are probably due to the destruction of neurons indigenous to the area, since iontophoretic injections of the neurotoxin kainic acid reproduce the effects of electrolytic damage.

Lesions in the lateral preoptic area have been reported to selectively impair drinking in response to salt loads. Recent experiments have suggested that damage to the LPO may also reduce the drinking response to high doses of polyethylene glycol and delay water intake after systemic angiotensin. Water intake after low salt loads or low doses of PG was normal in these studies. The involvement of the LPO in cellular dehydration thirst is further indicated by the fact that some cells in the area modulate their firing rate in response to systemic salt loads. Local microinjections of hypertonic saline or sucrose elicit drinking in rats and rabbits, although positive placements seem to be hard to find.

The tissues surrounding the anteroventral third ventricle (AV3V) have attracted much attention in recent years. Rats with lesions in this region are adipsic and extremely hypernatremic (as well as hyperthermic). Those animals that do not die within a few days after surgery eventually recover essentially normal ad libitum drinking, but persisting deficits are prominent. These animals drink little in response to deprivation, hypertonic saline, isoproterenol, and systemic as well as central angiotensin. Only the drinking response to PG-induced hypovolemia appears to be spared. Microinjections of angiotensin or hypertonic saline or sucrose into the AV3V elicit drinking.

AV3V lesions and microinjections typically invade neighboring tissues, and one might ask to what extent the AV3V syndrome may be due to this incidental damage. Impaired responding to systemic salt loads as well as hypernatremia have been reported after neurotoxin lesions in the medial preoptic region. In the same series of experiments, electrolytic lesions strictly confined to the lining of the third ventricle and immediately adjacent tissues had no effect on water intake in a variety of tests.

In sheep and goats, lesions of the organum vasculosum of the lamina terminalis produce the adipsia and hypernatremia observed in rats with AV3V lesions and impair drinking responses to systemic salt loads as well as to angiotensin. In dogs, ad libitum water intake is intact after selective damage to the OVLT, but drinking as well as vasopressin secretion in response to hypertonic saline is specifically impaired.

Selective damage to the nucleus medianus has been reported to produce transient adipsia (followed, in some animals, by hyperdipsia). Drinking in response to systemic salt loads as well as PG was impaired but only when the tests were conducted at night.

The subfornical organ may be the most sensitive brain site for angiotensin and carbachol. Lesions of this tiny structure severely reduce or abolish drinking responses to both dipsogens as well as to systemic polyethylene glycol and isoproterenol.

Some septal lesions result in hyperdipsia and consistently enhanced responding to extracellular thirst stimuli. Drinking responses to hypertonic saline, on the other hand, are normal. Electrical stimulation of the septum has been reported to inhibit drinking responses to cellular as well as extracellular thirst stimuli.

Chapter 8

Brain Mechanisms II: Intracranial Angiotensin

Dipsogenic Effects of Intracranial Renin–Angiotensin

The pioneering research of Fitzsimons (Fitzsimons and Simons, 1968, 1969; Fitzsimons, 1969a,b, 1970a,b, 1971a,b,c) and others (Gross *et al.*, 1965; Maebashi and Yoshinaga, 1967; Peskar *et al.*, 1970) demonstrated that water deprivation, as well as experimental procedures that lower blood pressure or volume, activates the renin–angiotensin system. Fitzsimons (1969a, 1970a) proposed two hypotheses, which are not mutually exclusive, to explain its role in extracellular thirst. Angiotensin might stimulate thirst-related brain mechanisms: (a) indirectly, by modulating the sensitivity of baroreceptors in the great veins and atria of the heart, which are sensitive to changes in blood pressure and volume, or (b) directly, by acting as a neurotransmitter or neuromodulator in the brain.

As we have seen in Chapter V, there is much experimental support for the proposed involvement of stretch receptors in the low-pressure return to the heart in extracellular thirst. Some extracellular thirst stimuli, such as polyethylene glycol-induced hypovolemia, may rely primarily if not exclusively, on this input system.

Just what influence circulating angiotensin may have on the receptors of this system has been difficult to establish. The procedures that block the release or conversion of angiotensin (e.g., nephrectomy, high doses of conversion blockers, etc.) have major direct effects on peripheral blood pressure. This, in turn, influences the activity of the left atrial mechanoreceptors that provide the brain with information about blood volume and pressure via vagal afferents. It has been difficult to isolate a component of this response that represents a a direct action of angiotensin on the receptors of this system.

Fitzsimon's hypothesis that angiotensin might act directly on the brain, on the other hand, was promptly supported by a flurry of reports that intracranial injections of angiotensin, in doses several orders of magnitude smaller than those shown to be effective systemically, elicit drinking as well as vasopressin release

(Booth, 1968; Epstein *et al.*, 1970; Severs *et al.*, 1970, Andersson and Westbye, 1970; Keil *et al.*, 1975; Hoffman and Phillips, 1977) (Fig. 8.1).

More recent research has added sodium appetite to the list of effects seen, at least in the rat, after intracranial angiotensin injections (Avrith and Fitzsimons, 1980; Bryant *et al.*, 1980; Epstein, 1982; Fluharty and Epstein, 1983; Fluharty and Manaker, 1983).

Intracranial angiotensin II (A-II) injections also result in systemic hypertension (Severs *et al.*, 1970; Hoffman and Phillips, 1976b, 1977), but the dipsogenic action of central angiotensin appears to be independent of its pressor effect (Kucharczyk and Mogenson, 1976; Fitzsimons and Kucharczyk, 1978; Simpson *et al.*, 1978b; Fitzsimons, 1979).

The dipsogenic properties of intracranial angiotensin have proven to be ubiquitous. A partial list of the species that drink in response to intracranial angiotensin includes the rat (Epstein *et al.*, 1970), cat (Sturgeon *et al.*, 1973), dog (Rolls and Ramsay, 1975), monkey (Setler, 1971), baboon (Lotter *et al.*, 1980), goat (Andersson and Westbye, 1970), sheep (Abraham *et al.*, 1975), gerbil (Block *et al.*, 1974), opossum (Elfont *et al.*, 1980), pigeon (Evered and Fitzsimons, 1976a,b), chicken (Snapir *et al.*, 1976), Japanese quail (Takei, 1977), Peking duck (deCaro *et al.*, 1980b), and iguana (Fitzsimons and Kaufman, 1977).

Early investigations of the dipsogenic properties of intracranial angiotensin

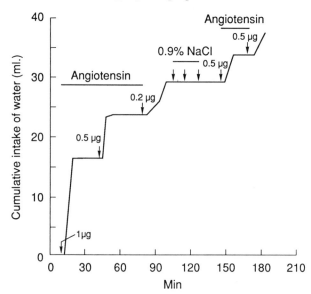

Fig. 8.1.   Drinking elicited in the rat by microinjections of angiotensin II into the lateral hypothalamus of the rat. After: Epstein, A. N., Fitzsimons, J. T., and Rolls, (nee Simons), B. J. (1970). Drinking induced by injection of angiotensin into the brain of the rat. *J. Physiol.* **210**, 457–474. With permission of the authors and the Physiological Society, Oxford, England.

used microgram doses, which now appear excessive. Subsequent efforts to determine the most sensitive central site(s) have demonstrated significant drinking after threshold doses of angiotensin in the nanogram or picogram ranges (Epstein and Hsiao, 1975; Hsiao et al., 1977; Simpson, 1975; Simpson et al., 1978a,b; Phillips, 1978). Contemporary investigators typically report optimal effects after 10–100 ng of A-II. It has been argued (e.g., Abraham et al., 1975) that even the lower doses result in local concentrations that are higher than those reached in plasma following the iv injection of dipsogenic doses of A-II. This is an important consideration for intraparenchymal injections. Angiotensin II injected icv becomes diluted by a substantial quantity of cerebrospinal fluid before reaching target tissues located, presumably, in circumventricular organs.

The dipsogenic properties of intracranial angiotensin are well established at this time. However, a number of questions about the effect have as yet been only partially resolved. Neurons in at least two different regions of the brain may be able to respond to changes in plasma angiotensin. Angiotensin receptors have been identified in many additional regions of the brain, suggesting that this peptide may act as a neurotransmitter or neuromodulator. Such an interpretation is supported by the fact that all components of the renin–angiotensin system are present in brain parenchyma. Renin and angiotensin have been detected in neurons but the distribution of converting enzyme has a different distribution, leading some investigators (Ganong, 1984) to suggest that A-II may be directly produced from substrate without angiotensin I (A-I) as an intermediate. Lastly, there are some puzzling differences between the effects of increased plasma angiotensin and intracranial injections and infusions (even though many of the same cardiovascular, hormonal, and behavioral mechanisms are involved).

Antidipsogenic Effects of A-II Synthesis Inhibitors and Receptor Blockers

Effects on Drinking to Intracranial Renin or Angiotensin

Intracranial injections of pepstatin, an inhibitor of the renin–angiotensinogen reaction that prevents the formation of A-I, have been shown to reduce the drinking response of rats to renin or renin substrate administered through the same cannula (Fig. 8.2). The drinking response to A-I or A-II was not significantly impaired (Epstein et al., 1974; Fitzsimons et al., 1978a) (Fig. 8.3).

Intrahypothalamic or icv injections of SQ-20881, an inhibitor of the converting enzyme responsible for the transformation of A-I to A-II, have been reported to significantly reduce drinking responses to renin, renin substrate, and A-I injected through the same cannula in rats (Severs et al., 1973; Epstein et al., 1974; Fitzsimons et al., 1978a) and pigeons (Evered and Fitzsimons, 1976b;

Fitzsimons and Evered, 1977). The drinking response to A-II was slightly increased in these experiments. The inhibitory effects of intrahypothalamic as well as icv injections of SQ-20881 on drinking responses to A-I administered via the same route have not been replicated in some laboratories (Burkhardt *et al.*, 1975; Swanson *et al.*, 1973a,b; Bryant and Falk, 1973). The reasons for this discrepancy are not entirely clear. It has been suggested (Fitzsimons, 1979) that the ratio of antagonist to agonist (A-I) may have been too low to prevent the conversion of significant quantities of A-I into A-II in the experiments that failed to demonstrate significant inhibitory effects.

Injections of saralasin, a specific competitive antagonist of angiotensin, into the preoptic area of the rat reduce or abolish the drinking response to renin, renin substrate, A-I, and A-II (but not carbachol) administered through the same cannula (Epstein *et al.*, 1974; Fitzsimons, 1975; Fitzsimons *et al.*, 1978a).

Intracerebroventricular injections of saralasin also significantly attenuate drinking responses to icv renin, A-I, and A-II in the rat (Summy-Long and Severs, 1974) and cat (Cooling and Day, 1975). Intracerebroventricular saralasin produces similar inhibitory effects on drinking responses to systemic (sc or iv) injections of A-II (Johnson and Schwob, 1975; Cooling and Day, 1975). Systemic injections of saralasin did not block the drinking response to sc angiotensin in some of these experiments (Johnson and Schwob, 1975). Intracerebroventricular infusions of saralasin also inhibit furosemide-induced sodium appetite (as well as waterdrinking response to icv A-II) in rats (Weiss, 1986).

Very high doses of saralasin administered iv have been reported to reduce the drinking response to icv angiotensin (Hoffman and Phillips, 1976a). This effect may be due to increased blood pressure, which may promote the transport of saralasin into brain (Phillips *et al.*, 1977b).

Intracranial injections of anti-angiotensin-II serum block the drinking response

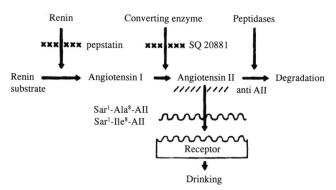

Fig. 8.2. The sites of action of angiotensin antiserum and of peptide antagonists of the renin angiotensin system. From: Fitzsimons, J. T. (1979). "The Physiology of Thirst and Sodium Appetite." Cambridge University Press, Cambridge. Reproduced with permission of the author and Cambridge University Press.

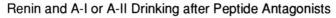

Renin and A-I or A-II Drinking after Peptide Antagonists

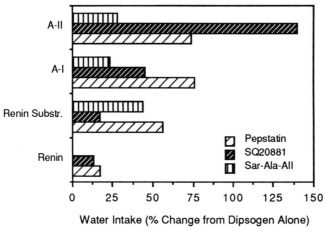

Water Intake (% Change from Dipsogen Alone)

Fig. 8.3. Effects of three peptide antagonists (see Fig. 8.2 for site of action) on water intake after renin, renin substrate, A-I, and A-II. Pepstatin (8.75×10^{-9} mol) was tested against 10^{-11} mol A-I or A-II or renin substrate or 1 mU of renin. SQ 20881 (10×10^{-9} mol) and Sar^1-Ala^8-A-II (5×10^{-14}) was tested against 10×10^{-12} mol of A-I or A-II or renin substrate or 10 mU of renin. Data from: Fitzsimons, J. T., Epstein, A. N., and Johnson, A. K. (1978a). Peptide antagonists of the renin-angiotensin system in the characterization of the receptors for angiotensin-induced thirst. *Brain Res.* **153**, 319–331.

of A-II and reduce the response to A-I and renin substrate administered through the same cannula (Epstein *et al.*, 1973).

Effects on Drinking Elicited by Cellular and Extracellular Thirst Stimuli

Intracerebroventricular injections of saralasin, at doses that inhibit drinking to icv angiotensin, have no significant effect on drinking responses to sc poly-ethylene glycol or sc hypertonic saline (Summy-Long and Severs, 1974; Ramsey and Reid, 1975). Intracranial (Schwob and Johnson, 1976) but not iv (Tang and Falk, 1974) injections of saralasin do inhibit the drinking response to systemic isoproterenol.

In agreement with the saralasin effects just noted, it has been shown that icv injections of angiotensin antiserum do not inhibit drinking responses to sc injec-tions of polyethylene glycol or hypertonic saline (Severs *et al.*, 1978).

Effects on Drinking after Deprivation

Most investigators have failed to observe significant effects of the competitive angiotensin inhibitor saralasin on water intake elicited by deprivation in rats (e.g., Phillips and Hoffman, 1977; Lee *et al.*, 1981), dogs (Ramsay and Reid, 1975), or sheep (Abraham *et al.*, 1975, 1976). Normal drinking after 48 h of water deprivation has also been observed in rats receiving continuous iv infusions of saralasin in addition to bolus icv injection of the compound (Severs *et al.*, 1977).

Malvin *et al.* (1977) have reported delayed deprivation-induced drinking in 30-h deprived rats following continuous infusions of saralasin for 75 min prior to access to water. However, the pattern of drinking (periods of complete suppression alternating with periods of apparently normal drinking) suggests nonspecific effects rather than a reduction in thirst commensurate with the relatively small (~25%) contribution of extracellular thirst under the deprivation conditions of the experiment.

A significant reduction of deprivation-induced drinking has been reported (Hoffman *et al.*, 1978; Severs *et al.*, 1978) following icv injections of the A-II receptor blocker saralasin combined with the cholinergic receptor blocker atropine. Neither compound was able to block drinking when administered alone. The synergistic action of the two receptor antagonists suggests that two different neural pathways may be involved in the powerful dipsogenic effects of A-II and carbachol, in spite of the many apparent similarities of icv injections of the two compound. Both pathways may independently contribute to deprivation-induced thirst.

Pressor Effects of Intracranial Angiotensin

The principal function of the renin–angiotensin system is the regulation of blood volume and pressure. The dipsogenic properties of intracranial angiotensin appear to be independent (although closely associated in most instances) of its direct and indirect effects on blood pressure (but see Simpson *et al.*, 1978b; 1979; and Fitzsimons and Kucharczyk, 1978). It nonetheless appears useful at this point to briefly consider the pressor effects of intracranial A-II and related compounds.

Intracerebroventricular injections of A-II increase blood pressure mainly by causing the release of vasopressin. (Severs *et al.*, 1970; Keil *et al.*, 1975; Hoffman *et al.*, 1977; Brody *et al.*, 1978). Intracerebroventricular A-II also stimulates the sympathetic nervous system directly, but this does not appear to be essential for the development of hypertension in the rat since chemical sympathectomy does not prevent the effect (Falcon *et al.*, 1976). Unlike iv angiotensin, which produces an immediate blood pressure rise of short duration, the increase seen after icvV A-II is delayed and persisting (Phillips *et al.*, 1977a) (Fig. 8.4).

ICV injections of angiotensin antagonists such as saralasin have been shown to lower blood pressure in a variety of strains of genetically hypertensive rats

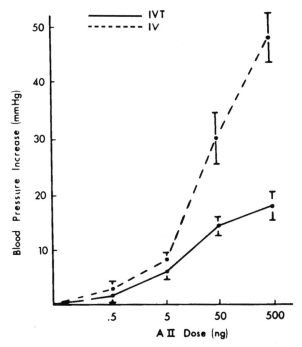

Fig. 8.4. Effects of angiotensin II administered intravenously (IV) or intracerebroventricularly (IVT) on blood pressure in the cat. From: Phillips, M. I., Felix, D., Hoffman, W. E., and Ganten, D. (1977a). Angiotensin-sensitive sites in the brain ventricular system. *In:* "Soc. Neurosci. Symposia." (W. M. Cowan, and J. A. Ferrrendelli eds.) pp. 308–339. Society for Neuroscience, Bethesda. Reproduced with permission of the authors and the Society for Neuroscience.

(Ganten *et al.*, 1975, 1978; Phillips *et al.*, 1975, 1977b; Sweet *et al.*, 1977; Schoelkens *et al.*, 1976).

In the rat, the pressor effects of icv angiotensin appear to be due primarily to its action on neurons in the subfornical organ (SFO) and the anteroventral third ventricle (AV3V) organum vasculosum of the laminae terminalis (OVLT) and nucleus medianus. Microinjections of very small quantities of A-II into either region release vasopressin and produce systemic pressor response (Simpson *et al.*, 1978b; Mangiapane and Simpson, 1980a; Johnson *et al.*, 1978, 1980). Intracerebroventricular injections restricted to the anterior third ventricle by cold-cream plugs also produce the effect (Phillips, 1978) .

Lesions in the SFO (Mangiapane and Simpson, 1980b) or AV3V (Mangiapane *et al.*, 1983; Brody *et al.*, 1978; Buggy *et al.*, 1977a; Thrasher and Ramsay, 1986) reduce the pressor responses normally produced by systemic injections of angiotensin. Transection of the reciprocal connections between the SFO and AV3V (Lind *et al.*, 1982; Miselis, 1981; Miselis *et al.*, 1979) produce similar effects (Lind *et al.*, 1983; Lind and Johnson, 1982a; Knepel *et al.*, 1982).

Lesions in the AV3V have also been reported to abolish antidiuretic and pressor responses to icv A-II (Johnson *et al.*, 1978).

These lesions also produce chronic elevations of plasma renin concentrations (Shrager and Johnson, 1980), although plasma renin activity appears to be unaffected, possibly due to decreased substrate induced and/or released (Hartle *et al.*, 1979).

Lesions in the AV3V also block or reverse various types of experimental hypertension (Buggy *et al.*, 1977a,b; Brody *et al.*, 1978; Brody and Johnson, 1980; Gordon *et al.*, 1982; Haywood *et al.*, 1983) that are thought to be initiated by increased plasma levels of angiotensin (Haber, 1976).

Efferents from the AV3V have been shown to project to vasopressin- and oxytocin-containing cells in the supraoptic and paraventricular nuclei (Miselis, 1981; Silverman *et al.*, 1981). These neurosecretory organs also receive neural input from the SFO (Shapiro and Miselis, 1978; Miselis, 1981, 1986). Some of these fibers traverse the AV3V and are thus interrupted by lesions in this area (Lind *et al.*, 1982). This probably contributes to the impaired vasopressin secretion seen after AV3V damage. There is some evidence that at least some of these projections may be angiotensinergic (Mitchell *et al.*, 1984).

Angiotensin-sensitive neurons have been found in the supraoptic nucleus (Sakai *et al.*, 1974; Nicoll and Barker, 1971). This suggests that vasopressin release may be due in part to the activation of these neurons by angiotensinergic efferents from the OVLT and nucleus medianum (Miselis *et al.*, 1979). This route may be especially important for the observed pressor responses to icv angiotensin. [Note, however, that Phillips *et al.*, (1977a) have suggested that A-II in cerebrospinal fluid (CSF) might gain direct access to vasopressin-secreting neurons or their projections.]

Projections from the AV3V region to the cardiovascular control centers of the lower brainstem have been shown to pass through the ventromedial hypothalamus (VMH) (Conrad and Pfaff, 1976; Swanson *et al.*, 1978). Lesions in the VMH have been shown to prevent the systemic pressor effects of intracranial injections of angiotensin (Johnson *et al.*, 1981a).

In the dog, cat, and rabbit, the area postrema in the lower brainstem has been identified as the primary central site of action for systemic pressor responses to blood-borne angiotensin (Ferrario *et al.*, 1972). In the rat, A-II injections into the vertebral arteries that supply the lower brainstem are no more effective than intraaortic injections, and ablation of this region does not prevent the development of experimental renal hypertension (Buggy *et al.*, 1978b). This suggests that in the rat the lower brainstem cardiovascular centers may receive neural rather than hormonal (A-II) inputs from A-II–sensitive neurons in the AV3V and/or SFO.

It is noteworthy, in this context, that the AV3V and specifically the nucleus medianus receive prominent afferents from several brainstem cardiovascular centers, including the paraventricular nucleus of the hypothalamus, the parabrachial nucleus, the nucleus of the solitary tract (NST), and the ventrolateral medulla (Saper and Levisohn, 1983). Neural information reaches the NST via cranial nerves IX and X. From here, catecholaminergic projections ascend to the region of the AV3V (Saper *et al.*, 1983). There is some evidence that these ascending noradrenergic projections play a major role in the regulation of blood pressure and vasopressin release (Lightman *et al.*, 1984). The NST also projects to the parabrachial nucleus, which in turn enervates the nucleus medianus (Saper and Loewy, 1980).

Localization of Angiotensin-Sensitive Brain Mechanisms

Most of the early investigations (e.g., Booth, 1968; Fitzsimons, 1971a; Epstein *et al.*, 1970; Sharpe and Swanson, 1974; Burckhardt *et al.*, 1975; Johnson, 1975; Kucharczyk and Mogenson, 1976) injected angiotensin into the parenchyma of the brain and reported sensitive sites in regions of the brainstem (such as the preoptic region, lateral hypothalamus, and septum) that had been implicated in the control of thirst by earlier lesion studies. However, A-II injections into other sites such as the mesencephalic grey and anterior thalamus of the rat (Swanson and Sharpe, 1973; Swanson *et al.*, 1973a,b) and monkey (Sharpe and Swanson, 1974) also produced drinking. The success of these intraparenchymal injections is difficult to interpret because angiotensin does not cross the blood-brain barrier under normal circumstances (Osborne *et al.*, 1971; Shrager *et al.*, 1975; Ganten *et al.*, 1975).

Most investigators in the field have therefore turned their attention to the circumventricular organs (CVOs) that have an arterial blood supply that is entirely or in part on the blood side of the blood-brain barrier. The fenestrated capillaries of the CVOs permit large peptides such as angiotensin to act on neurons that project to numerous other regions of the brain (Weindl, 1973; Van Houten *et al.*, 1980).

Investigators of the dipsogenic and pressor effects of angiotensin have concentrated on two of the CVOs: (a) the subfornical organ (SFO) and (b) the region of the anteroventral third ventricle (AV3V), which includes the organum vasculosum of the lamina terminalis (OVLT), the nucleus medianus of the preoptic region (nMPO), and immediately adjacent portions of the periventricular region and medial preoptic (MPO) area (Fig. 8.5).

The Subfornical Organ (SFO)

The subfornical organ is a small circumventricular organ that protrudes into the ventricular spaces near the junction of the lateral and third ventricles. The arterial blood supply of the SFO is on the blood side of the blood-brain-barrier and thus

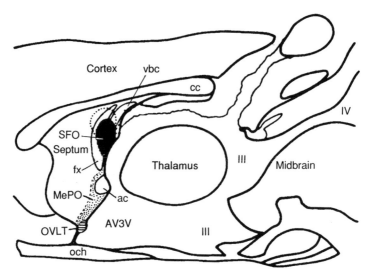

Fig. 8.5. Tissues adjacent to the anterior aspects of the third ventricle, which have been implicated in the regulation of thirst and body fluid balance. SFO, subfornical organ (black); MePO, nucleus media-nus of the preoptic region (stippled); OVLT, organum vasculosum of the laminae terminalis (striped); AV3V, anteroventral third ventricle; III and IV, third and fourth ventricle. After: Lind, R. W., Thunhorst, R. L., and Johnson, A. K. (1984). The subfornical organ and the integration of multiple factors in thirst. *Physiol. Behav.* **32,** 69–74. With permission of the authors and Pergamon Press.

provides access to neural tissue of the brain for larger peptides, such as angiotensin, which are excluded elsewhere (Spoerri, 1963).

The SFO contains many neurons that respond to iv injections or iontophoretic applications of A-II. This response is blocked by topical application of the competitive A-II blocker saralasin (Felix, 1976; Felix and Akert, 1974; Phillips and Felix, 1976; Felix *et al.*, 1986) (Fig. 8.6).

Simpson and Routtenberg (1973) first reported that microinjections of A-II into the subfornical organ elicited significant drinking in rats at nanogram doses that were lower than those found to be effective when injected icv. Subsequent, more detailed analyses of the phenomenon indicated that microinjections of picogram doses of A-II, which were lower than those found effective elsewhere in the brain, into the SFO could elicit significant drinking in the rat (Simpson *et al.*, 1978a,b; Mangiapane and Simpson, 1980a) (Fig. 8.7).

Abdelaal *et al.* (1974b) have reported that destruction of the subfornical organ significantly reduced the drinking response of the rat to systemically administered angiotensin II. This observation has been replicated in rats (Simpson and Routtenberg, 1975, 1978; Simpson *et al.*, 1978a; Buggy and Fisher, 1976; Hosutt *et al.*, 1981), dogs (Thrasher *et al.*, 1982a), opossums (Elfont *et al.*, 1980), and pigeons (Massi *et al.*, 1986b). In rats as well as opossums, SFO lesions block the drinking response to systemic A-II completely, and apparently

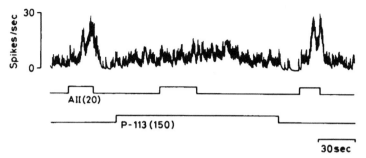

Fig. 8.6. The response of neurons in the subfornical organ to iontophoretically applied angiotensin II before, during, and after the administration of the blocking analogue saralasin (P–113). From: Phillips, M. I., Felix, D., Hoffman, W. E., and Ganten, D. (1977a). Angiotensin-sensitive sites in the brain ventricular system. *In:* "Soc. Neurosci. Symposia." (W. M. Cowan, and J. A. Ferrrendelli (Eds.) pp. 308–339. Society for Neuroscience, Bethesda Md. Reproduced with permission of the authors and the Society for Neuroscience.

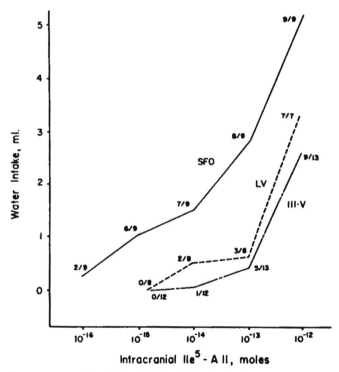

Fig. 8.7. Dose-response relationship for drinking during 15 min after the injection of Ile[5] angiotensin II into the subfornical organ (SFO), the dorsal third ventricle (III-V), or lateral ventricle (LV) at the level of the interventricular foramen. From: Simpson, J. B., Epstein, A. N., and Camardo, J. S. (1978a). Localization of receptors for dipsogenic action of angiotensin II in the subfornical organ of rat. *J. Comp. Physiol. Psychol.* **92**, 581–608. Reproduced with permission of the authors and the American Psychological Association.

permanently, when the latter is administered in near-threshold doses (Simpson *et al.*, 1978a; Elfont *et al.*, 1980). In rats, the drinking response to systemic (sc) renin has been reported attenuated but not abolished after SFO lesions (Johnson and Buggy, 1977). In sheep, the dipsogenic effect of A-II is not affected by SFO lesions (McKinley *et al.*, 1986). Transections of the efferent connections of the SFO also have been reported to block drinking responses to systemic A-II in the rat (Eng and Miselis, 1981; Lind and Johnson, 1982a,b)

The specificity of the SFO lesion effect is emphasized by the results of experiments that have shown that microinjections of the competitive angiotensin receptor blocker saralasin into the SFO reduce drinking responses to systemic (iv) angiotensin in a dose-dependent manner (Simpson *et al.*, 1978a).

A reduced drinking response to polyethylene glycol-induced hypovolemia (thought to be independent of renal angiotensin) and isoproterenol (which releases renin from the kidney) has also been reported after SFO lesions in the rat (Simpson *et al.*, 1978a). The impaired response to PG is seen only with low to moderate doses. When a high concentration of the coloid is administered or the PG test is preceded by injections of caffeine, rats with SFO lesions drink as much as controls (Hosutt *et al.*, 1981) (Fig. 8.8).

Subfornical organ lesions also reduce the drinking response to systemic salt loads. Hosutt *et al.* (1981) have reported that this impairment is seen only after

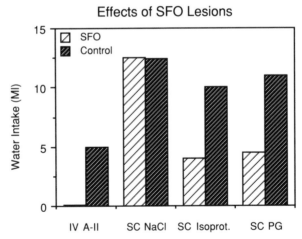

Fig. 8.8. Effects of SFO lesions on drinking to various dipsogens. Drinking response to iv infusions of 16–128 ng/μl/min of angiotensin II continued for 17.5 min was completely abolished. The response to sc injections of 2 ml of 2 *M* NaCl was intact, but drinking response to two extracellular thirst stimuli, isoproterenol (2-h intake after 160 μg/kg, sc) and polyethylene glycol (PG) (7-h intake after 5 ml of a 20% solution, sc) was impaired. Data from: Simpson, J. B., Epstein, A. N., and Camardo, J. S. (1978a). Localization of receptors for dipsogenic action of angiotensin II in the subfornical organ of rat. *J. Comp. Physiol. Psychol.* **92**, 581–608.

low doses of hypertonic NaCl. Essentially normal drinking after high salt loads has been reported by several investigators (Eng and Miselis, 1981; Simpson et al., 1978a). Others (Lind et al., 1984) have reported that SFO lesions produce significant deficits after high as well as low doses.

Deefferentation of the SFO also has been reported to reduce the drinking response to high as well as low doses of hypertonic NaCl (Lind and Johnson, 1982a,b). It has been suggested (Lind et al., 1984) that the more effective SFO lesions involve the ventral stalk, which carries all known efferent connections of the SFO (Lind et al., 1982; Miselis, 1981; Miselis et al., 1979). On balance, these results suggest that the SFO may exert a general influence on thirst, although the response to blood-borne A-II appears to be most severely affected by damage to this structure.

Simpson and Routtenberg (1973) have reported that SFO lesions also reduced or abolished the drinking response to A-II injections into the preoptic region and suggested that the effects of intracranial injections might depend on ventricular diffusion of A-II to the SFO. Several investigators (Phillips et al., 1974; Buggy et al., 1975) have replicated the basic finding that SFO lesions reduce the drinking response to intraparenchymal as well as icv intracranial injections of A-II. However, others have reported only small decreases, no inhibitory effects at all, or rapid recovery in rats (Lind et al., 1984; Buggy and Fisher, 1976; Buggy et al., 1975; Hoffman and Phillips, 1976b) as well as other species (Massi et al., 1986b; Findlay et al., 1980).

It is noteworthy that lesions of the SFO, which many believe to be one of the principal targets of blood-borne A-II, eliminate drinking induced by systemic A-II injections but have little or no effect on ad libitum or deprivation-induced drinking (Simpson and Routtenberg, 1972, 1973, 1975; Kucharczyk et al., 1976; Thrasher et al., 1982a; Lind et al., 1984).

The AV3V, OVLT, and Nucleus Medianus

Reports of drinking responses to intracranial A-II in animals with SFO lesions have given rise to the hypothesis that SFO lesions may interfere with the dipsogenic properties of intracranial A-II not because the SFO is itself the exclusive target organ for the peptide but because its destruction temporarily obstructs the flow of CSF through the narrow foramen that interconnects the lateral and third ventricles.

The hypothesis has been tested (Buggy et al., 1975; Buggy and Fisher, 1976; Buggy and Johnson, 1978; Hoffman and Phillips, 1976b,c) in a series of experiments that determined the drinking response to icv A-II after the flow of CSF was temporarily blocked by plugs of cold cream.

A plug inserted into the dorsal aspects of the third ventricle near the foramen of Monroe (which essentially encapsulated the SFO) abolished drinking responses to A-II injected into the preoptic area or lateral ventricle but had no effect on the dipsogenic effects of angiotensin injected into the ventral portion of the anterior third ventricle.

When cold cream plugs were placed into that region, all intracranial A-II drinking was abolished even though the injected material had free access to the SFO. These findings suggest that access of angiotensin to the subfornical organ may be neither necessary nor sufficient for drinking responses to intracranial A-II.

Johnson and Buggy (1977) have reported that the same plugs that reduce or abolish drinking to ICV A-II actually facilitate drinking responses to systemic (sc) injections of angiotensin, indicating that systemic A-II gains access to central receptor mechanisms not via CSF but via the circulation. This conclusion is supported by a number of recent investigations that have shown that intact angiotensin cannot be transported from the general circulation into cerebrospinal fluid (Schelling et al., 1976; Ganten et al., 1976).

Lesions in the AV3V, which include the OVLT as well as the median nucleus of the preoptic region, have been reported to produce transient adipsia followed by an apparently permanent inhibition of the dipsogenic as well as pressor effects of systemic, icv, or intrapreoptic A-II. The complete pattern has so far been reported in detail only in the rat (Johnson and Buggy, 1977, 1978; Buggy et al., 1977a,b; Buggy and Johnson, 1977a,b, 1978). However, the basic lesion effects of transient adipsia followed by unresponsiveness to systemic angiotensin have also been observed in dogs (Thrasher et al., 1982b; Thrasher and Ramsay, 1986) and sheep (McKinley et al., 1982, 1986).

Such lesions also attenuate or abolish drinking responses to cellular dehydration in the rat (Buggy and Johnson, 1977a,b; Johnson and Buggy, 1978), dog (Thrasher et al., 1982b; Thrasher and Ramsay, 1986) and sheep (McKinley et al., 1982, 1986), but do not decrease the dipsogenic effects of hypovolemia in the rat (Buggy and Johnson, 1977a,b) or dog (Thrasher and Ramsay, 1986).

In the dog, OVLT lesions induce an acute diuresis, not compensated by appropriate changes in ad libitum water intake, so that a significant rise in plasma osmolality occurs. This recovers within a few weeks, but a reduced ability to drink or release vasopressin in response to hypertonic saline (or A-II) remains (Thrasher et al., 1982b).

It has been suggested (Thrasher et al., 1982b; Thrasher and Ramsay, 1986; McKinley et al., 1982) that the region of the OVLT may contain thirst-related osmoreceptors (although it cannot be the sole osmoregulatory mechanisms, since lesions in the area reduce but do not abolish drinking to hypertonic saline).

This should not be interpreted to imply that osmosensitive mechanisms provide the final common path for A-II drinking. It is well established that the drinking response to threshold doses of intracranial or iv A-II "sums" with the drinking response to threshold doses of sc or iv hypertonic saline (Fitzsimons and Simons, 1969; Fitzsimons, 1970b; Hsiao et al., 1977). This interaction clearly indicates the existence of independent mechanisms.

The hypothesis that the OVLT may contain osmoreceptor mechanisms is supported by several reports that neurons in the periventricular aspects of the preoptic region respond, apparently selectively, to hypertonic saline in the mouth or injected intravenously (indeed, some cells respond to both classes of stimuli) (Nicolaidis, 1968, 1969a,b, 1970a,b; Sessler and Sahli, 1981; Nicoll and Barker, 1971). Nicolaidis (1970a,b) has also observed single cell responses in this region to experimentally induced hypovolemia and has suggested that the area may function as an integrative mechanism for various types of thirst stimuli.

There is some controversy concerning the specific location of the neural elements responsible for the inhibitory effects of OVLT lesions. Phillips and Hoffman (1977) have shown that surgical knife cuts that approach the OVLT from the olfactory bulbs (and hence produce little direct damage to the preoptic area proper) abolish drinking to ICV A-II in rats, suggesting that the diffuse OVLT system itself may be involved.

Johnson (1983) has reported a loss of A-II drinking in the rat after lesions that appeared to be restricted to the nucleus medianus. Various other impairments in the rat's ability to regulate fluid intake have been reported after lesions that were presumably restricted to the nucleus medianus (e.g., Brody and Johnson, 1980; Mangiapane et al., 1983). In the dog, Thrasher and colleagues (Thrasher et al., 1982b) have reported that lesions in the region of the OVLT did not affect water intake unless they were large enough to include the nucleus medianus.

Large lesions near the anterior border of the third ventricle of goats (Andersson et al., 1975) and dogs (Witt et al., 1952) also have been reported to produce adipsia. The specific involvement of the OVLT or nucleus medianus in these lesions is difficult to estimate. Further anatomical study of this complex region is clearly needed before we can hope to understand its apparently multifaceted influence on thirst and water intake.

The region of the anteroventral third ventricle (AV3V) and the organum vasculosum of the lamina terminalis (OVLT) has been further implicated in thirst regulation in a variety of additional experimental paradigms.

There are several reports (Nicolaidis and Fitzsimons, 1975; Phillips and Hoffman, 1977) that injections of angiotensin into the region of the OVLT of rats produce more drinking than the same doses injected directly into the SFO (Fig. 8.9). Indeed, Phillips (1978; Phillips et al., 1977a) has reported that microinjections of as little as 50 fg of A-II in the region of the OVLT of rats produced significant drinking as well as blood pressure effects.

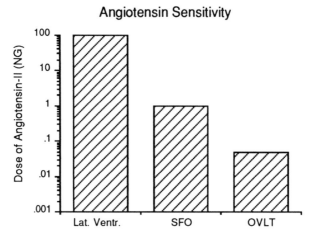

Fig. 8.9. Average threshold dose of angiotensin II required to elicit 5 ml of drinking. After: Phillips, M. I., Felix, D., Hoffman, W. E., and Ganten, D. (1977a). Angiotensin-sensitive sites in the brain ventricular system. *In:* "Soc. Neurosci. Symposia." (W. M. Cowan, and J. A. Ferrrendelli eds.) pp. 308–339. Society for Neuroscience, Bethesda Md. With permission of the authors and the Society for Neuroscience.

The Preoptic Area

The first attempt to localize the central site of action of angiotensin by intracranial microinjections (Epstein *et al.*, 1970) demonstrated that the most effective intraparenchymal injection sites were in the preoptic region of the rostral diencephalon. The basic observation that injections of angiotensin into the preoptic area promptly elicit significant drinking has been replicated in the rat (Kucharczyk and Mogenson, 1976; Swanson *et al.*, 1978), dog (Fitzsimons and Kucharczyk, 1978), and monkey (Sharpe and Swanson, 1974). Although the experimental observation is not in doubt, the interpretation of the phenomenon has been the subject of controversy.

Because angiotensin does not under normal circumstances cross the blood–brain barrier and the preoptic area is not part of the system of circumventricular organs that possess only weak or essentially no blood–brain barrier to angiotensin, it is difficult to see how A-II of renal origin could gain access to neurons in the preoptic region.

The Ventricular Diffusion Hypothesis
Some of the early studies of the dipsogenic effects of intracranial angiotensin obtained excellent results with A-II injections into the lateral or third ventricles of a variety of species (McFarland and Rolls, 1972; Rolls *et al.*, 1972; Andersson and Ericksson, 1971; Cooling and Day, 1975). These observations suggested

that components of the renin–angiotensin system might enter cerebrospinal fluid and act on cells in or immediately adjacent to the ventricular lining.

There appears to be no renin and no renin-generating activity in CSF (Ganong, 1984; Ganten *et al.*, 1978). However, A-I and A-II have been detected in significant quantities, although different measuring techniques have not always produced comparable effects (Ganong, 1984). The angiotensin found in CSF does not appear to be of peripheral (i.e., renal) origin, since radioactively labeled angiotensin II is taken up from the circulation by circumventricular organs but does not enter CSF (Phillips, 1978) or the rest of the brain (Van Houten *et al.*, 1980). These observations would appear to rule out a physiological role for CSF-borne angiotensin as well as the possibility that CSF angiotensin can gain access to cells in the preoptic region. They do not, of course, exclude the possibility that the dipsogenic and pressor effects of intracranial A-II may be due to ventricular transport to SFO, OVLT, or both.

Johnson and Epstein (1975; see also Johnson, 1975) have supported the ventricular diffusion hypothesis by a systematic analysis of effective intraparenchymal angiotensin infusion sites. It indicated that positive sites in the preoptic region and adjacent aspects of the forebrain (which had been identified as most sensitive to A-II) either were located very near the walls of the cerebral ventricles or resulted from cannula placements that traversed a ventricle before reaching the target site. When the approach of the implant was changed so that the cannula no longer traversed a ventricle, previously sensitive sites became negative. Conversely, negative sites were converted into sensitive regions by approaching them via a ventricle.

When the injections were made directly into the lateral ventricles in these experiments, the lowest doses of angiotensin (1.0 ng) that had been effective at the most sensitive preoptic sites produced reliable drinking. Moreover, autoradiographic studies showed that tritiated angiotensin rapidly spread into the ventricular system when cannulae in sensitive sites traversed a ventricle, and failed to enter CSF from cannulae in negative sites that were angled so as to bypass the ventricular system (see also Epstein and Hsiao, 1975).

Other investigators have reported strong drinking responses from cannulae in the preoptic area that were not immediately adjacent to ventricles and did not traverse the ventricular system. Injections of radioactive substance into these placements did not result in significant radioactivity in CSF, and an analysis of the distribution of placements indicated that the effectiveness of the injections was not correlated with proximity to the third ventricle (Richardson and Mogenson, 1981; Swanson *et al.*, 1978).

It has also been reported (Assaf and Mogenson, 1976) that intraventricular injections of the competitive angiotensin inhibitor saralasin did not reduce the dipsogenic effects of subsequent intrapreoptic area injections of A-II when the preoptic implants were angled so as to avoid the ventricular system. Preoptic cannulae that did pass through a ventricle were more effective when only A-II was administered but lost the advantage (but not a residual robust drinking effect) after icv saralasin injections.

Evidence for a Separate Preoptic A-II System

Some investigators (notably Mogenson and Kucharczyk, 1978; see also Mogenson et al., 1977; Kucharczyk et al., 1976; Phillips and Hoffman, 1977; Severs et al., 1978) have maintained that there are several angiotensin-sensitive thirst-related systems. One of these is thought to originate in the preoptic region and project to the ventral tegmental area and central grey of the midbrain (Swanson et al., 1978). This hypothesis receives experimental support from the following experimental observations:

1. Microinjections of angiotensin into the preoptic region increase the discharge rate of roughly 30% of single neurons in the lateral hypothalamus (as well as lower portions of the brainstem) (Black et al., 1973; Mogenson et al., 1977).
2. Unilateral lesions in the lateral hypothalamus reduce the drinking response to ipsilateral A-II injections into the preoptic region but have little effect on the dipsogenic effects of contralateral injections (Black et al., 1974; see also Mogenson and Kucharczyk, 1975).
3. Bilateral lesions in the midlateral hypothalamus reliably reduce the drinking response to preoptic injections of A-II without affecting the response to SFO or icv injections (Kucharczyk et al., 1976) (Fig. 8.10).

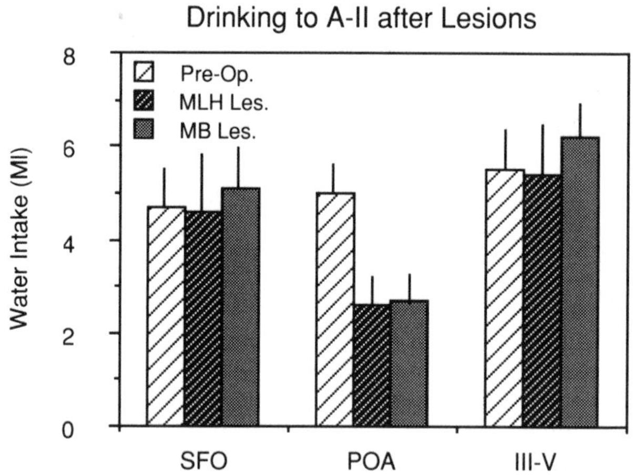

Fig. 8.10. Effects of lesions in the midlateral hypothalamus (MLH) or rostroventral mesencephalon (MB) on water intake 15 min after injections of angiotensin II into the subfornical organ (SFO) (10 ng), preoptic area (POA) (50 ng), or anterior third ventricle (III-V) (50 ng). After: Kucharczyk, J., Assaf, S. Y., and Mogenson, G. J. (1976). Differential effects of brain lesions on thirst induced by the administration of angiotensin II to the preoptic region, subfornical organ and anterior third ventricle. *Brain Res.* **108**, 327–337. With permission of the authors and Elsevier, Amsterdam.

4. In the dog as well as the monkey, the preoptic region appears to be more sensitive to low doses of A-II than the ventricular system (although no more sensitive than the subfornical organ) (Fitzsimons and Kucharczyk, 1978; Sharpe and Swanson, 1974). Fitzsimons and Kucharczyk (1978) have argued that their analyses of dose–response curves and response latencies for icv, SFO, and preoptic injections indicated that the the the drinking response to pre-optic area A-II could not be mediated by ventricular diffusion to the SFO.

Since there is no known mechanism by which blood-borne or even CSF-borne angiotensin could gain access to neurons of the preoptic area, one might want to entertain the possibility that afferents to the preoptic region may secrete an-giotensin or a closely related peptide as a neurotransmitter or neuromodulator. This implies endogenous brain renin–angiotensin mechanisms, which have been the subject of much recent investigation and controversy. It is impossible to do justice to this complex question in the context of this discussion, but a brief summary of some relevant observations may provide a useful perspective.

A Separate Brain Renin–Angiotensin System

All components of the renin–angiotensin system, including renin substrate, con-verting enzyme, A-I and A-II, angiotensinases which inactivate A-II, and specif-ic angiotensin receptors, have been found in brain, notably in the hypothalamus. Moreover, iontophoretic application of angiotensin to nerve cells in several areas of the brain modulates their firing rate.

Angiotensin II–containing nerve terminals and A-II binding sites have been demonstrated in the subfornical organ (SFO), the OVLT and nucleus medianus, supraoptic nucleus, paraventricular nucleus, and circumventricular regions of the posterior hypothalamus (Sirett et al., 1977; Ganten et al., 1978; Zimmerman et al., 1980; Brownfield et al., 1982; Lind and Johnson, 1982c; Felix et al., 1982, 1986; Healy and Prinz, 1984; Gehlert et al., 1986; Mendelson et al., 1984). The functional significance of this brain isorenin-angiotensin system is, as yet, ob-scure (see for review Ganong, 1984; Unger et al., 1986; Phillips, 1987).

If changes in circulating angiotensin do indeed influence water intake and/or conservation by modulating the activity of neural mechanisms in regions of the brain such as the hypothalamus and preoptic region, the existence of a well-demonstrated blood–brain barrier indicates that the hormone almost certainly must act on neurons in one or more of the circumventricular organs. These may then communicate with thirst-related mechanisms in the brainstem via neural projections that may use angiotensin as a neurotransmitter or neuromodulator.

Apparently specific neural responses to topically applied A-II or changes in circulating A-II have been reported from at least two circumventricular organs, the subfornical organ (SFO) (Ishibashi et al., 1985; Nicolaidis et al., 1983; Phillips and Felix, 1976; Felix and Akert, 1974) and the organum vasculosum of the lamina terminalis (OVLT) (Nicolaidis and Jeulin, 1984; Jeulin and Nicolaidis, 1986; Thornton *et al.*, 1985). Neurons in these areas also increase their firing rate (or glucose uptake) after water deprivation, experimentally induced hypovolemia, hypotension, or cellular dehydration (Nicolaidis, 1970a,b; Nicolaidis *et al.*, 1981, 1983).

There are, nonetheless, a number of observations that are not easily understood unless one assumes a fully functional brain renin-angiotensin system. Among these are numerous reports of drinking in the rat, cat, dog, and pigeon after intracranial injections of systemically ineffective doses of renin substrate (Evered and Fitzsimons, 1976b; Hoffman *et al.*, 1977), renin (Epstein *et al.*, 1970; Fitzsimons, 1971a; Brophy and Levitt, 1974; Burckhardt *et al.*, 1975; Evered and Fitzsimons, 1976b; Fitzsimons and Kucharczyk, 1978; Fitzsimons *et al.*, 1978a; Reid and Ramsay, 1975; Simpson *et al.*, 1978c), or angiotensin I (Swanson *et al.*, 1973b; Reid and Ramsay, 1975; Evered and Fitzsimons, 1976; Fitzsimons *et al.*, 1978b) (see Fig. 8.3). Presumably, these compounds must undergo conversion to A-II in order to become dipsogenic, and this implies that the mechanisms for such conversions are present in brain.

That different substrates may be responsible for systemically and centrally administered angiotensin is also indicated by the fact that SFO lesions have frequently been reported to have differential effects. There is good agreement that SFO lesions significantly reduce and, in some experiments, completely abolish the drinking response to systemic A-II in rats (Abdelaal *et al.*, 1974b; Simpson and Routtenberg, 1975, 1978; Simpson *et al.*, 1978a; Buggy and Fisher, 1976; Hosutt *et al.*, 1981), dogs (Thrasher *et al.*, 1982a), opossums (Elfont *et al.*, 1980), and pigeons (Massi *et al.*, 1986b). In rats as well as opossums, SFO lesions block the drinking response to systemic A-II completely, and apparently permanently, when the latter is administered in near-threshold doses (Simpson *et al.*, 1978a; Elfont *et al.*, 1980).

Some investigators have reported that SFO lesions also reduce the drinking response to intraparenchymal as well as icv intracranial injections of A-II (Simpson and Routtenberg, 1973; Phillips *et al.*, 1974; Buggy *et al.*, 1975). However, others have reported only small decreases, no inhibitory effects at all, or rapid recovery of the drinking response to intracranial angiotensin in rats (Lind *et al.*, 1984; Buggy and Fisher, 1976; Buggy *et al.*, 1975; Hoffman and Phillips, 1976b) as well as other species (Massi *et al.*, 1986b; Findlay *et al.*, 1980).

Mechanisms of Action

Angiotensin-II Interactions with Catecholaminergic or Cholinergic Brain Pathways

Any direct action of circulating angiotensin on brain neurons is most easily understood when one considers angiotensin as a neurotransmitter or neuromodulator. Although the presently available evidence can be interpreted differently (e.g., an indirect action on neurons secondary to local vasoconstriction), much of the data that have been cited to support the existence of an endogenous isorenin–angiotensin system (see for review Ganong, 1984; Unger et al., 1986) are compatible with this interpretation. There is, furthermore, a rapidly increasing body of evidence suggesting that many peripherally active peptides may have central neurotransmitter or neuromodulator functions (e.g., Barker, 1976).

Angiotensin has many of the properties of a neurotransmitter or modulator. In the brain, it is found in synaptic terminals, shows high affinity and reversible binding to neuronal receptors, and excites or inhibits some neurons when applied iontophoretically in minute quantities (Raizada et al., 1981; Palovcik and Phillips, 1984; Nicolaidis and Jeulin, 1984; Nicolaidis et al., 1983; Phillips and Felix, 1976; Dickinson and Ferrario, 1974). A specific interaction of A-II and central catecholaminergic pathways is suggested by a variety of observations, as follows.

Intracerebroventricular injections of the neurotoxin 6-hydroxydopamine (6-OHDA), which selectively destroys central catecholaminergic neurons, attenuate or abolish the drinking response to icv A-II, without affecting the drinking response to carbachol (Fitzsimons and Setler, 1975). The effect may be due, at least in part, to the destruction of noradrenergic cells in the region of the OVLT and nucleus medianus. Microinjections of 6-OHDA into this region have been shown to reduce the drinking response to both icv and systemic A-II (Bellin et al., 1984a). This impairment was reversed by transplants of noradrenergic cells into the 6-OHDA-denervated region (Bellin et al., 1984b).

Intracerebroventricular injections of the beta-adrenergic blocker propranolol (Cooling and Day, 1975) or the alpha-adrenergic blocker phentolamine (Cooling and Day, 1975; Severs et al., 1971b) also block the drinking response to icv angiotensin in cats and rats. Microinjections of these adrenergic blockers into brain parenchyma (preoptic area, septal area) do not block the drinking response to A-II applied via the same cannula (Lehr and Goldman, 1973; Fitzsimons and Setler, 1975; Covian et al., 1972).

These observations suggest that alpha- as well as beta-adrenergic neurons may play an essential role in the organization of drinking responses to icv injections of angiotensin. These pathways do not appear to mediate the drinking response to A-II injections into the preoptic area. This is of potential significance to the controversy (addressed above) concerning the etiology of the drinking response to intraparenchymal (especial intrapreoptic) injections of A-II.

Microinjections of the dopamine agonists haloperidol or spiroperidol into the preoptic area (Fitzsimons and Setler, 1971, 1975) or septal area (Peres et al., 1974) of rats block the drinking response to subsequent injections of A-II through the same cannula. This suggests that dopaminergic neurons may be part of an angiotensin-sensitive system in these areas. [However, see Swanson et al. (1973b) for a report of negative results obtained under seemingly comparable circumstances.]

A relation between A-II and cholinergic brain neurons is suggested by the fact that the SFO appears to be an especially sensitive site for both carbachol- and A-II–induced drinking (Simpson and Routtenberg, 1972, 1973; Simpson et al., 1976, 1978a) as well as vasopressin release and peripheral pressor effects (Simpson et al., 1979; Mangiapane and Simpson, 1980a, 1983). Lesions of the SFO have been reported to abolish the drinking response to both compounds (although the inhibitory effects on central A-II drinking is controversial as discussed above) (Simpson and Routtenberg, 1972, 1973; Simpson et al., 1978a).

The drinking response of rats to icv angiotensin has been reported to be unaffected by low icv doses of the cholinergic antagonist atropine (Fitzsimons and Setler, 1975) but to be reduced or abolished by high doses (Fitzsimons and Setler, 1975; Severs et al., 1970, 1978). Intracerebroventricular atropine has also been reported to abolish the drinking response to icv A-II in the dog (Ramsay and Reid, 1975) but to have no effect in the cat (Cooling and Day 1975), an animal that also does not drink in response to intracranial carbachol (MacPhail and Miller, 1968). The inhibitory effects of icv atropine are consistent with the SFO lesion data in supporting the hypothesis that icv angiotensin may act directly or indirectly on cholinergic components of the SFO.

Electrophysiological investigations have demonstrated the existence of neurons in the subfornical organ as well as preoptic area that are sensitive to iontophoretic applications of A-II as well as acetylcholine. The activity of these neurons appears to be specifically inhibited by atropine (Felix and Akert, 1974; Felix, 1976; Felix et al., 1986; Felix and Schlegel, 1978). Unfortunately , these elegant electrophysiological studies were done exclusively in the cat, a species that does not show carbachol-induced drinking (McPhail and Miller, 1968).

The dipsogenic effects of intraparenchymal injections of angiotensin, on the other hand, do not appear to be mediated by cholinergic or cholinoceptive neurons. This is indicated by the consistent finding that microinjections of atropine into the hypothalamus, preoptic region, or septal area, at doses that inhibit the powerful drinking response to carbachol (Grossman, 1962a,b), do not reduce the drinking response to subsequent injection of A-II into the same brain tissue (Giardina and Fisher, 1971; Covian et al., 1972; Swanson et al., 1973a,b).

The Vascular Hypothesis

Nicolaidis and Fitzsimons (1975) have suggested that the central effects of angiotensin may be related to its vasoconstrictor properties. According to this hypothesis the subfornical organ (SFO) and the organum vasculosum of the lamina terminalis (OVLT) may act as volume receptor organs that are sensitive to the amount of blood circulating through them. Reduced blood flow during general hypovolemia or vasoconstriction due to angiotensin could be sensed by stretch receptors, located most probably in the blood vessels supplying the SFO and OVLT.

Fitzsimons (1979) has enumerated the following observations in support of the vascular hypothesis:

1. The SFO and OVLT appear to be the most A-II–sensitive brain structures.
2. The peptide specificity requirement of the dipsogenic receptor is similar to that of myotropic receptors.
3. The dipsogenic receptor responds like the A-II vascular receptor to various antagonists of the renin–angiotensin system.
4. Compounds that have little in common except a constrictor action on blood vessels elicit drinking when injected into the brain.
5. Vasoplegic drugs interfere with A-II drinking response (Fig. 8.11).
6. The drinking responses to various vasoactive drugs interact, suggesting that they activate the same mechanism.

Angiotensin-II Interactions with Periventricular Sodium Receptors

Andersson (1971, 1978; Andersson *et al.*, 1982) has suggested that the renin-angiotensin system, which he regards as a relatively insignificant influence on thirst under normal circumstances, may act via CSF to potentiate the activity of circumventricular sodium receptors. According to his hypothesis, angiotensin could exert this facilitatory effect by promoting the movement of sodium from

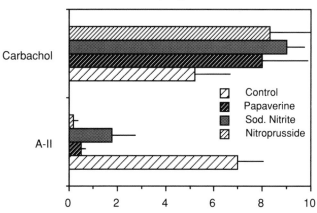

Fig. 8.11. Drinking response to 100 ng of angiotensin II or 300 ng of carbachol injected into the subfornical organ. On control tests, this was preceded by $1-4$ µl of 0.9% saline. On the experimental tests, one of three vasoplegic drugs was injected through the same cannula before the A-II or carbachol injections. The drugs were papaverine ($53-318 \times 10^{-3}$ mol), sodium nitrite ($20-40 \times 10^{-9}$ mol), and sodium nitroprusside ($10-100 \times 10^{-9}$ mol). After: Nicolaidis, S., and Fitzsimons, J. T. (1975). La dépendance de la prise d'eau induite par l'angiotensine II envers la fonction vasomotrice cérébrale locale chez le rat. *Comptes Rendus de L'Académie des Sciences,* **281D**, 1417–1420. With permission of the authors and L'Académie des Sciences, Paris.

CSF into brain tissue, by sensitizing the sodium receptor, or by facilitating the entry of sodium into brain receptors.

Andersson's hypothesis of brain angiotensin action is based on the following data base: icv infusions of angiotensin alone or hypertonic saline alone produce a small amount of drinking as well as antidiuresis and natriuresis in the goat. When the same dose of angiotensin was administered together with hypertonic saline, a large amount of drinking occurred that was far greater than the sum of the responses to saline and angiotensin given alone. The antidiuretic and natriuretic effects of the combined treatment were also disproportionally greater than the response to either alone. When angiotensin was infused in isotonic glucose, its dipsogenic, antidiuretic, and natriuretic effects were all but nonexistent (Andersson and Westbye, 1970; Andersson and Eriksson, 1971; Andersson et al., 1972). Intracerebroventricular A-II injections have also been reported to potentiate antidiuretic hormone release in response to intracarotid infusions of hypertonic saline (Olsson and Kalmodin, 1974).

As we have seen earlier, the goat may indeed have evolved circumventricular receptors that are specifically sensitive to sodium. Andersson's demonstration of interactive angiotensin–sodium effects further supports his hypothesis that they play a central role in water intake and conservation in this species.

In the rat, icv as well as intraparenchymal injections of angiotensin appear to be equally effective when administered in hypertonic saline or sucrose, isotonic saline, or distilled water. This indicates that sodium receptors are not involved in the rat brain's response to angiotensin (Fitzsimons, 1973; Swanson, et al., 1973a).

It should be noted that the more general hypothesis that angiotensin can gain access to brain receptor sites via the cerebrospinal fluid has not been rejected (see Phillips et al., 1977a; Phillips, 1978). It is, in fact, favored by some contemporary investigators (e.g., Ganong, 1984) even though the functional significance of the proposed icv transport mechanism is not at all clear. The preponderance of the available evidence (Ganten et al., 1976; Schelling et al., 1976; Simpson et al., 1978b; Ramsay and Reid, 1975) indicates that circulating A-II does not gain access to CSF. Earlier studies by Volicer and Loew (1971) and Johnson (1975) did obtain evidence of penetration, using very high doses of angiotensin. Phillips and colleagues (1978; Phillips et al., 1977a) have suggested that these strongly hypertensive doses may exert sufficient capillary pressure to promote the movement of A-II through the choroid plexi. It is not clear whether this mechanism could be a significant factor under normal circumstances.

Review and Conclusions

Intracranial injections of angiotensin in nano- and even picogram doses elicit drinking as well as systemic pressor responses within seconds or minutes after the injection. The effects are robust but typically of short duration. A delayed and persisting sodium appetite has also been reported after intracranial infusions of A-II.

The dipsogenic effects of intracranial injections of components of the renin angiotensin system are reduced or abolished when the formation of A-II is blocked or its action inhibited.

Intracranial pepstatin, which prevents the formation of A-I, inhibits the dipsogenic effects of renin and renin substrate but does not reduce the response to A-I or A-II.

SQ 20881, which blocks the formation of A-II, inhibits the drinking response to renin, renin substrate, and A-I (administered through the same intraparenchymal or icv cannula) without reducing the response to A-II.

Intraparenchymal or icv injections of the specific A-II antagonist saralasin inhibit the dipsogenic properties of all components of the renin angiotensin system (including A-II) administered through the same cannula. Intracranial saralasin also reduces the drinking response to systemic A-II and drinking after systemic isoproterenol.

Intracranial injections of antiangiotensin serum have effects on water intake that are similar to those of saralasin.

It has been suggested that there may be several angiotensin-sensitive sites in the brain. Some of these (such as the subfornical organ) may be sensitive only to blood-borne A-II. It seems likely that A-II activates neurons in the SFO that project angiotensinergic projections to the periventricular tissues of the AV3V (Lind and Johnson, 1981; Johnson, 1985). Electrophysiological recordings of neuron responses to iontophoretically applied A-II suggest that the effect of A-II on SFO neurons may be due to a neurotransmitter or neuromodulator action. However, an indirect effect due to vasoconstriction may also be responsible for an indirect activation of cells in this region.

Other areas (such as the OVLT) may be capable of responding to endogenous as well as blood-borne components of the renin–angiotensin system. There is evidence that tanycytes connected by tight junctions on the OVLT and the adjacent nucleus medianus transport angiotensin from cerebrospinal fluid to the region of the OVLT where gap junctions of the nucleus medianus allow entry of the peptide (Phillips et al., 1978; Landas et al., 1980). Phillips (1987) has reviewed this evidence and concluded that the OVLT itself may be sensitive to both blood-borne and CSF-borne angiotensin, whereas the nucleus medianus may respond specifically to A-II in CSF.

The area receives afferents from the SFO, as well as other brainstem regions such as the paraventricular nucleus, parabrachial nucleus, nucleus of the solitary tract, and ventrolateral medulla (Saper and Levisohn, 1983; Miselis, 1981; Miselis et al., 1979) known to contribute to the regulation of cardiovascular functions.

Still other regions such as the preoptic area (Kucharczyk et al., 1976) may be sensitive, under normal circumstances, only to the products of a separate brain isorenin–angiotensin system, which may act as neuromodulators or neurotransmitters in the region. Such a conclusion is suggested by the fact that A-II injections into parenchyma not immediately adjacent to the ventricular system elicit drinking and continue to do so after brain lesions that abolish the drinking response to A-II injections into SFO or anterior third ventricle (Kucharczyk *et al.*, 1976).

The blood–brain barrier (BBB) prevents diffusion of systemic angiotensin to brain A-II (and possibly A-III) receptors in brain parenchyma under normal circumstances. As long as blood A-II levels are low, the hormone acts only on receptors in circumventricular organs that are on the blood side of the BBB or are protected by a barrier that is ineffective against A-II and related peptides. Only when blood A-II levels are very high (or the BBB less resistant because of high blood pressure) can the peptide invade brain parenchyma and act on receptors not normally available (Phillips, 1987). This could account for the many differences between the effects of systemic and central A-II administrations while taking into consideration the fact that these differences disappear under special circumstances.

The relevant evidence is quite persuasive for the suggested role of the SFO in drinking responses to systemic A-II. The region of the OVLT and nucleus medianus has also been persuasively implicated, but it is as yet not certain whether the region participates directly in the response to blood-borne A-II, or A-II in CSF or secondarily to neural inputs from the SFO. The area does appear to be sensitive to changes in CSF A-II, but the physiological significance of this remains to be elucidated. Whether an endogenous isorenin–angiotensin system in the preoptic area or elsewhere is active in the regulation of water intake remains to be demonstrated.

Recent neuroanatomical studies (Miselis *et al.*, 1979; Miselis 1981, 1986) have traced efferents from the SFO to the OVLT and adjacent preoptic area, a pathway that possibly complements a projection from the preoptic area through the medial forebrain bundle to regions of the midbrain apparently involved in the central pressor responses to angiotensin (Swanson *et al.*, 1978). Reciprocal projections from this area to the SFO (Lind *et al.*, 1982) complete a circuit that may play a pivotal role in thirst.

Chapter 9

Brain Mechanisms III: Neuropharmacology

Introduction

The relatively brief history of the neuropharmacology of thirst mirrors recent developments in neuropharmacology as a whole.

When it became apparent in the late 1950s and early 1960s that mammalian brains contained more than one neurotransmitter, it seemed plausible that functionally related neural pathways might be characterized by a common neurotransmitter. The hypothesis has been exhaustively studied, particularly with respect to the biogenic amines and, more recently, various peptides. We now have a vast literature that indicates that major brain functions such as sleep, arousal, hunger, etc. may be mediated, at least in part, by neural pathways that are pharmacologically as well as anatomically identifiable. Thirst researchers were at the forefront of this effort.

By 1960, water intake (accompanied by decreased urine flow and increased urine concentration) was shown to be elicited, apparently selectively, by intracranial injections of acetylcholine and other cholinergic agonists such as carbachol (Grossman, 1960). The effect appeared to be behaviorally as well as pharmacologically specific. Shortly thereafter, it was shown that microinjections of alpha-adrenergic agonists such as epinephrine and norepinephrine into portions of the hypothalamus inhibit water intake (Grossman, 1962a). In the early 1970s, drinking was also reported after intracranial injections of the transmitter histamine (Leibowitz, 1973b).

In the 1960s and early 1970s, numerous research projects were undertaken to elucidate the the effects of intracranial neurotransmitter injections on thirst and renal water and sodium conservation, in terms of their neural substrate, relationship to specific cellular and extracellular dipsogens, and significance for natural thirst and satiety. These investigations have produced a wealth of experimental data that have been helpful in our continuing quest for a more thorough understanding of the brain mechanisms which control drinking. However, many important questions have remained unanswered.

Traditional Neurotransmitters

Acetylcholine and Carbachol

Intracranial injections of acetylcholine elicit drinking in water-replete rats (Grossman, 1960, 1962a; Simpson and Routtenberg, 1974; Mangiapane and Simpson, 1983). More robust and prolonged effects are obtained by injections of cholinomimetics such as carbachol that are not subject to rapid metabolic decomposition and thus produce more sustained excitatory effects on cholinergic synapses than acetylcholine itself (Grossman, 1960, 1962a). Significant drinking is also elicited by central injections of cholinesterase inhibitors such as eserine which prolong the action of naturally occurring acetylcholine (Miller, 1965; Winson and Miller, 1970).

Carbachol-induced thirst has been shown to motivate water-rewarded operant behavior and to increase deprivation-induced drinking as well as drinking responses to ip injections of hypertonic saline (Grossman, 1962a; Miller, 1965; Block and Fisher, 1970; Franklin and Quartermain, 1970) (Fig. 9.1).

The dipsogenic properties of carbachol have been shown to be due to its action on muscarinic receptor mechanisms (Stein and Seifter, 1962). Carbachol-induced drinking is blocked by systemic or intracranial injections of atropine (Grossman, 1962b; Stein and Seifter, 1962; Miller, 1965). Centrally admin-

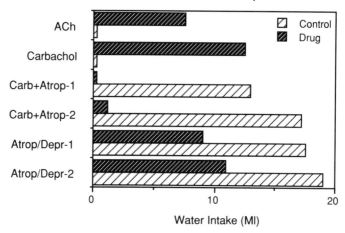

Fig. 9.1. Water intake 1 h after the intracranial administration of 5 µg of acetylcholine (ACh) or the synthetic cholinomimetic drug carbachol. Also shown are the effects of (1) systemic (25 mg/kg) or (2) central (15–20 µg/rat) pretreatment with atropine on drinking 1-h after carbachol and 1-h after 24 h of water deprivation. Data from: (1) Grossman, S. P. (1962a). Direct adrenergic and cholinergic stimulation of hypothalamic mechanisms. *Am. J. Physiol.* **202**, 872–882. (2) Grossman, S. P. (1962b). Effects of adrenergic and cholinergic blocking agents on hypothalamic mechanisms. *Am. J. Physiol.* **202**, 1230–1236. And (3) unpublished observations by S. P. Grossman.

istered atropine also has been shown to reduce deprivation-induced drinking as well as drinking responses to ip hypertonic saline (Grossman, 1962b; Block and Fisher, 1970). Intracranial injections of atropine do not, however, reduce the drinking response to angiotensin II or isoproterenol, administered via the same cannula (Giardina and Fisher, 1971). Systemic injections of the cholinergic blocker scopolamine, on the other hand, have been reported by produce a significant blockade of drinking responses to central angiotensin as well as isoproterenol (Fisher, 1973).

The dipsogenic properties of cholinomimetics are not secondary to diuresis. Intracranial carbachol injections actually decrease urine flow while increasing its concentration (Miller, 1965). The effect appears to be mediated by increased ADH secretion (Kühn, 1974). Intracranial carbachol also elicits systemic pressor responses (Hoffman and Phillips, 1976d; Mangiapane and Simpson, 1983), which may be mediated partly by increased ADH release (since hypophysectomy decreases the pressor response) and partly by increased sympathetic activity (since the alpha-adrenergic blocker phentolamine further reduces the effect in hypophysectomized animals (Hoffman and Phillips, 1976d).

The specific site of action for the dipsogenic effects of carbachol and related compounds has been the subject of controversy. Positive injection sites have been found throughout the upper brainstem, septum, and hippocampus (Fisher and Coury, 1962; Grossman, 1964). The resulting notion of a cholinergic limbic thirst pathway received support from studies showing that atropine injections at most sites along the postulated circuit could block the drinking response to carbachol administered at other injection sites (Levitt, 1971; Levitt and Fisher, 1966). Carbachol injections along the limbic circuit also alter neural activity at many sites along the proposed pathway (Buerger et al., 1973; Snyder and Levitt, 1975). However, lesions at various points along the limbic circuit do not suppress carbachol drinking, the single exception being the lateral hypothalamus (Levitt, 1971; Setler, 1977). It is possible that the lesion data merely attest to the diffuse nature of the proposed limbic circuit, but Routtenberg (1967, 1972) has proposed an alternative interpretation of the widespread and diffuse distribution of carbachol-sensitive sites. He suggested that carbachol might not act at the point of injection but diffuse via the ventricle to a common site of action. Routtenberg and colleagues have shown that injections of acetylcholine or carbachol directly into the subfornical organ elicit more drinking more promptly than comparable injections into the lateral hypothalamus or cerebral ventricle. Lesions of the SFO reduced (but did not abolish) drinking responses to icv carbachol in these experiments (Routtenberg and Simpson, 1971; Simpson and Routtenberg, 1972, 1973, 1974; Simpson et al., 1978).

It is generally accepted today that the SFO is a site of carbachol action but there is some evidence that thirst-related neurons in the AV3V region and/or preoptic area may also be cholinergic. Swanson and Sharpe (1973), for instance, concluded on the basis of an extensive mapping study, using injection volumes of only 0.1 µl, that the most sensitive drinking sites were in the rostromedial diencephalon. The efficacy of carbachol injections into this area has been reported to be unaffected by SFO lesions. Also, icv injections of carbachol lose their dipsogenic effects when the AV3V region is covered by a cold cream plug that denies the drug access to the region (Buggy and Fisher, 1976; Buggy, 1978).

In the rat, carbachol drinking is a very robust and reliable phenomenon and it seems certain that at least some thirst-related brain pathways are cholinergic in this species. Interest in the phenomenon has nonetheless waned in recent years because other species show only weak responses (or none at all) to intracranial carbachol. Comparatively small effects after high doses have been reported in the dog (Ramsay and Reed, 1975) and rabbit (Sommer et al., 1967). In the monkey nicotine has been reported to elicit drinking, suggesting somewhat different cholinergic influences on thirst (Myers, 1969; Myers et al., 1973). Some species (such as the cat) display extreme autonomic reactions, extreme behavioral arousal or sleep, which are essentially incompatible with drinking (Hernandez-Peon et al., 1962; Myers, 1964; Myers and Sharpe, 1968).

Catecholamines

Systemic injections of beta-adrenergic compounds elicit drinking (Lehr et al., 1967). Intracranial injections have similar effects (Lehr et al., 1967). However, it has become clear that the doses required intracranially are as large as those effective systemically (Lehr, 1973), suggesting that the effects are due to a systemic action of the drug (Fisher, 1973).

Intracranial injections of alpha-adrenergic compounds such as norepinephrine or epinephrine, on the other hand, have pronounced *inhibitory* effects on drinking at doses as low as 1 ng, which are far lower than those effective systemically (Leibowitz, 1973b, 1980). Inhibitory effects of intrahypothalamic injections of norepinephrine (NE) were first described in water-deprived rats by Grossman (1962a). The effect has been replicated in several laboratories (Hendler and Blake, 1969; Hutchinson and Renfrew, 1967; Lovett and Singer, 1971; Leibowitz, 1970, 1971a) and may be due to a drug action on neurons in the the region of the periventricular nucleus (PVN) (Leibowitz, 1973b,c). The inhibitory effects of NE appear to be due to an action on alpha-adrenergic receptors since it is duplicated by epinephrine (E) and blocked by alpha-adrenergic blockers (such as phentolamine) but not by beta-adrenergic blockers (such as propranolol) (Leibowitz, 1972, 1973b,c, 1980; Setler, 1975).

Intrahypothalamic injections of NE also reduce drinking responses to systemic hypertonic saline or central carbachol (Singer and Kelly, 1972; Setler, 1975; Leibowitz, 1980). There is some disagreement in the literature on whether the inhibitory effects of intracranial NE include drinking elicited by extracellular thirst stimuli. Leibowitz (see Leibowitz, 1980, for review) has reported that NE injections into the PVN reduce by approximately 50% water intake elicited by systemic hypertonic saline or polyethylene glycol as well as intracranial carbachol or angiotensin. Setler (1975) has reported marked effects of NE injections into the preoptic area on deprivation-induced drinking and drinking responses to systemic salt loads or intracranial carbachol. However, Setler found no decrease in water intake after systemic isoproterenol or polyethylene glycol or intracranial angiotensin (Fig. 9.2). It is possible that the disagreement reflects differences in the injection site, although the partial overlap of their results remains puzzling.

Injections of NE into the lateral or third ventricle or into the supraoptic nucleus (SON) have been reported to release vasopressin, decrease urine output, and increase urine osmolality, the effects being inhibited by alpha adrenergic blocking agents such as phentolamine or phenoxybenzamine (Kühn, 1974; Garay and Leibowitz, 1974; Morris et al., 1976, 1977; Urano and Kobayashi, 1978). The release of vasopressin and consequent renal conservation of water is not readily understood in terms of an activation of satiety-related mechanisms. It seems more likely that the release of vasopressin may reflect an action of NE on neurons in the supraoptic nucleus (SON) that is not related to the inhibition of drinking that appears to be due to an action of NE on neurons in the region of the periventricular nucleus (PVN) of the medial hypothalamus. Opposite effects

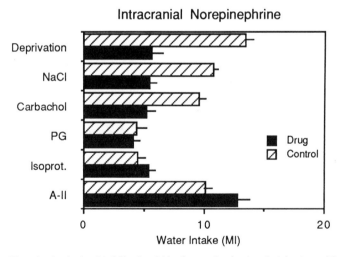

Fig. 9.2. Water intake during 1 h following 24 h of water deprivation, ip injections of 2 ml of 2 M NaCl, intrapreoptic injections of 300 ng of carbachol; ip injections of 2 ml of 50% solutions of polyethylene glycol (PG); sc injections of 50 mg/kg of isoproterenol; or 100 ng of angiotensin II injected into the preoptic area. On "drug" tests, the animals were pretreated with 32.5 nmol of norepinephrine. Data from: Setler, P. E. (1973). The role of catecholamines in thirst. *In:* "The Neuropsychology of Thirst" (A. N. Epstein, H. R. Kissileff, and E. Stellar, eds.) pp. 279–290. V. H. Winston and Sons, Washington.

(i.e., increased urine output and decreased osmolality) have been reported after intrahypothalamic (Blundell and Herberg, 1973) as well as icv (Wolny *et al.*, 1974) injections of NE, but the use of extremely high doses in these experiments suggests that these may not be physiological responses.

Systemic (sc) injections of dopamine receptor blockers such as haloperidol reduce water intake caused by deprivation, hypertonic saline, polyethylene glycol, or isoproterenol (Block and Fisher, 1975; Rowland and Engle, 1975; Cooper and Gilbert, 1986). It is interesting to note that concurrent systemic injections of haloperidol and a cholinergic blocker have been reported to block extracellular thirst completely. Interestingly, there was no evidence of additivity with respect to deprivation- or salt-induced drinking in these experiments even though both were reduced about equally (Fisher, 1973; Block and Fisher, 1975).

Intracerebroventricular injections of dopamine receptor blockers inhibit A-II–induced drinking (Setler, 1977; Rowland and Engle, 1977). Intracranial injections of dopamine or related agonists produce little (Setler, 1977; Fisher, 1973) or no (Leibowitz and Rossakis, 1979a,b) effects on water intake in thirsty or water replete animals.

Histamine

Systemic injections of histamine elicit drinking in the rat (Gerald and Maikel, 1972; Leibowitz, 1973a,b). The dipsogenic effects of histamine correlate temporally with a rapid decrease in blood pressure and subsequent increase in plasma renin activity (Leenen *et al.*, 1975), suggesting the involvement of the renin–angiotensin system. However, histamine-induced drinking is only slightly reduced by nephrectomy or systemic injections of the beta-adrenergic antagonist propranolol (Gutman and Krausz, 1973). Systemic histamine injections also reduce urine output, partly because of direct effects on renal functions and partly due to the release of vasopressin (see Leibowitz, 1979, for a comprehensive review).

Histamine injections into the supraoptic nucleus or periventricular nucleus also elicit drinking as well as antidiuresis at doses (as low as 60 ng) far smaller than those shown to produce significant vascular or renal effects when injected systemically (Leibowitz, 1973a,b, 1979) (Fig. 9.3). The relationship between the systemic and central effects of histamine is unclear. Although they appear to be all but identical, the results of an autoradiographic study indicate that only small quantities of histamine cross the blood–brain barrier (Snyder *et al.*, 1964).

Histamine-sensitive mechanisms have been specifically implicated in feeding-associated drinking (Kraly, 1986). Systemic injections of the H-1 antagonist dexbrompheniramine in combination with the H-2 antagonist cimetidine have been reported to prevent the drinking response to histamine (Kraly, 1983) and to reduce periprandial drinking (Kraly, 1983; Kraly and Specht, 1984), although

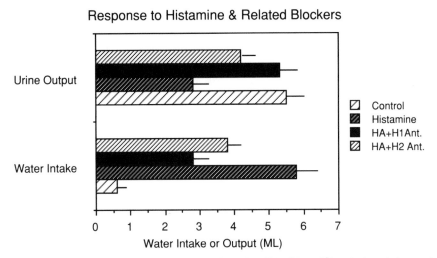

Fig. 9.3. Water intake and urine excretion after histamine (HA) (25 nmol) into the hypothalamus of the rat. Optimal drinking responses to histamtine were obtained from the region of the paraventricular nucleus, and optimal antidiuretic responses from the region of the supraoptic nucleus. The drinking response to HA was partially blocked by compounds that block H_1 or H_2 receptors. The antidiuretic response was reduced by H_2 blockers as well as alpha-adrenergic blockers (not shown). Data from: Leibowitz, S. F. (1979). Histamine: Modifications of behavioral and physiological components of body fluid homeostasis. *In:* "Histamine Receptors." (T. O. Yellin, ed.) pp. 219–253. Spectrum Press, New York.

they have no significant inhibitory effect on deprivation-induced water intake at comparable doses (Kraly, 1983; Kraly *et al*, 1983; Kraly and Specht, 1984).

Peptides

Peptides are compounds consisting of two or more amino acids joined so that the carboxyl group of one unites with the amino group of the other with a resultant loss of one molecule of water. This link is called the "peptide bond."

Peptides were first isolated from the gut and secretory organs such as the pancreas and pituitary. In the late 1960s and early 1970s investigators learned that the release of pituitary hormones is under the control of peptide "releasing factors" produced in the hypothalamus. It was not until the late 1970s and early 1980s that technological advances (radioimmunoassays, immunohistochemistry, and, more recently, recombinant DNA techniques) demonstrated that many of the peptides found in the periphery (as well as some not found peripherally) also exist in nerve cells of the brain.

At this time as many as 50 endogenous neuropeptides have been found in mammalian brains, and there is rapidly increasing evidence that these compounds may act as neurotransmitters, neuromodulators, or neurohormones that serve as intercellular messengers. In many instances, more than one neuropeptide are secreted from one neuron and it is not uncommon to find that traditional transmitters such as norepinephrine, serotonin, dopamine, or acetylcholine are secreted from the same neuron as neuropeptides. The resulting interactions vastly complicate the picture for the neuroscientist trying to understand the exchange of information in the brain.

The relationship between peripheral and brain peptides is presently the subject of controversy. Because of technical difficulties, it has been very difficult to prove unequivocally that peripherally produced peptides do or do not cross the blood–brain barrier (or the CSF–brain barrier). Recent research suggests that some peptides may enter the brain in significant quantities while others do not. We have encountered the problem in our discussion of the effects of blood-borne angiotensin on thirst and discussed an explanation (transport at circumventricular organs) that has been used to explain the apparently central effects of other systemically administered peptides (Phillips, 1987; Van Houten et al., 1979). It has been pointed out, however, that the ependymal barrier associated with circumventricular organs is a substantial hindrance for peptide transport. The alternative explanation in terms of a separate brain isorenin–angiotensin system may, of course also apply to other peptides.

Amphibian Peptides

In recent years, a number of peptides have been extracted from amphibian skin that closely resemble peptides found in mammalian brain and/or intestinal organs. Many of these compounds have pronounced inhibitory effects on water intake when injected intraventricularly in the rat.

The first group consists of tachykinins such as eledoisin, physalaemin, and substance P, which inhibit, in a dose-related manner, drinking responses to icv angiotensin or carbachol, as well as sc hypertonic saline and water deprivation, the latter requiring far higher doses than the former (deCaro et al., 1977, 1978a,b). The tachykinin kassinin is apparently unique in its ability to inhibit cellular thirst selectively (deCaro and Micossi, 1986). The tachikinins also inhibit sodium appetite in sodium-depleted rats (Massi et al., 1986a) (Fig. 9.4).

The tachykinins also release ADH and thus reduce diuresis (Cantalamessa et al., 1984). Their effects on water intake appear to be behaviorally specific, since the tachykinins do not reduce food intake even at higher doses than those required to inhibit drinking (Massi et al., 1986c). The tachykinins appear to act centrally since they do not affect water intake when administered systemically.

This conclusion is supported by the results of recent mapping studies (Massi et al., 1988), which have shown that intracranial injections of eledoisin, physalaemin, and substance P inhibit the drinking response to A-II most effectively

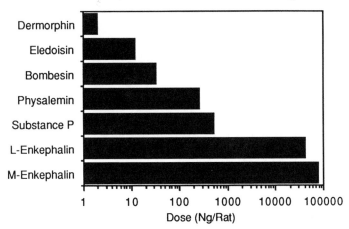

Fig. 9.4. Tachykinins, bombesins, and opioid peptides, administered icv, produce inhibitory effects on drinking, but their effectiveness varies considerably depending on the nature of the thirst stimulus. In the example shown here, all are shown to reduce drinking to intracranial A-II but the dosage required to obtained a 50 ±10% reduction in water intake varies enormously. Data from: DeCaro, G. (1986). Effects of peptides of the "gut-brain-skin triangle" on drinking behaviour of rats and birds. *In:* "The Physiology of Thirst and Sodium Appetite." (G. deCaro, A. N. Epstein, and M. Massi eds.) pp. 213–226. Plenum Press, New York.

when administered into the medial preoptic area, anterior hypothalamus, or subfornical organ. Other brainstem injection sites produced smaller effects, and most appeared to be differentially sensitive to the three tachikinins.

The second family of drugs in this group are the bombesins (bombesin, ranatensin, and litorin). When administered icv in nanogram doses, these compounds potently antagonize angiotensin-induced drinking. At considerably higher doses, they also attenuate drinking responses to icv carbachol, water deprivation, and cellular dehydration (deCaro *et al.*, 1980a, 1984a; Cantalamessa, 1982a).

Many of the bombesins also inhibit food intake and locomotor activity, but only in doses that are several times higher than those required to produce a selective inhibition of drinking. A specific drug action on thirst-related mechanisms is also suggested by the fact that some of the peptides of this group appear to selectively inhibit drinking responses to specific classes of thirst stimuli (e.g., bombesin and ranatensin, but not litorin, inhibit angiotensin-induced drinking; bombesin and litorin, but not ranatensin, are effective against deprivation-induced thirst). As in the case of the tachykinins discussed above, systemic administration of the bombesins has no effect on water intake.

It is interesting to note that the tachykinins and bombesins do not exert inhibitory effects in pigeons and ducks but act, in fact, as potent dipsogens when administered icv or ip (although they are somewhat less effective than angiotensin) (Evered *et al.*, 1977; deCaro *et al.*, 1978c, 1980b). Although the dipsogenic effect of the bombesins appears similar to that of icv angiotensin, different receptor mechanisms appear to be involved. Intracerebroventricular injections of angiotensin antagonists block the drinking response to A-II but have no effect on drinking in response to bombesin or the tachykinin eledoisin in the pigeon (deCaro *et al.*, 1982).

Lesions of the subfornical organ of the pigeon abolished drinking responses to ip angiotensin but had only relatively small inhibitory effects on the response to icv angiotensin injections. The lesions did not reduce the dipsogenic effects of icv or systemic injections of bombesin or the tachykinins litorin, ranatensin, or physalaemin (Massi *et al.*, 1986b).

Endogenous Opioids and Related Compounds

Enkephalins

Intracerebroventricular injections of rather high doses of the naturally occurring brain opioid peptides leucine-enkephalin or methionine-enkephalin have been shown to produce an initial inhibitory effect on drinking, followed by a persisting polydipsia, accompanied by an increase in plasma renin activity that appears to be mediated by beta-adrenergic stimulation of renal mechanisms (Cantalamessa *et al.*, 1982b).

Dermorphin, a peptide that is structurally related to the endogenous opioids, has been shown to be an extremely effective inhibitor of angiotensin-induced drinking at icv doses as low as 0.5–1.0 ng (deCaro, 1984b). That this may reflect a specific interaction with brain mechanisms involved with drinking responses to A-II is suggested by the observation (see deCaro, 1986) that dermorphine-like immunoreactivity has been found only in the subfornical organ (SFO), the organum vasculosum of the lamina terminalis (OVLT), and arcuate nucleus (in marked contrast to enkephalins, which are known to be diffusely distributed throughout many areas of the rat brain). A specific action of dermorphin on tissues of the SFO is further indicated by the observation that direct injections of dermorphin into this small structure were far more effective in blocking A-II drinking responses than icv injections of comparable doses (deCaro *et al.*, 1983; Perfumi *et al.*, 1986).

Morphine

Subcutaneous injections of morphine have also been reported to produce an initial suppression of water intake followed by hyperdipsia (and hyperphagia), which persisted for several hours but was followed by a prolonged (18 h) period of reduced water (as well as food) intake (Arslan *et al.*, 1986). The effects of morphine on water intake were antagonized by naltrexone, whereas food intake did not show consistent effects of this opioid receptor blocker.

Opiod Receptor Blockers

Systemic administration of opioid receptor blockers such as naloxone and naltrexone attenuates ad libitum water intake as well as drinking after deprivation (Brown and Holtzman, 1979; Sanger, 1983; Leander and Hynes, 1983), salt loads, hypovolemia, or angiotensin (Rowland, 1982). Intracranial injections of these compounds have been shown to be effective, suggesting a direct drug action of brain opiate receptors (Czech *et al.*, 1983). Naloxone also appears to reduce salt appetite (Cooper and Turkish, 1983; Cooper and Gilbert, 1984, although this effect is often difficult to separate from the general hypodipsic effect of these compounds.

Benzodiazepines

Drugs of the benzodiazepine family, including chlordiazepoxide, diazepam, flurazepam, orazepam, midazolam, and oxazepam, are widely used as sedatives and minor tranquilizers. The benzodiazepines increase deprivation-induced thirst as well as drinking after experimentally induced hypovolemia or cellular dehydration (Cooper, 1983a,b).

The dipsogenic effects of these compounds is reversed or prevented by the administration of benzodiazepine receptor blockers, which do not, however, themselves attenuate deprivation-induced drinking (Copper, 1982a, 1986). Opioid receptor blockers such as naloxone and naltrexone, which do reduce deprivation-induced thirst, also block chlordiazepoxide-induced hyperdipsia (Cooper, 1982b,c), suggesting a link between the dipsogenic properties of the benzodiazepines and brain opioid mechanisms.

Prostaglandins

Prostaglandins are members of a large and varied family of compounds that originate from essential fatty acids in all tissues including the brain. They influence a wide range of physiological functions at least in part by acting as local hormones or paracrines (Elattar, 1978).

In the central nervous system, the synthesis of prostaglandins has been shown to be affected by a variety of stimuli including neurotransmitters, hormones, analeptics, pyrogens, trauma, and ischemia. The prostaglandins are thus ideally suited to act as modulators of neural activity and as messengers for the interaction between neural and nonneural events.

Because their absolute concentrations are extremely low under normal circumstances and they are rapidly inactivated (by facilitated transport into the general circulation), it has been very difficult to specify their functions or to obtain a detailed understanding of their mechanism of action in the brain. Their role in temperature regulation is understood best and has served as a model for hypotheses concerning other functions. According to widely accepted theory, fever results when pyrogens stimulate the synthesis of prostaglandin E-2 in the rostral hypothalamus. Prostaglandin E_2 (PGE_2) then resets the setpoint around which body temperature is regulated (Stitt, 1986; Cooper, 1987). The theory is supported by the observation that icv (Feldberg and Saxena, 1971, 1975) as well as intraparenchymal injections of very low doses of PGE increase body temperature. It is interesting to note that the PGE-sensitive structures include such thirst-related structures as the preoptic region (Williams et al., 1977; Lipton et al., 1973), OLVT (Stitt, 1986), and ventral septal area (Ruwe et al., 1985).

Prostaglandins may affect the regulation of the body's water and sodium balance in a variety of ways, including direct effects on renal glomeruli (Gross and Bartter, 1973), systemic vasodilator effects (Aiken and Vane, 1973), central pyrexic effects (Feldberg, 1975; Fluharty, 1981), etc. Most interesting, in the present context, is the possibility that prostaglandins of the E series may oppose the dipsogenic effects of angiotensin II peripherally and/or centrally.

ICV Injections

In the rat, icv injections of nanogram doses of prostaglandin E_1 or E_2 attenuate drinking responses to central as well as systemic angiotensin II. At substantially higher doses, deprivation-induced drinking as well as drinking after intracranial carbachol or PG-induced hypovolemia are also reduced. Cellular dehydration thirst, on the other hand, appears to be unaffected (Nicolaidis and Fitzsimons, 1975; Kenney and Epstein, 1978; Perez-Guaita and Chiaraviglio, 1980; Kenney 1980, 1986; Fluharty, 1981) (Fig. 9.5).

Intracerebroventricular injections of prostaglandins also elevate core temperature. The effect appears to be correlated with their antidipsogenic effects under some (Fluharty, 1981) but not all (Kenney and Epstein, 1978; Kenney, 1986) conditions.

It has been suggested (Fluharty, 1981; Kenney, 1986) that the pyrexic response to icv prostaglandins may contribute to their antidipsogenic effects, especially when used at higher doses, which attenuate drinking in response to several different extracellular dipsogens. The persistence of osmotic thirst suggests, however, that more specific inhibitory influences are also generated. This con-

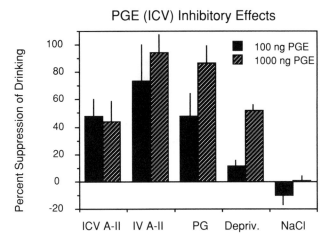

Fig. 9.5. Inhibition of the drinking response to deprivation and various dipsogens after icv injections of 100 or 1000 ng/rat of prostaglandin E. Data from: (1) Kenney, N. J. (1986). Suppression of water intake by the E prostaglandins. *In:* "The Physiology of Thirst and Sodium Appetite." (G. deCaro, A. N. Epstein, and M. Massi eds.) pp. 227–238 : Plenum Press, New York. And (2) Kenney, N. J., and Epstein, A. N. (1978). The antidipsogenic role of the E-prostaglandins *J. Comp. Physiol. Psychol.* **92**, 204–219.

clusion is supported by the fact that food intake is not reduced by antidipsogenic icv injections of prostaglandin, provided the animals are hydrated so that no prandial drinking is required (Kenney and Epstein, 1978).

The fact that intracranial injections of prostaglandins of the E series inhibit drinking to A-II as well as other extracellular dipsogens known to activate the renin–angiotensin system, without reducing cellular dehydration thirst that does not affect plasma A-II (Abdelaal *et al.*, 1976), led to the working hypothesis (Kenney and Epstein, 1978) that angiotensin and prostaglandin E might act in an antagonistic fashion on brain mechanisms concerned with extracellular thirst.

According to this view, increases in plasma or CSF A-II activate extracellular thirst mechanisms in the subfornical (or other circumventricular) organ and thus elicit drinking. Angiotensin also stimulates the the synthesis of prostaglandin E, which terminates thirst either by a direct antagonism of A-II or by acting on different neural mechanisms that exert inhibitory "satiety" influences.

The proposed antagonism between angiotensin II and prostaglandin E could also involve opposing vasomotor effects. Increased plasma angiotensin levels result in peripheral vasoconstriction, and it has been suggested (Epstein and Simpson, 1974; Nicolaidis and Fitzsimons, 1975) that angiotensin might activate thirst-related brain mechanisms by constricting vessels in some circumventricular organ such as the SFO. Prostaglandin E is a peripheral vasodilator in most species and has been shown to antagonize the renal vasoconstrictor action of

A-II. Intracerebroventricular injections of prostaglandin E have been shown to increase rather than decrease arterial blood pressure (Hoffman and Schmid, 1979; Kenney and Perara, 1980), much like A-II itself (Severs and Daniels-Severs, 1973). However, this does not rule out the proposed interaction in a structure such as the SFO, which is on the blood side of the blood–brain barrier. Direct experimental evidence is not available as of this time.

The hypothesis that prostaglandin E is released by angiotensin in the brain and opposes its dipsogenic properties leads to the prediction that inhibition of the biosynthesis of prostaglandin should enhance the drinking response to intracranial A-II (as well as experimental dipsogens that release A-II). Experiments designed to test this straightforward prediction have produced inconsistent results. Phillips and Hoffman (1977) have reported that icv injections of the prostaglandin synthesis inhibitor meclofenamate significantly increased the duration and magnitude of the drinking response to icv A-II administered concurrently.

Kenney (1980) reported that icv injections of bradykinin, a naturally occurring peptide that increases prostaglandin synthesis (McGiff et al., 1972), reduced the drinking response to icv A-II, suggesting that enhanced synthesis of endogenous brain prostaglandins may produce antidipsogenic effects. Fluharty (1981; see also Fluharty and Epstein, 1980) supported such an interpretation by showing that icv injections of the prostaglandin precursor arachidonic acid produced antidipsogenic as well as pyrexic effects similar to those seen after icv prostaglandin E_2. Both of these effects were blocked by icv pretreatment with the prostaglandin synthesis inhibitor indomethacin. The interpretation of these results is, unfortunately, complicated by the fact that the same doses of indomethacin failed to affect the drinking response to icv injections of a wide range of doses of angiotensin II.

Attempts to enhance the drinking response to icv A-II by systemic injections of prostaglandin synthesis inhibitors, which might more readily gain access to the vasculature of circumventricular organs than icv injections, have met with similarly mixed success. Perez-Guiata and Chiaraviglio (1980) reported that ip injections of indomethacin increased drinking in response to icv A-II and also enhanced water intake in deprived rats. Kenney and Moe (1981), on the other hand, observed no significant effects of chronic oral indomethacin administration on the drinking response to icv A-II, even though plasma levels of prostaglandin E_2 were markedly reduced by the treatment, and ad libitum water intake and the drinking response to iv A-II were augmented (discussed below).

Before pursuing the interaction between prostaglandins of the E series and systemic A-II, it should be noted that these compounds do not produce antidipsogenic effects in all species.

In the goat, icv injections of prostaglandin E_1 have been reported to increase water intake, especially when infused with hypertonic saline or in combination with angiotensin (Andersson and Leksell, 1975; Leksell, 1976). Brief bursts of drinking in response to icv prostaglandin E_2 have also been observed in the rat (although these injections reliably counteract the dipsogenic effects of icv A-II), but the effect has been described as often weak and variable (Nicolaidis and Fitzsimons, 1975).

Systemic Injections

Systemic (ip) injections of prostaglandin E_1 or E_2 in microgram doses produce transient inhibitory effects on deprivation-related drinking and suppress drinking responses to iv angiotensin II. Unlike icv injections of prostaglandins, systemic administration of even low doses significantly reduces drinking elicited by cellular dehydration (which is not affected by icv injections of prostaglandins even at high doses), and drinking elicited by PG-induced hypovolemia is reduced only by very high doses (Fig. 9.6). The systemic route of administration also reduces body temperature, in contrast to icv injections, which are pyrexic (Kenney *et al.*, 1981; Goldstein *et al.*, 1979).

Both systemic and central prostaglandin E reduces A-II–induced water intake. This suggests that the prostaglandin antagonism of A-II drinking may be due to an action on vascular or neural mechanisms that are accessible by systemic as well as icv injections. The effects of icv and systemic PGEs on other experimen-

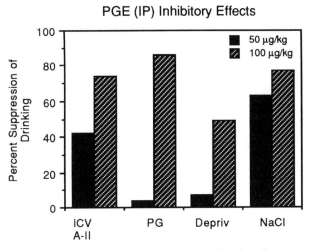

Fig. 9.6. Inhibition of the drinking response to deprivation and various dipsogens after systemic (IP) injections of 50 or 100 μg/kg of prostaglandin E. Data from: (1) Kenney, N. J. (1980). A case study of the neuroendocrine control of goal-directed behavior: the interaction between angiotensin II and prostaglandin E_1 in the control of water intake. *In:* "Neural Mechanisms of Goal-Directed Behavior and Learning." (R. F. Thompson, L. H. Hicks, and V. B. Shvyrkov, eds.) pp. 437–446. Academic Press, New York. And (2) Kenney, N. J. (1986). Suppression of water intake by the E prostaglandins. *In:* "The Physiology of Thirst and Sodium Appetite." (G. deCaro, A. N. Epstein, and M. Massi eds.) pp. 227–238. Plenum Press, New York.

tal dipsogens, on the other hand, are quite different. The antidipsogenic effect of the prostaglandins on cellular dehydration thirst may reflect their action on brain mechanisms accessible from plasma but not CSF. The fact that icv injections of the prostaglandins are more effective than systemic administration in reducing PG-induced drinking is congruent with the hypothesis that hypovolemia may activate a peripheral neural mechanisms as well as the renin–angiotensin system.

The differential efficacy of systemically administered prostaglandins in inhibiting drinking to different dipsogens suggests that the reduced water intake may not be merely the result of general malaise. The fact that ip injections of large, generally antidipsogenic doses of prostaglandin E do not support the formation of a conditioned taste aversion (Kenney et al., 1981) supports this conclusion.

Intraperitoneal injections of the prostaglandin synthesis inhibitor indomethacin have been reported to elicit drinking in water replete rats. This effect was abolished by nephrectomy but not by ureteric ligation, suggesting an important role for the renin–angiotensin system (Feuerstein et al., 1978). Large doses of indomethacin have also been reported to increase water intake after 10 h of deprivation (Perez-Guiata and Chiaraviglio, 1980). These observations are compatible with the hypothesis that prostaglandins of the E series may play a role in the inhibition of thirst under normal conditions.

Other data indicate, however, that much more information is needed before we can hope to understand their role in the regulation of water intake. For instance, chronic oral administrations of prostaglandin synthesis inhibitors such as indomethacin or acetylsalicylic acid do not modify ad libitum water intake, although they increase the drinking response to A-II as well as hypertonic saline. The magnitude of the drinking response to PG-induced hypovolemia was not significantly affected in these experiments, although the latency of the first draft was decreased (Kenney and Moe, 1981, 1982).

Review and Conclusions

The past quarter century has seen a staggering amount of research designed to elucidate the pharmacology of brain mechanisms concerned with thirst and various cellular and extracellular influences on it.

The research of the 1960s and early 1970s demonstrated that the cholinomimetic compound carbachol is an extremely potent dipsogen when administered icv or directly into many sites in the upper brainstem, septum, and hippocampus. Injections of the acetylcholine receptor blocker atropine into the same sites blocks the effects of carbachol and decreases deprivation- or salt-induced drinking. The effects of carbachol and related receptor blockers on water intake appear to be due at least in part to a drug action on neurons in the subfornical organ and in the region of the anteroventral third ventricle or preoptic region. Destruction of the SFO as well as cold-cream blockade of access to the AV3V suppress cholinergic drinking. Stimulation of cholinergic neurons in the supraoptic nucleus of the preoptic region releases vasopressin. The resultant reduction in urine flow complements carbachol-induced thirst.

The cholinergic pathways appear to be concerned primarily if not exclusively with cellular thirst. They may be opposed by an inhibitory or "satiety" mechanism that relies on the activation of alpha-adrenergic receptors in the region of the paraventricular nucleus of the hypothalamus. Microinjections of norepinephrine or epinephrine into this region inhibit deprivation- and salt-induced drinking as well as drinking responses to intracranial carbachol. Norepinephrine (NE) injected icv or directly into the supraoptic nucleus releases vasopressin and thus decreases urine output. The effects of intracranial NE on drinking and urine output are inhibited by pretreatment with alpha-adrenergic blockers.

Histamine injections into the supraoptic or periventricular nuclei elicit drinking and antidiuresis. Systemic administration of much larger doses also elicit drinking as well as decreased blood pressure and renin release. The latter does not appear to be primarily responsible for the dipsogenic effects of systemic histamine, since histamine-induced drinking is decreased only slightly by nephrectomy. Histamine may act specifically on feeding-related drinking because systemic injections of histamine receptor blockers abolish the effects of histamine and reduce periprandial drinking without affecting water intake after deprivation.

Peptides were first isolated from the gut and various glands of mammals and from amphibian skin. More recently, many similar or identical peptides have been detected in brain tissue. Many of them have been shown to be released from nerve endings, and it appears likely that they exert neuromodulator or neurotransmitter functions. The relationship between the peptides found in the periphery and those detected centrally is the subject of contemporary controversy, since most cannot cross the blood–brain barrier except, perhaps, at certain circumventricular organs.

Several classes of peptides obtained from amphibian skin have been shown to have pronounced effects on water intake when administered in very small doses icv or directly into the anterior hypothalamus, medial preoptic area, or subfornical organ. Tachykinins such as eledoisin, physalemin, and substance P inhibit water intake in response to both cellular and extracellular thirst stimuli. They are most effective against drinking induced by icv A-II, somewhat less effective against icv carbachol, and least effective in blocking drinking elicited by systemic salt loads or water deprivation. Another amphibian peptide, kassinin, appears to inhibit cellular thirst selectively.

A second group, the bombesins, also produces inhibitory effects on water intake. However, individual members of this family seem to affect the response to certain thirst stimuli quite selectively. For instance, icv ranatensin or bombesin (but not litorin) blocks drinking to icv A-II. Litorin, but not ranatensin, blocks deprivation-induced thirst effectively. Dermorphin, a distant relative of the endogenous opioids, is extremely effective in blocking icv angiotensin II, especially when administered directly into the subfornical organ.

Intracerebroventricular injections of the naturally occurring brain opioids leucine- or methionine-enkephalin produce an initial inhibitory effect on drinking followed by a sustained hyperdipsia. Similar effects have been reported after systemic injections of the plant-derived drug morphine. Systemic injections of opioid receptor blockers such as naloxone have been shown to inhibit drinking responses to cellular as well as extracellular thirst stimuli. The effects may be centrally mediated, since icv injections of the blockers are also effective.

Prostaglandins are ubiquitous fatty acid derivatives found in brain as well as peripheral tissues. Some are believed to act in the central nervous system as neurotransmitters or neuromodulators. Prostaglandins of the E series (PGE_1 and PGE_2) reduce drinking responses to icv as well as systemic angiotensin II. At higher doses, they also reduce drinking after intracranial carbachol or systemic polyethylene glycol. Cellular dehydration thirst is apparently not affected. Systemic injections of PGEs do reduce drinking responses after salt loads as well as iv A-II at relatively low doses, whereas hypovolemic thirst is affected only at significantly higher doses. Intracerebroventricular prostaglandins also produce pyrexic effects, which may contribute to their antidipsogenic action, particular at higher doses.

Intracerebroventricular injections of prostaglandin precursors or agents that enhance PGE synthesis have been reported to produce antidipsogenic effects similar to those seen after PGE itself. Conversely, drinking responses to A-II is enhanced by icv meclofenamate, a drug that inhibits PGE synthesis. However, other PGE synthesis inhibitors apparently do not produce significant facilitatory effects when administered icv, although systemic injections of larger doses elicit water intake in replete rats and increase drinking in deprived animals. When these drugs are administered chronically, ad libitum water intake does not appear to be affected. It is clear that we do not yet understand the influence of PGEs on normal drinking or the mechanisms of their actions on thirst-related brain pathways.

Chapter 10

Sodium Appetite

Introduction

Sodium plays a major role in (a) the maintenance of blood volume, pressure, and osmolarity; (b) the regulation of the movement of water between the cellular and extracellular compartments; and (c) cellular metabolism and function. It is essential that the sodium concentration of the body's fluids be closely regulated.

Sodium is continually lost from skin, kidney, salivary glands, and gastrointestinal tract. When plasma sodium levels fall, the renin–angiotensin system is activated. This, in turn results in the increased release of the mineralocorticoid aldosterone from the adrenal cortex (Spielman and Davis, 1974). This hormone conserves sodium by reducing its excretion in urine, saliva, and perspiration (Ganong, 1971). In rats and perhaps other species as well, aldosterone also acts in concert with angiotensin to stimulate a specific salt appetite, which assures that sodium levels are replenished before unacceptable deviations from the normal sodium concentration of the body fluids (approximately 0.9%) can threaten survival (Fluharty and Epstein, 1983; Stricker, 1983; Moe *et al.*, 1984).

A specific appetite for sodium is found in many species. Many herbivores do not obtain sufficient sodium in their diet under some ecological conditions and travel great distances to find salt licks or salt pools. As long as the supply is adequate, the diet of carnivores contains an excess of sodium. The regulation of the sodium content of body fluids becomes then entirely a matter of renal excretion. Omnivores occupy an intermediate position, their specific salt needs fluctuating with regional and/or seasonal variations in the diet (see Denton, 1982, for an extensive review).

Humans, of course, notoriously ingest far more sodium than they require. In addition to the plentiful supply of salt in basic foods, salt is used generously in the preparation of processed foods, and to top it off, we pour salt onto just about everything during a meal. Indeed, most of us eat so much salt that the complex system that regulates salt excretion cannot keep up. As a consequence, hypernatremia becomes a significant factor in hypertension.

Salt appetite has been studied experimentally most extensively in the laboratory rat. This animal displays an innate preference for salt even when it is sodium
replete (Richter, 1936, 1956; Epstein and Stellar, 1955; Nachman, 1962; Wolf,
1969). In the adult rat, the threshold for the expression of the animal's salt
preference is ~0.06% NaCl, the most preferred concentration is in the region of
0.9%, and saline begins to be aversive (i.e., more water than saline is selected in
a two-bottle preference test) at a concentration of 1.5% NaCl.

When an acute or chronic sodium deficiency occurs, a true sodium appetite
develops that greatly expands the range of acceptable salt solutions (from a low
of 0.003% to a high of 5.0% or more). This condition appears to be innate
(Berridge et al., 1984) and has been shown to motivate a variety of learned
behaviors that have previously led to salt (Richter, 1936, 1956; Kriekhaus and
Wolf, 1968; McCutcheon and Levy, 1972; Schulkin et al., 1985).

The taste of salt is a significant component of the series of events that reduce
salt appetite. There are several reports in the literature indicating that salt appetite
is not appeased by stomach loads of hypertonic saline (e.g., Nachman and
Valentino, 1966; DiCara and Wilson, 1974).

Other investigators have emphasized postingestional factors on the basis of
observations such as the following: (a) The salt appetite seen after formalin
injections abates after sufficient saline has been injected intragastrically to restore
the animal's sodium balance (Quartermain et al., 1967; Levy and McCutcheon,
1974). (b) Adrenalectomized rats doubled their intake of hypertonic saline when
treated with an exchange ion that prevented the absorption of about half of the
ingested sodium (Epstein and Stellar, 1955). (c) Chronic intragastric infusions of
saline reduce salt appetite (Kissileff and Hoeffer, 1975). (d) Infusions of isotonic
saline into the hepatic portal vein reduces NaCl consumption in rats maintained
on salt-deficient diets and treated with the natriuretic agent furosemide (Tordoff
et al., 1986). (e) When postabsorptive influences are eliminated by draining
orally ingested saline through an esophageal fistula, salt appetite is not reduced
(Mook, 1969).

The results of more recent investigation indicate that there may be both oral
and postingestional satiety cues that come into play at different times. In the
short term, gastric loads of saline that bypass oral salt receptors are less satiating
than sodium solutions ingested by mouth. However, the effectiveness of stomach
loads increases when the tests are extended and matches the satiety effects of oral
ingestion after about 16 h (Wolf et al., 1984) (Fig. 10.1). Infusions of hypertonic
saline into the hepatic portal vein have also been shown to reduce subsequent
saline ingestion in furosemide-treated rats maintained on a salt-deficient diet.
The magnitude of this effect was comparable to that produced by oral ingestion
of a comparable quantity of hypertonic saline (Tordoff et al., 1987).

That taste is, indeed, a significant component of satiety for salt appetite is
indicated by the results of investigations (Nachman, 1963; Falk, 1965b; Jalowiec
et al., 1966; Schulkin, 1982) that have demonstrated that sodium-deficient rats

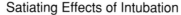

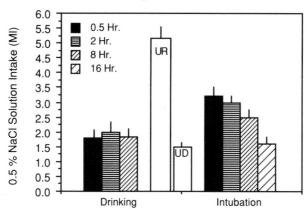

Fig. 10.1. An illustration of the influence of taste and postingestional factors in the satiation of sodium appetite. The animals were maintained on a salt-deficient diet for 2 days and injected with 2.5, 5.0, or 10.0 mg of the natriuretic drug furosemide at the beginning of the second day. Repletion of body sodium was achieved by gavage of 5 ml of 3% saline or by allowing the rats to drink 5 ml of a 3% NaCl solution. Saline (0.5%) was made available for 10 min or 0.5, 2, 8, or (in the case of gavage) 16 h afterwards. UD, undepleted control; UR, unrepleted control. Data from: Wolf, G., Schulkin, J., and Simon, P. E. (1984). Multiple factors in the satiation of salt appetite. *Behav. Neurosci.* **98**, 661–673.

will select salty-tasting solutions that contain potassium (KCl) or lithium (LiCl) but no sodium and prefer saltier solutions of other salts over less salty-tasting NaCl solutions.

Adrenal Mineralocorticoids

Chronic sodium depletion can arises naturally as a consequence of dietary deficiency. It can be produced experimentally by adrenalectomy, which results in an uncontrolled loss of sodium from the kidney (as well as other tissues such as salivary glands and colon) due to the absence of the adrenal mineralocorticoids aldosterone and deoxycorticosterone (DOC) (Richter, 1936). Salt appetite returns to normal following replacement therapy with the adrenal mineralocorticoids (Richter, 1941).

A seemingly paradoxical salt appetite develops when large, pharmacological doses of of the mineralocorticoids aldosterone or deoxycorticosterone (frequently in the form of deoxycorticosterone acetate, DOCA) are administered over several days to intact rats (Richter, 1941; Rice and Richter, 1943; Braun-Menéndez, 1952) or adrenalectomized rats (Wolf, 1965; Wolf and Handal, 1966; Fregley and Waters, 1966a,b) (Fig. 10.2). Low doses have opposite,

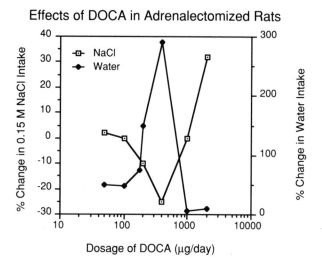

Fig. 10.2. Change in 0.15 *M* saline and water intake in adrenalectomized rats in response to deoxycorticosterone acetate (DOCA). Data from: Fregly, M. J., and Waters, W. I. (1966a). Effect of mineralocorticoids on spontaneous sodium chloride appetite of adrenalectomized rats. *Physiol. Behav.* **1**, 65–74.

inhibitory effects (for a discussion of species differences, see Denton, 1982). Adrenal glucocorticoids (cortisone, corticosterone) do not stimulate sodium appetite but potentiate the response to DOCA (Wolf, 1965; Braun-Menéndez, 1952).

Rats treated with mineralocorticoids ingest large quantities of saline and accept even strongly hypertonic solutions avidly (Wolf and Quartermain, 1966; Schulkin *et al.*, 1985). The salt appetite appears to be innate, since experience with salty solutions is not a prerequisite for its expression following the initial exposure to mineralocorticoids (Schulkin, 1978).

The fact that excessive sodium loss, produced by adrenalectomy, as well as sodium retention, produced by mineralocorticoid treatment, produce similar effects on salt appetite has posed a perplexing problem to investigators in the field. We have only recently begun to gain some insights into the complex mechanisms involved.

The Renin–Angiotensin System

A loss of sodium from the body results in hypovolemia and renin release. The increased release of A-II stimulates the secretion of aldosterone by the adrenal gland, and this mineralocorticoid, in turn, promotes tubular reabsorption of sodium in the kidney. Efforts to demonstrate a comparable role of angiotensin in sodium appetite that develops as a consequence of hyponatremia (Richter, 1936) and is eventually responsible for reversing it have resulted in a complex and as yet incomplete picture. Renin has been an integral part of the overall puzzle of salt appetite, at least in part because renin release is increased in the adrenalectomized rat but reduced after DOCA.

Extracellular thirst stimuli such as hemorrhage, caval ligation, peritoneal glucose dialysis, and polyethylene glycol-induced hypovolemia elicit a sodium appetite that is delayed by many hours and persists, often for weeks or even months after the hyponatremia has been reversed (Falk, 1966; Falk and Lipton, 1967; Fitzsimons, 1969a; Stricker and Jalowiec, 1970; Fitzsimons and Wirth, 1978; Falk and Tang, 1980) (Fig. 10.3). Hyponatremia (due to water loading) alone does not elicit salt appetite in rats (Stricker, 1973), and stomach loads of sodium, administered after the salt appetite has developed, do not terminate it (Falk and Lipton, 1967).

These and related observations have given rise to the suggestion that hyponatremia or hypovolemia/hypotension may be essential for the initiation of hor-

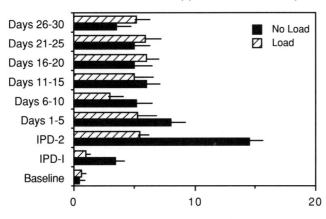

Fig. 10.3. Intake of a $0.5\ M$ NaCl solution during daily test periods after two 4-h intraperitoneal dialyses (IPD) (spaced 2 days apart), which resulted in hypernatremia. Although the animals consumed more salt than needed to replenish the sodium withdrawn during IPD–1, the salt intake after IPD was far greater after IPD–2 and persisted for the subsequent 30-day observation period. Sodium appetite persisted even in animals that received a 4% body weight stomach load of $0.5\ M$ saline (nearly twice the amount removed by dialysis) at the end of each ip dialysis. Data from: Falk, J. L., and Lipton, J. M. (1967). Temporal factors in the genesis of NaCl appetite by intraperitoneal dialysis. *J. Comp. Physiol. Psychol.* **63**, 247–251.

monal events that arouse salt appetite but not for the maintenance of the salt-seeking behavior, which may continue (because of the persistence of hormonal influences) long after the original deficiency has been repaired.

Attempts to elucidate the role of the kidney have shown that nephrectomy produces an aversion to all saline solutions above the absolute taste threshold. Ureteric ligation that leaves an intact kidney produces similar effects, indicating that the absence of renin is not the determining factor (Fitzsimons and Stricker, 1971). Nephrectomy, as well as ureteric ligation, also abolishes the salt appetite of adrenalectomized as well as formalin-treated intact rats.

Intraperitoneal injections of kidney extract or renin that are clearly dipsogenic in the rat produce only a very small and delayed effect on saline ingestion (Fitzsimons, 1969a). More substantial effects have been reported after iv infusions of A-II (Findlay and Epstein, 1980). The salt appetite of adrenalectomized or formalin-treated rats is not affected by ip injections of renin that are dipsogenic in the intact rat (Fitzsimons and Stricker, 1971; Fitzsimons and Wirth, 1978). Intracranial injections of angiotensin, on the other hand, have been reported to restore sodium appetite in sodium depleted nephrectomized rats (Chiaraviglio, 1976) (discussed below). Significant increases in saline intake have also been reported in DOCA-treated adrenalectomized animals after subcutaneous infusions of low doses of A-II that resulted in elevations of plasma A-II that appear to be within the range of values seen after sodium deprivation (Dalhouse et al., 1986).

Intracranial Angiotensin

Early studies of the effects of icv injections of renin or A-II showed that the single-choice preference-aversion function after icv renin was no different from that of 24-h water-deprived animals (Fitzsimons, 1971b). In a two-bottle choice test, a wide range of doses of icv angiotensin also produced a pattern of water and saline ingestion that was not different from that of rats that were water-deprived overnight (Fitzsimons and Wirth, 1978).

Other investigators (Fisher and Buggy, 1975) have noted a gradual shift from water to isotonic saline after intracranial injections of angiotensin or have observed small (Covian et al., 1972) or inconsistent (Radio et al., 1972) effects on sodium appetite after single intracranial injections or short-term infusions of angiotensin.

Significant increases in sodium intake have been reported after long term intracranial infusions of angiotensin. Fisher and Buggy (1975) infused 500 ng of angiotensin icv every 8 min for 8 h (for a total dose of 30 μg) and reported significant intake of hypertonic saline. More recently, Avrith and Fitzsimons (1980, 1983) as well as Bryant et al. (1980) have elicited significant, sustained saline intake during slow intracranial infusions of far smaller doses of angiotensin-II. In some of these experiments, infusions of somewhat larger doses of renin, or renin substrate or angiotensin, produced a salt appetite that persisted for many hours and even days, presumably because angiotensin continued to be produced from components of the cerebral renin–angiotensin system (Avrith and Fitzsimons, 1983; Bryant *et al.*,1980) (Fig. 10.4).

Some questions have been raised about the sodium appetite seen after icv infusions of angiotensin because relatively large total doses are required and intracranial angiotensin has been shown to cause natriuresis, which could act as the primary stimulus for sodium appetite (Severs *et al.*, 1971a). Some investigators have suggested that icv angiotensin infusions produce an initial relatively brief phase of saline ingestion, which precedes natriuresis, as well as a more pronounced and prolonged episode that could be due to urinary salt loss (Fluharty and Manaker, 1983).

This interpretation finds little support in Avrith and Fitzsimons's (1983) observation that a single icv injections of renin causes sufficient ingestion of hypertonic saline during the first hour to induce a positive Na balance, which is maintained for the subsequent 24 h.

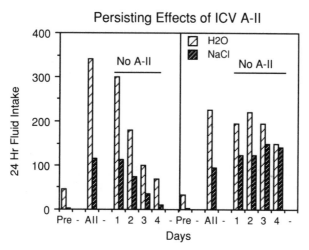

Fig. 10.4. Two "star" performers from an experiment by Bryant et al. (1980), which demonstrated that icv infusions of 100 ng/min of angiotensin II, continued for 4 days, produced significant increases in 0.5 *M* NaCl solution as well as water intake (the means for the 4 days are shown in the two left columns of each group). Water and saline intake remained elevated during the following 4 days (shown in the four sets of columns on the right of each group). After: Bryant, R. W., Epstein, A. N., Fitzsimons, J. T., and Fluharty, S. J. (1980). Arousal of a specific and persistent sodium appetite in the rat with continuous intracerebroventricular infusion of angiotensin II. *J. Physiol.* **301**, 365–382. With permission of the authors and the Physiological Society, Oxford, England.

Angiotensin Converting Enzyme Inhibitors

That central angiotensin plays a significant role in salt appetite has further been suggested by the results of recent investigations of the powerful angiotensin-converting enzyme inhibitor captopril (Horovitz, 1981). The effects of this drug on extracellular thirst and sodium appetite can be understood (Fitzsimons, 1986) when one considers the following.

When captopril is administered systemically in low doses, the enzyme-converting inhibitor does not enter the brain in significant quantities (Cohen and Kurz, 1982). Peripherally, it prevents the conversion from A-I to A-II. The resulting loss of angiotensin II from the circulation removes inhibitory feedback to the endogenous renin-secreting mechanisms and thus facilitates renin release and A-I formation (Schiffrin et al., 1981). The increased availability of A-I promotes its transport into the brain, where it is converted into A-II (since the converting-enzyme inhibitor is excluded from brain at low doses). The elevated brain levels of A-II, in turn, elicit water intake and salt appetite.

When captopril is administered systemically in high doses the converting enzyme inhibitor can enter the brain in significant quantities (Evered et al., 1980; Cohen and Kurz, 1982). This prevents the conversion of A-I to A-II in brain and thus functionally inactivates the excess A-I, which is transported into brain as a consequence of the peripheral effects of captopril (described in the preceding paragraph) or renin-releasing extracellular thirst stimuli.

As predicted by this model, systemic injections of low doses of captopril elicit some water drinking and enhance water intake in response to extracellular thirst stimuli (Mann et al., 1986; Elfont and Fitzsimons, 1983; Barney et al., 1980; Katovich et al., 1979; Lehr et al., 1973). These facilitatory effects of captopril appear to be renin-dependent, since they are abolished by nephrectomy (Elfont and Fitzsimons, 1981).

Low doses of captopril administered orally, sc, or iv also increase sodium appetite in salt-depleted rats (subjected to furosemide-induced natriuresis and maintained on a low-salt diet) and adrenalectomized rats (Fregly, 1980; Moe and Epstein, 1986; Epstein, 1986) (Fig. 10.5). These facilitatory effects of captopril are abolished when the blood–brain barrier is surgically compromised (e.g., shortly after the implantation of an icv cannula) or when captopril is concurrently administered icv in amounts known to block the A-I to A-II conversion centrally (Fig. 10.6). Captopril-induced salt appetite thus appears to be due to a movement of excess A-I into regions of the brain that are not protected by low systemic doses of the enzyme-converting inhibitor.

The captopril-induced salt appetite is not readily seen during short-term tests, but the phenomenon is unequivocal when extended observations are used, as is true for other types of renin-dependent salt appetite (Elfont et al., 1984; Moe and Epstein, 1986).

High systemic doses of captopril (or low systemic doses combined with small

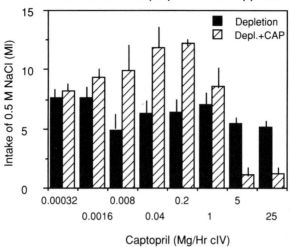

Fig. 10.5. Intake of 0.5 *M* NaCl solution in a 2-h test by rats maintained on a sodium deficient diet overnight and given two sc furosemide injections (5 mg/0.5 ml separated by 2, 16, and 18 h before the test). Captopril was infused intravenously at the indicated dose. Data from: Moe, K. E., and Epstein, A. N. (1986). Sodium appetite during captopril blockade of endogenous angiotensin formation. *In:* "The Physiology of Thirst and Sodium Appetite." (G. deCaro, A. N. Epstein, and M. Massi, eds.) pp. 431–439. Plenum Press, New York.

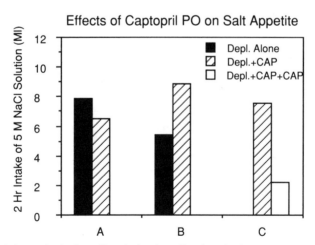

Fig. 10.6. Salt appetite in the sodium-depleted rat. Two-hour intake of 0.5 *M* NaCl solution in sodium-depleted (furosemide-treated, maintained on salt-deficient diet overnight) rats: (a) 1–2 weeks postsurgery when the blood–brain barrier was damaged due to cannula implantation; (b,c) 2–4 weeks after surgery when the blood–brain barrier again precluded the movement of captopril (CAP) into the brain. The hatched columns represent animals that had 0.1 mg/ml of captopril in the drinking water overnight. The light column represents animals that received icv infusions of CAP (1.2 μg/h) in addition to CAP in the drinking water. After: Moe, K. E., and Epstein, A. N. (1986). Sodium appetite during captopril blockade of endogenous angiotensin formation. *In:* "The Physiology of Thirst and Sodium Appetite." (G. deCaro, A. N. Epstein, and M. Massi, eds.) pp. 431–439. Plenum Press, New York. With permission of the authors and of Plenum Press.

icv injections) attenuate water intake elicited by polyethylene glycol (Mann *et al.*, 1986) or partial occlusion of the abdominal aorta between the renal veins (which causes the left kidney, distal to the occlusion, to secrete abnormally large amounts of renin) (Costales *et al.*, 1986; Fitzsimons, 1986).

High systemic doses of captopril (or low systemic doses combined with small icv injections) also reduce the salt appetite elicited by ligation of the vena cava (Costales *et al.*, 1986; Fitzsimons, 1986), furosemide-induced natriuresis combined with a low-salt diet (Moe and Epstein, 1986; Epstein, 1986), or adrenalectomy (Epstein, 1986). Single injections of captopril had no significant effects on ad libitum water intake in these experiments, although the animals drank more water overnight when captopril was put into their water supply (Moe and Epstein, 1986).

Continuous icv infusions of captopril in sodium-depleted rats (subjected to furosemide-induced natriuresis and maintained on a low-salt diet) have been reported to inhibit sodium intake in a dose-dependent manner without affecting ad libitum water intake (Weiss, 1986). DOCA-induced salt appetite, which is known to be independent of the renin–angiotensin system since DOCA inhibits renin release (Pettinger *et al.*, 1971), was not affected by icv captopril in these experiments.

Intracerebroventricular infusions of a blocking analogue of angiotensin, SAR (Sar-1-Ile-8-angiotensin II), have been reported to inhibit furosemide-induced sodium appetite (as well as water drinking in response to icv A-II) in rats (Weiss, 1986).

Angiotensin–Mineralocorticoid Interactions

Fluharty and Epstein (1983) have reported that continuous icv infusions of angiotensin did not stimulate significant salt ingestion in sodium-replete rats unless the dosage was increased to 100 pg/min. However, when small doses of DOCA (which did not elicit sodium appetite when given alone) were concurrently injected subcutaneously, icv angiotensin infusions stimulated significant ingestion of 3% saline at doses as low as 1 pg/min. Similar facilitatory interactions were observed when rats were pretreated with sc DOCA (Fluharty and Epstein, 1983) or aldosterone (Sakai, 1986) for several days prior to pulsed icv injection of A-II (Fig. 10.7).

DOCA-primed rats given icv injections of angiotensin have also been shown to emit a learned instrumental behavior for saline rewards, supporting the interpretation that the treatment elicits a compelling salt drive (Zhang *et al.*, 1984).

Epstein (1983, 1986) has suggested, on the basis of these and related observations, that angiotensin and aldosterone, which interact in the periphery to control the conservation of sodium by the kidney and other tissues, may also act syn-

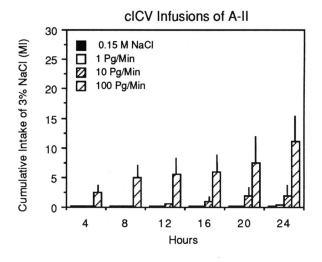

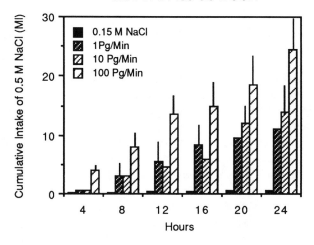

Fig. 10.7. Salt appetite in the sodium-replete rat. Cumulative intake of 0.5 *M* NaCl solution during 24 h of continuous intracerebroventricular (cicv) infusions of various doses of angiotensin II alone (top) or in combination with deoxycorticosterone acetate (DOCA), given sc just before the 24-h icv infusion of angiotensin. Both water and saline but not food were available ad libitum. Data from: Fluharty, S. J., and Epstein, A. N. (1983). Sodium appetite elicited by intracerebroventricular infusion of angiotensin II in the rat: II. Synergistic interaction with systemic mineralocorticoids. *Behav. Neurosci.* **97**, 746–758.

ergistically in the brain to give rise to the salt appetite that directs the behavioral responses needed to replenish the sodium balance of the body's fluids. Only when elevated to pathological levels can either hormone alone give rise to sodium appetite. Thus, in the adrenalectomized animal, renin levels are elevated and elicit sodium appetite even though aldosterone is absent. Conversely, prolonged exposure to pharmacological doses of DOCA is capable of eliciting salt ingestion even though the doses inhibit renin secretion.

Fuller and Fitzsimons (1986) have reported increases in sodium intake in intact, adrenalectomized, and deoxycorticosterone-pretreated rats after intracranial injections of low doses of angiotensin II. The DOC-treated rats displayed by far the largest increase in saline intake, a finding that supports Epstein's interaction hypothesis. (These animals also showed a pronounced natriuresis after the angiotensin injections, which may have contributed to the salt appetite. However, icv injections of carbachol also resulted in significant natriuresis but failed to elicit significant saline intake.) Adrenalectomized rats ingested smaller but significant quantities of hypertonic saline after intracranial angiotensin and did not display a natriuretic response to the injection.

Intact rats drank only little hypertonic saline after icv angiotensin in these experiments, leading Fuller and Fitzsimons to suggest that the synergistic interaction between adrenal mineralocorticoids and angiotensin that Epstein (1983) has proposed may become apparent only when large amounts of the adrenal hormones are present.

Stricker (1983) has suggested that a synergistic action of aldosterone and angiotensin may account for the typically delayed sodium appetite seen in rats after sc or ip injections of polyethylene glycol. Stricker et al. (1979) have shown that this treatment results in hypersecretion of aldosterone as well as renin which peaks at about the time sodium appetite appears. Prior maintenance on low-salt diets has no effect on PG-induced renin secretion but increases the aldosterone release. The low-salt diets also potentiate the PG-induced salt appetite.

This appears to be due to a permissive action of aldosterone, which may be due to its interaction with A-II in the brain. That aldosterone is not necessary for normal salt appetite after PG is indicated by Stricker's (1983) observation of a normal pattern of delayed salt ingestion after PG treatments administered to adrenalectomized rats treated with low doses of DOCA. A permissive action is indicated by the further observation that hypophysectomy that abolished the PG-stimulated aldosterone secretion (without affecting renin release) also abolished the facilitatory effects of the low-salt diets on PG-stimulated salt intake.

That the presence of larger than normal concentrations of aldosterone might act specifically to permit angiotensin to act, presumably on the brain, to evoke salt appetite is suggested by a further experiment of this series (Stricker, 1983). Captopril, which blocks the conversion of A-I to A-II in the periphery but not centrally (and thus makes excess amounts of A-I available for conversion to A-II

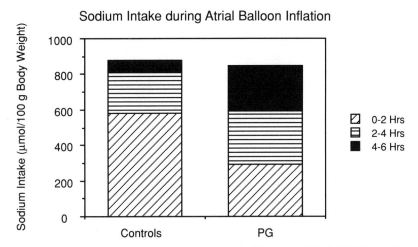

Fig. 10.8. Intake of 2.7% NaCl solution by rats after ip dialysis with 15 ml of 25% polyethylene glycol (PG). Balloons in the junction between the right superior vena cava and atrium were inflated during the first 2 h of the experiment. Data from: Kaufman, S. (1986a). Control mechanisms of salt appetite. *In:* "The Physiology of Thirst and Sodium Appetite." (G. deCaro, A. N. Epstein, and M. Massi, eds.) pp. 459–463. Plenum Press, New York.

in brain), was found to enhance PG-stimulated sodium appetite even when water was not available, so that sodium concentrations were above normal levels.

Atrial Stretch Receptors

There is some evidence that peripheral neural mechanisms may also play a role in salt appetite. Kaufman (1986a,b), for instance, has shown that inflation of balloons placed into the junction of the right atrium of the heart and the vena cava, 17 h after the administration of PG, reduces the sodium intake of rats previously maintained on a salt-deficient diet. When the balloons were deflated after 2 h, the experimental animals increased their saline intake so that at the end of a 6-h test no significant differences between the experimental and control groups remained (Fig. 10.8).

Rats that developed a salt appetite after being maintained on a low-salt diet and treated with the mineralocorticoid DOCA for 8 consecutive days also drank less of a hypertonic saline solution during the inflation of right atrium/superior vena cava balloons. Kaufman (1986a) suggested that these results further support the hypothesis that the effects of the balloon procedure reflect direct stimulation of neural receptors, since long-term DOCA treatments are known to result in a return to normal sodium levels and a suppression of the renin–angiotensin system (the so-called "mineralocortical escape").

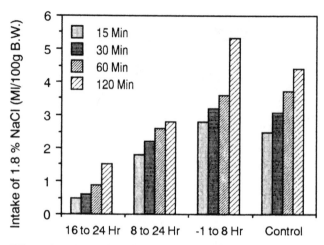

Fig. 10.9.   Effects of continuous icv infusions of 1 μl/h of hypertonic saline on 2-h 1.8% NaCl solution intake. Group "16 to 24 Hr" received 8 h of icv infusion beginning 16 h after ip glucose dialysis (10% of body weight of a 5% glucose solution). Group "8 to 24 Hr" received 16 h of icv infusions beginning 8 h after IPGD. Group "−1 to 8 Hr" received 8 h of icv infusions beginning 1 h before the end of the dialysis treatment. The tonicity of the ICV infusions was adjusted to assure comparable additions of NaCl to CSF. Data from: Chiaraviglio, E. and Pérez-Guaita, M. F. (1986). Effect of cerebroventricular infusion of hypertonic sodium solutions on sodium intake in rats. *In:* "The Physiology of Thirst and Sodium Appetite." (G. deCaro, A. N. Epstein, and M. Massi, eds.) pp. 503–508. Plenum Press, New York.

Peritoneal Glucose Dialysis

A delayed sodium appetite, which persists in spite of prompt replacement therapy, has been observed after intraperitoneal dialysis with isotonic glucose that produces an acute sodium deficiency. Serum sodium decreases significantly within 30 min and reaches its lowest level in about 2–3 h. Salt appetite, on the other hand, appears only after delays of 8–12 h or more (Falk and Tang, 1980; Falk and Lipton, 1967; Tang and Falk, 1979; Ferreyra and Chiaraviglio, 1977).

Cerebrospinal fluid (CSF) levels of sodium decrease roughly in parallel with serum sodium after ip dialysis. Intracerebroventricular (icv) infusions of hypertonic saline during the first 8 h after the dialysis have been reported to have no effect on sodium intake 24 h after dialysis. Similar infusions, begun 8 or 16 h after dialysis, when sodium appetite normally begins to appear, significantly decreased sodium intake in a similar test (Chiaraviglio and Pérez-Guaita, 1986) (Fig. 10.9).

Extracellular Thirst and Salt Appetite

Although it is clear that sodium deficiency initiates events that result in a pronounced and persisting salt appetite, the intermediary mechanisms are poorly understood. Many of the procedures that give rise to extracellular thirst *without inducing hyponatremia* (vascular dilution eventually occurs if the animals are permitted to drink) elicit salt appetite, including caval ligation and hemorrhage (Fitzsimons, 1969a, 1971c), polyethylene glycol (Stricker and Jalowiec, 1970; Stricker, 1973), and systemic or central angiotensin injections (Bryant *et al.*, 1980; Findlay and Epstein, 1980; Fluharty and Epstein, 1983).

Isoproterenol has been reported not to elicit salt appetite in short-term experiments (Fitzsimons and Wirth, 1978). Long-term observations, which might be important in view of the generally delayed salt-appetite seen after other extracellular challenges, have not yet been performed.

In nearly all cases, the salt appetite is delayed, typically by many hours, and persists for several days, weeks, and, according to a recent report, sometimes indefinitely (Frankmann *et al.*, 1986) even when the precipitating sodium deficiency is reversed promptly (Fig. 10.10).

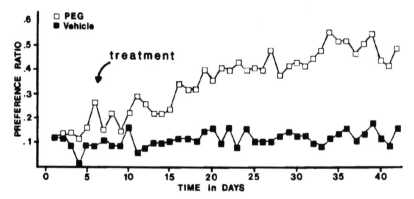

Fig. 10.10. Persisting effects of a single sc injection of 16.7 ml of 20% polyethylene glycol (PEG) on the daily intake of 0.3 M NaCl solution and water, both available ad libitum. Following the PEG treatment, the preference ratio for saline steadily increased, mainly because the animals consumed far greater amounts of 0.3 M NaCl. (Saline intake increased from a baseline of 5 ml/day to 30 ml over the first 2–3 weeks after the PEG injection.) Plasma sodium concentration, osmolality, and hematocrit were normal in spite of the increased intake 5 weeks after the injections. From: Frankmann, S. P., Dorsa, D. M., Sakai, R. R., and Simpson, J. B. (1986). A single experience with hyperoncotic colloid dialysis persistently alters water and sodium intake. *In:* "The Physiology of Thirst and Sodium Appetite." (G deCaro, A. N. Epstein, and M. Massi, eds.) pp. 115–121. Plenum Press, New York. Reproduced with permission of the authors and Plenum Press.

The nature of the stimulus that triggers the delayed salt appetite after sub-cutaneous injections of polyethylene glycol (PG) has been the subject of much speculation and experimentation (see Stricker, 1980, 1981).

The treatment sequesters isotonic fluid in a subcutaneous or peritoneal edema. The ingestion of water alone (which is the initial response to PG treatments) thus cannot reverse the resulting vascular hypovolemia. The osmolality and volume of the body's fluids can return to normal values only after sufficient salt has been ingested to retain the ingested water in the extracellular fluid reservoir.

It may be efficient to drink some water before ingesting salt after PG in order to avoid cellular dehydration, but there is no obvious reason for the very long delays actually observed under most conditions and, as yet, no firm understand-ing of the events that trigger salt appetite in many diverse experimental situa-tions. The appearance of the sodium appetite is associated with a significant plasma volume deficit, but this cannot be a sufficient stimulus for salt ingestion since it is present, and indeed maximal, long before salt appetite appears.

When both water and saline are available during the first hours after PG, rats drink mainly water and achieve significant osmotic dilution at the time a switch to saline ingestion occurs. Little or no sodium is ingested when saline and water are not available until 8 hs after PG (a procedure that avoids plasma dilution prior to the time salt appetite would normally develop). These observations strongly implicate vascular dilution (which may be a satiety signal for hypovolemic thirst) in the genesis of sodium appetite. However, acute osmotic dilution by itself does not significantly increase saline ingestion (Stricker and Wolf, 1966), suggesting that the puzzle must have further complications.

The volume deficit itself appears to be important for the development of salt appetite. Yet the temporal relations do not support an immediate, causal relation-ship. Volume deficits are present long before salt appetite develops, and they accrue more rapidly after higher concentrations of PG. Yet the onset of the sodium appetite appears to be unrelated to PG concentration (Stricker and Ja-lowiec, 1970; Stricker, 1980). Very high doses of PG have, in fact, been re-ported to elicit water drinking without producing a delayed sodium appetite at all (Stricker, 1971b, 1973).

It has been suggested (Stricker, 1981) that salt appetite after PG might be delayed because the vascular bed has access to salt reserves in the interstitial fluid and because hypovolemic thirst initially overrides the early manifestations of salt appetite.

According to this interpretation, the ingestion of water during the first 5 h after PG results in rapid osmotic dilution and a consequent reduction of thirst. This permits the behavioral manifestation of salt appetite and thus causes the ingestion of hypertonic saline during phase two, which, in turn, reduces osmotic dilution and reinstates hypovolemic thirst. During phase two, the animal thus "cycles" between draughts of saline and draughts of water, the proportion between the two fluids being a function of the tonicity of the saline solution. Sodium appetite becomes more and more prominent in phase three when the original stimulus for thirst, vascular hypovolemia, has been eliminated. At this stage, water and sodium are ingested in a proportion that results in a mixture that approximates isotonicity.

That the interstitial fluid may provide a resupply of sodium during the early stage of PG-induced hypovolemia is suggested by the following experimental findings. (a) Subcutaneous injections of low concentrations of formalin arouse salt appetite far more rapidly than PG injections that have comparable effects on plasma volume (Stricker, 1966; Jalowiec and Stricker, 1970a). Formalin interferes with cellular salt metabolism and thus reduces extracellular salt concentration as well as volume. It also makes interstitial fluid relatively inaccessible to the circulation because it reduces plasma oncotic pressure. (b) Rats maintained on a salt-deficient diet for several days prior to subcutaneous injections of PG drink saline promptly and copiously, skipping most of the first stage of water ingestion normally seen after this treatment. The pattern of salt and water ingestion in these experiments was affected by the duration of the preinjection salt deprivation in a manner consistent with the proposed interpretation (Stricker, 1981). (c) Adrenalectomy, which also results in sodium deficiency, has also been shown to potentiate PG-induced sodium appetite (Stricker, 1981).

The proposed interpretation is compatible with Denton's (1966) suggestion that salt appetite may be the result of activation of receptors in the brain that monitor the availability of salt in extracellular fluid (see also Stricker, 1981). Denton and colleagues (Weissinger et al., 1979, 1982) have supported this interpretation by demonstrating that a decrease in the sodium concentration of the cerebrospinal fluid of goats acutely elicits sodium appetite. The efficacy of intraventricular injections suggests that sodium receptors in or near the ventricular lining may monitor CSF sodium concentration.

Similar observations are not as yet available for the rat, and there are a number of observations that suggest that salt appetite is not simply related to the concentration of plasma sodium in this species. For instance, the sodium intake of rats that are hyponatremic as a result of adrenalectomy (Fitzsimons and Wirth, 1976) or peritoneal glucose dialysis (Falk and Lipton, 1967) persists after the sodium deficiency has been reversed by subcutaneous or intragastric injections of saline . Also, hypophysectomy that prevents the hypersecretion of aldosterone normally seen after PG injections (Stricker et al., 1979) abolishes the facilitatory effects of low-salt maintenance diets on PG-induced salt appetite (Stricker, 1983).

Epstein's (1986) hypothesis that hyponatremia triggers endocrine events (increased release of renin–angiotensin and aldosterone), which develop slowly and may persist after the sodium deficiency has been repaired, can potentially deal with most of the difficulties in this area. However, Stricker and Verbalis (1987) have pointed out that while renin–angiotensin and aldosterone levels increase in parallel with sodium appetite after PG treatments in rats, salt appetite persists after the precipitating hypovolemia has abated and plasma renin *and* aldosterone levels have returned to normal (Stricker, 1981; Stricker *et al.*, 1979).

Stricker and Verbalis (1986) have shown that hypovolemia stimulates the release of the neurohypophyseal hormones arginine vasopressin (AVP) and oxytocin (OT). Osmotic dilution, which preceeds salt ingestion after PG, inhibits the secretion of these hormones. This led to the hypothesis that salt appetite may be inhibited by vasopressinergic or oxytocinergic neurons, which are found almost exclusively in the supraoptic and/or paraventricular nuclei.

A series of tests of this hypothesis (Stricker and Verbalis, 1987) showed that plasma levels of oxytocin were low in sodium-deficient adrenalectomized rats as well as in intact animals treated daily with high doses of deoxycorticosterone. AVP levels were unaffected. Experimental treatments that reduced plasma levels of oxytocin (lithium chloride, copper sulfate, or hypertonic saline) reduced the saline intake of adrenalectomized rats maintained on a salt-deficient diet. These treatments also delayed salt ingestion in PG-treated rats.

Systemic infusions of synthetic oxytocin increased both water and saline ingestion after PG, indicating that the plasma levels of oxytocin do not appear to be the primary stimulus for sodium appetite. Stricker and Verbalis noted that the oxytocin infusions caused a significant increase in renal sodium loss. They suggested that the apparently paradoxical increase in saline (and water) intake seen after oxytocin may have resulted from a consequent facilitatory effect on the renin–angiotensin/aldosterone system. This explanation unfortunately does not readily account for the fact that infusions of a specific oxytocin receptor antagonist significantly reduced the PG-induced intake of both saline and water, since oxytocin is natriuretic only when present in very high concentrations (Balment *et al.*, 1980).

Although the oxytocin story may not yet be entirely understood, Stricker and Verbalis (1987) have used it as the basis of an interesting hypothesis. It proposes, in essence, that sodium appetite may be under the control of two distinct influences: (a) an excitatory input mediated, at least in part, by increased activity in the renin–angiotensin/aldosterone system, and (b) an inhibitory input mediated by oxytocinergic neurons of the paraventricular nucleus. According to this scheme, hypovolemia initially activates both systems. Sodium appetite cannot be expressed until the ingestion of water results in osmotic dilution, which reduces the activity of the inhibitory oxytocinergic system.

Stricker and Verbalis suggest further that reduced activity in this inhibitory system may account for the persistence of saline ingestion after PG-induced hypovolemia has been repaired as well as the salt appetite observed in adrenalectomized or DOCA-treated animals. The proposed mechanism of lowered activity of an inhibitory system might coexist with a positive input from either the renin–angiotensin system (in the adrenalectomized rat) or the aldosterone system (in the DOCA-treated rat), as Epstein (1986) has suggested.

Brain Mechanisms

Introduction

Sodium appetite appears to be under the control of neural mechanisms in the upper brainstem and associated limbic system structures. It is unaffected by complete neodecortication (Wolf *et al.*, 1970; Wirsig and Grill, 1982) but cannot be elicited in a decerebrate preparation that does show evidence of control over food intake (Grill *et al.*, 1986). The effect seen in decerebrate animals may be due to the transection of gustatory afferents. Lesions of the parabrachial nucleus (Hill and Almli, 1983) or rostral nucleus of the solitary tract (Schulkin *et al.*, 1985) impair or abolish salt appetite. Similar effects have been reported after lesions in portions of the hypothalamus, zona incerta, and ventral thalamus, which receive parabrachial efferents (discussed below). It is interesting to note that decerebrate rats do reduce urine sodium output when placed on a salt-deficient diet and excrete excess sodium after a salt load (Grill *et al.*, 1986). It would appear that the renal and behavioral control of body fluid sodium are mediated by different brain mechanisms.

Several reports of intact salt appetite after hippocampal lesions indicate that phylogenetically older and more primitive cortical mechanisms also do not contribute to the regulation of salt intake (Murphy and Brown, 1970; Magarinos *et al.*, 1986).

The septum that stands at the junction between cortical and subcortical mechanisms is not essential for the expression of salt appetite (Chiaraviglio, 1969) but appears to exert inhibitory influences, which may interact with opposite amygdaloid influences (discussed below).

Hypothalamus

The hypothalamus has been a focus of research in this field ever since Andersson and McCann (1956) reported that electrical stimulation of the perifornical hypothalamus caused goats to avidly lick a block of salt. Similar results have been reported, more recently, in sheep (McKenzie and Denton, 1974).

There are several reports that ventromedial hypothalamic (VMH) lesions abolish salt preference in experimentally sodium-depleted rats (Nováková and Cort, 1966; Quartermain *et al.*, 1969), a surprising finding in view of the well-documented fact that such lesions increase the intake of palatable foods.

Lesions in the dorsolateral hypothalamus have been reported to have no effect or even to enhance the preference for mildly sapid sodium solutions (Wolf, 1964; Wolf and Quartermain, 1967). However, these lesions result in an apparently complete and permanent loss of the salt appetite that is normally produced by adrenalectomy (Wolf and Quartermain, 1967), mineralocorticoid treatments (Wolf, 1964), or peritoneal dialysis (Wolf, 1964). There is no evidence of spontaneous recovery (Ahern *et al.*, 1978) or benefit from preoperative experience with saline under need-free conditions (Wolf, 1971). However, a significant reduction of the impairment has been reported as a result of preoperative experience with saline under conditions of sodium depletion (Wolf and Schulkin, 1980; Ruger and Schulkin, 1980; Wolf *et al.*, 1983). The critical variable appears to be preoperative experience with the drive itself, rather than the ingestion of hypertonic solutions per se (Schulkin and Fluharty, 1985).

Lesions in the anterior hypothalamus (Mercer *et al.*, 1978), particularly the tissues surrounding the anterior third ventricle (Bealer and Johnson, 1979), decrease sodium preference in the rat but do not abolish sodium appetite after sodium deprivation, adrenalectomy, or formalin-induced hypovolemia and hyponatremia.

Zona Incerta

Rats with lesions in the rostromedial zona incerta do not display the basic sodium preference typical of the species (Grossman and Grossman, 1978; Walsh and

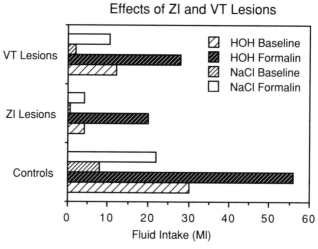

Fig. 10.11. Effects of electrolytic lesions in the rostromedial zona incerta (ZI) or ventral thalamus (VT) on the 24-h baseline intake of water and 0.5 *M* NaCl in a two-bottle choice test. Also shown is the 24-h intake of water and 5 *M* NaCl after sc injections of 2.5 ml of 1.5% formalin. Data from: Walsh, L. L., and Grossman, S. P. (1977). Electrolytic lesions and knife cuts in the region of the zona incerta impair sodium appetite. *Physiol. Behav.* **18**, 587–596.

Grossman, 1977). They also drink significantly less saline than controls after sc injections of formalin (Walsh and Grossman, 1977) or polyethylene glycol (Grossman and Grossman, 1978), even though they consume normal or nearly normal quantities of water (Fig. 10.11).

Similar effects on sodium preference and sodium appetite after formalin have been reported after knife cuts in the horizontal plane that transected the dorsal or ventral connections of the zona incerta (Walsh and Grossman, 1977).

Electrical stimulation of ventral aspects of the zona incerta has been reported to elicit drinking of saline solutions (Gentil *et al.*, 1971).

Ventromedial Thalamus

Deficits in sodium preference and/or appetite have also been reported in rats after lesions in the ventromedial thalamus in the region of the gustatory nucleus (Walsh and Grossman, 1977; Wolf and DiCara, 1971; Wolf, 1968; Oakley and Pfaffmann, 1962) (Fig. 10.11), after brainstem lesions just caudal to the gustatory nucleus (Chiaraviglio, 1972), and after lesions in portions of the striatum that receive projections from the medial thalamus (Neill and Linn, 1975). Preoperative experience with the taste of saline solutions has been reported to protect rats from the inhibitory effects of ventromedial thalamic lesions (Ahern *et al.*, 1978; Hartzell *et al.*, 1985).

An earlier report of intact sodium appetite after preoptic, zona incerta, and tegmental lesions (Wolf, 1967) appears to be in disagreement with the more recent literature. The reasons for this are not immediately apparent, although some of the partial deficits discovered in the past decade may not have seemed noteworthy to early investigators when compared to the devastating deficits seen after lateral hypothalamic lesions.

Septal Area, Nucleus Medianus, and Amygdala

Lesions in the septal area have been reported to produce a persisting increase in the intake of saline solutions that are within the normally preferred range (Negro-Vilar *et al.*, 1967; Grace, 1968; Chiaraviglio, 1969; Saad *et al.*, 1972). Electrical stimulation of the region conversely produces a decreased intake of 0.9% or 1.5% saline (Gentil *et al.*, 1971).

Rats with septal lesions also drink more saline in response to polyethylene glycol, provided the animal is sodium-deprived prior to the PG test (Stricker, 1984).

Lesions of the ventral portion of the nucleus medianus also produces increased saline (as well as water) intake, mainly at night (Gardiner and Stricker, 1985a,b; Gardiner et al., 1986). Lesions in the region of the nucleus medianus also reduce the secretion of oxytocin and vasopressin in response to cellular dehydration (Gardiner et al., 1985; Mangiapane et al., 1983). This is significant in the context of the present discussion because sodium deficiency has been shown to be associated with low plasma levels of oxytocin. Treatments that stimulate pituitary oxytocin secretion conversely inhibit sodium appetite (Stricker and Verbalis, 1987). Whether direct damage to this structure or an interruption of of its connections with the septum might be responsible for the effects of septal damage on water and saline intake remains to be established. The latter conclusion is tempting in view of the fact that lesions in the region of the nucleus medianus produce hyperdipsia much like some septal lesions do (Gardiner and Stricker, 1985a). It is interesting to note, in this context, that knife cuts that transect ventral subfornical organ projections to the region of the anteroventral third ventricle and nucleus medianus have no effect on salt appetite induced by DOCA or sodium-free diets (Schulkin et al., 1983).

The amygdaloid complex has also been implicated in sodium appetite. Lesions in the corticomedial amygdala have been reported to increase saline intake, whereas lesions in the basolateral aspects of the amygdala decrease it (Gentil et al., 1968; Nachman and Ashe, 1974). Electrical stimulation in both regions have opposite effects on sodium intake (Gentil et al., 1971).

Lesions of medial aspects of the amygdala decrease depletion-induced NaCl intake. More restricted damage to aspects of the medial amygala has been reported to reduce aldosterone-induced salt appetite without affecting salt intake after adrenalectomy or acute sodium depletion (Zolovick et al., 1977; Schulkin et al., 1989).

Septal lesions made in rats that drink excessive amounts of saline as a result of amygdala lesions have been shown to further increase sodium intake. Amygdala lesions made in animals that overconsume sodium as a result of septal lesions had no significant additional effects (Saad et al., 1972).

Total destruction of the amygdaloid complex produced a severe but not complete inhibition of sodium appetite elicited by mineralocorticoid or natriuretic agents (Cox et al., 1978). Destruction of the the stria terminalis or the ventral amygdalofugal pathway, which constitute the principal efferent connections of the region with the septum and lower brainstem, also reduces saline intake in sodium-deprived rats. Only the lesions of the ventral amygdalofugal pathway reduced sodium intake in sated animals (Chiaraviglio, 1971).

The overall pattern of stimulation and lesion effects in the septum and amygdala has led several investigators to the conclusion that both of these limbic system structures may affect salt appetite only indirectly by modulating "primary" control mechanisms in the hypothalamus and/or zona incerta (e.g., Gentil et al., 1968; Chiaraviglio, 1971; Saad et al., 1972; Cox et al., 1978).

Review and Conclusions

Sodium is the body's most important electrolyte. It plays an essential role in the regulation of body fluids as well as cellular metabolism. Because there is a continual obligatory sodium loss its resupply must be assured. Many species rely on dietary intake alone; others must actively seek out and ingest sodium.

Some species, such as the rat and perhaps humans, have an innate preference for sodium that is expressed even when the organism is sodium-replete. During acute or chronic sodium depletion, the range of preferred sodium concentrations expands. The proximal cause of this true sodium appetite is as yet not fully understood, although recent experimental findings have implicated several interacting mechanisms.

Sodium deficiency can be experimentally induced by low-salt diets, adrenalectomy, or, acutely, by peritoneal glucose dialysis. In all cases sodium appetite develops. In the adrenalectomized animal, salt appetite disappears when the hyponatremia is reversed by administration of the adrenal mineralocorticoids aldosterone or DOCA.

Hyponatremia appears to be a sufficient cause of salt appetite in these experiments. However, hyponatremia induced by water loading does not elicit salt appetite, and restoration of the organism's sodium balance via stomach loads or ingestion of salt does not terminate sodium appetite under many experimental conditions.

That sodium deficiency is not an essential condition for the development of salt appetite is shown in numerous experimental paradigms. For example, large doses of the adrenal mineralocorticoids that promote sodium retention elicit salt appetite in intact as well as adrenalectomized rats. Also, many extracellular thirst stimuli that result in hypovolemia and/or hypotension without disturbing the osmolality of extracellular (or cellular) fluid elicit salt appetite.

A further argument against the logically simplest explanation of sodium appetite arises from the fact that most experimental treatments that result in acute sodium deficiencies produce salt appetite that is expressed only after a delay of 8–12 h, and do so even when the sodium balance has been restored many hours earlier. Sodium appetite then persists, often for days or weeks (and in one recent experiment apparently indefinitely), even though the disturbances in vascular volume, pressure, and/or sodium concentration that gave rise to the sodium appetite have long been reversed.

Hyponatremia results in hypovolemia. Hypovolemia and/or hypotension release renin from the kidney. The resulting increase in angiotensin II stimulates the release of aldosterone from the adrenal gland, and this mineralocorticoid, in turn, promotes tubular reabsorption of sodium in the kidney. Hyponatremia or hypovolemia/hypotension may be essential for the initiation of these hormonal events, which, in turn, may be responsible for the arousal of salt appetite. Salt-seeking behavior may continue, because of the persistence of hormonal influence, long after the original salt and/or fluid deficiency has been repaired.

Extensive study of the renin–angiotensin system has produced a complex picture. Nephrectomy, as well ureteric ligation, produces an aversion to saline solutions and abolishes the salt appetite of adrenalectomized rats. The effectiveness of ureteric ligation suggests that renin may not be an essential factor in salt appetite. Systemic administrations of renin or A-II also produce only disappointingly small effects on salt appetite in intact rats and do not restore it in adrenalectomized or formalin-treated rats.

Single icv injections of A-II similarly have only small effects on salt appetite. However, larger doses of renin, or renin-substrate, can produce a salt appetite that persists for many hours and even days, presumably because angiotensin continues to be produced from components of the cerebral renin-angiotensin system. Slow, continuous infusions of A-II itself also elicit significant sodium intake. Continuous icv infusions of the converting enzyme inhibitor captopril inhibit sodium intake in sodium-depleted rats. Together, these observations indicate that salt appetite may be under the control of angiotensin-sensitive brain mechanisms that appear to be curiously insensitive to changes in plasma angiotensin.

Extremely low doses of angiotensin, administered icv, elicit salt appetite when DOCA is concurrently administered centrally or systemically. Similar facilitatory interactions have been observed when rats were pretreated with DOCA or aldosterone for several days prior to a pulsed icv injection of A-II.

Epstein has suggested, on the basis of these and related observations, that angiotensin and aldosterone, which interact in the periphery to control the conservation of sodium, may also act synergistically in the brain to give rise to the salt appetite that directs the behavioral responses needed to replenish the sodium balance of the body's fluids. According to this hypothesis, either hormone alone can give rise to sodium appetite only when its concentration reaches pathological levels. In the adrenalectomized animal, renin levels are elevated and elicit sodium appetite even though aldosterone is absent. Conversely, prolonged exposure to pharmacological doses of DOCA is capable of eliciting salt ingestion even though the doses inhibit renin secretion.

Stricker has shown that polyethylene glycol induced hypovolemia results in (a) a hypersecretion of aldosterone as well as renin, which peaks at about the time sodium appetite appears, and (b) release of the neurohypophysial hormones oxytocin and vasopressin. Plasma levels of oxytocin were low in sodium-deficient adrenalectomized rats as well as in intact animals treated daily with high doses of deoxycorticosterone. Arginine vasopressin levels were unaffected. Experimental treatments that reduced plasma levels of oxytocin reduced the saline intake of adrenalectomized rats maintained on a salt-deficient diet.

Stricker postulates on the basis of these and related observations that sodium appetite may be under the control of two distinct influences: (a) an excitatory input mediated, at least in part, by a synergistic increase in the activity of renin–angiotensin and aldosterone, and (b) an inhibitory input mediated by oxytocinergic neurons of the paraventricular nucleus. Hypovolemia initially activates both systems. Sodium appetite cannot be expressed until the ingestion of water results in osmotic dilution, which reduces the activity of the inhibitory oxytocinergic system.

This hypothesis accounts for the puzzling fact that volume deficits, which appear to be a common early component of all stimuli for salt appetite, develop long before salt ingestion begins. It does not, by itself, explain why salt appetite often persists for days, weeks or even months. There is, as yet, no independent evidence that the activity of the renin–angiotensin or aldosterone/DOCA systems or their target organs in the brain undergoes long-term changes in response to a single experience with systemic hypovolemia.

When one examines the literature that has attempted to elucidate the brain mechanisms responsible for salt appetite, a picture emerges that does not, as yet, readily complement the story of interacting hormonal messengers we have developed above.

As in the case of thirst itself, most of the early attention of neuroscientists was devoted to the hypothalamus. Both medial and lateral pathways appear to be involved in salt preference and/or salt appetite. (An interesting aspect of these data is the fact that brain lesions often affect salt preference and salt appetite differentially. One surprising example is provided by dorsolateral hypothalamic lesions, which abolish salt appetite elicited by adrenalectomy or mineralocorticoids but may actually enhance the preference for mildly salty solutions.) Impaired sodium appetite has also been reported after lesions in the zona incerta, ventromedial thalamus, and portions of the striatum that receive projections from the medial thalamus.

Lesions in the septal area increase salt preference and the salt appetite elicited by various experimental treatments. Damage to the corticomedial amygdala have similar effects, whereas damage to the basolateral amygdala, as well as total destruction of the region, abolishes salt appetite.

Notably absent from the list of structures that appear to exert significant influences over salt preference and/or appetite are most of the regions that have been implicated in thirst. Indeed, it appears that their role in salt appetite has not been systemically studied. The few available reports have not been encouraging. For example, lesions in the anterior hypothalamus/preoptic region and the AV3V itself have been shown to reduce salt preference but have no effect on the expression of salt appetite after various experimental treatments. Lesions in the ventral portions of the nucleus medianus increase saline (as well as water) intake at night and reduce oxytocin release—a possible link to Stricker's observation that sodium deficiency is associated with low plasma levels of oxytocin whereas treatments that stimulate oxytocin release inhibit sodium appetite.

There is, of course, ample evidence that intracranial angiotensin stimulates salt appetite, particularly when combined with icv or systemic DOCA or aldosterone. Yet there is little or no information on where in the brain angiotensin might act to produce these effects. The relatively small effects of systemic angiotensin on salt appetite (as well as the meager effects of lesions in brain areas known to contribute to A-II thirst) suggest that one may not be able to generalize a priori from the thirst-related brain mechanisms, which are being worked out rather well.

Chapter 11

Retrospect and Prospect

After reading this book or, indeed, almost any section of it, one cannot help but be impressed with the tremendous advances that have occurred in this field in recent decades. Without in any way denigrating the important contributions of early pioneers in this field, it is probably fair to say that 80–90% of our knowledge about thirst and salt appetite has been collected since the early 1960s. Moreover, it seems that the pace of discovery has been accelerating. It is increasingly difficult to keep up-to-date with all contemporary developments, the principal impetus for writing this little book. It is the aim of the following discussion to provide perspectives on past achievements and to point out some of the questions in need of future study. Both of these endeavors reflect personal bias—were this chapter written by someone else, different priorities might well emerge.

Early Questions and Their Contemporary Status

Oral Sensations

Prior to the turn of the century, what little scientific research was conducted was devoted to proving, or more likely disproving, the dry-mouth theory of thirst. By the early 1900s it was clear that Cannon's interpretation of thirst as an oral sensation could not be true. In every species tested, sham drinking was shown to continue after enough water was taken by mouth to satisfy the existing fluid deficits, were it allowed to be absorbed. However, contrary to Cannon's prediction, sham drinking does eventually stop and is, in fact, proportional to the deficit. Surgical or pharmacological inhibition of salivation does not, in a fundamental way, increase thirst (although prandial requirements may increase water intake to some extent) and denervation or pharmacological blockade of efferents from the mouth and throat do not abolish thirst. Interest in oral factors promptly waned, although W. B. Cannon continued to defend his theory until well into the 1930s.

It is interesting to note at this point that we still don't fully understand what role oral sensations do play under normal conditions. Recent investigations of human subjects have shown that oral sensations (including dryness and a "putrid" taste) do, in fact, arise during water deprivation and disappear promptly when water is ingested. It is possible, as Wolf suggested many years ago, that oral sensations become conditioned stimuli for thirst because of their close association with whatever the true thirst sensations are. It is ironic that we still cannot describe the nature of these sensations or the neural mechanisms responsible for our awareness of them, in spite of all the progress that has been made in recent years.

Contemporary research on intragastric or intravenous infusions of water suggests that their effect is not comparable to oral ingestion. In the rat, intragastric infusions, administered at a rate calculated to replace the water normally consumed by mouth, reduce oral intake only by 0.3–0.4 ml for each 1.0 ml infused. Even when quantities far in excess of normal oral intake are infused, rats drink as much as 30% of the water they would have ingested without receiving the intragastric load. The effectiveness of intravenous infusions reaches a similar asymptote in the rat. Comparable observations have been made in dogs and monkeys, although the size of the residual oral intake varies among species and depends to some extent on the nature of the experimental paradigm.

The basic observation that intragastric or iv preloads do not entirely abolish oral intake has been replicated in numerous investigations. What is not so clear is how one should interpret the observation. Some investigators have suggested that there is an irreducible oral water need that cannot be satisfied by systemic injections. It is interesting to note, in this context, that while rats can be trained to self-administer water intravenously, they inject 30% less intravenously than they would ingest orally. The amount of water injected is sufficient for survival—further evidence that ad libitum intake includes a sizeable oral component not required for the maintenance of normal salt and fluid levels. It would be important to know whether this oral "need" is the result of prandial requirements. Rats are generally maintained on dry and rather salty chow, and it is well known that their oral water intake decreases, often quite dramatically, during periods of food deprivation.

A quite different interpretation of the residual oral intake after ig or iv preloads has been offered by several investigators who have pointed out that in many experimental paradigms, deprivation precedes the preload and this depletes extracellular as well as cellular water to varying degrees, depending on the duration of the deprivation and the availability of food. Unfortunately, there have been large differences with respect to these and related variables between laboratories so that direct comparisons of results are often difficult. It seems probable, however, that under conditions approximating ad libitum intake, rats do display a sizeable oral "need" that does not seem to be related to residual extracellular thirst. Why nephrectomized rats should drink precisely enough to compensate for a salt load remains something of a puzzle in this context.

Paradigms that have used longer (usually overnight or more) periods of deprivation and ig injections immediately prior to the return of access to water typically have obtained evidence for residual drinking that may reflect extracellular influences, although the numbers (typically 25–30% of total intake is consumed orally after water loads that return plasma osmolality to normal levels) are disconcertingly similar to the "irreducible" oral need in the rat.

A significant influence of extracellular thirst, even after relatively brief periods of deprivation, is suggested by the observation that iv preloads of isotonic saline, which restore plasma volume without significant effect on osmolality, have been shown to reduce oral intake by 20–26% in the rat and dog. When iv infusions of isotonic saline that restore plasma volume were given in addition to intracarotid infusions of water (which restore the osmolality of the circulation of the brain), oral intake was abolished almost completely in experiments on the dog.

Cellular Dehydration Thirst

The second major issue that confronted thirst researchers in the first half of this century arose at the turn of the century from a dispute between A. Mayer, who believed that thirst was a result of an increase in the absolute osmotic pressure of the blood, and Wettendorff, who proposed that cellular dehydration initially maintains the volume and concentration of extracellular fluid.

Gilman's classic research in the 1930s proved that the administration of solutes that are rigidly excluded by cellular membranes and thus result in cellular dehydration produces thirst, whereas others such as glucose that readily enter cells do not. By the early 1950s, Adolph, Bellows, and other pioneers in the field had demonstrated that cellular dehydration produces thirst in humans and drinking in every species tested. However, the amounts of water ingested in response to hypertonic salt loads were reported to vary greatly between species as well as between members of the same species. The nature of the relationship between cellular dehydration and water intake was not fully understood until Fitzsimons's work on nephrectomized animals in the 1960s. The actual contribution of cellular dehydration to ad libitum drinking, or drinking after deprivation, was not elucidated until recently and remains, to some extent, the subject of controversy.

Among the issues that remain to be resolved is the central question of whether cellular dehydration is the principal (and perhaps only) physiological influence on drinking, at least in some species. A number of investigators have questioned whether extracellular hypovolemia, and the attendant activation of the renin–

angiotensin system, is an important aspect of the response to water deprivation under normal conditions, rather than being an emergency response to severe and sudden losses of blood volume (and/or pressure).

When water is readily available, many species, including the rat and humans, drink in anticipation of need, mostly in association with eating. Neither cellular nor extracellular thirst probably plays a significant role under these conditions. When water is available only intermittently, cellular as well as extracellular dehydration come into play. During early stages of deprivation vascular volume appears to be maintained at the expense of cellular water, but the increasing concentration of cellular fluid establishes osmotic forces that eventually counter the efflux of water from the cell. All of this is well understood in principle, but a far more precise quantitative understanding of the interplay of cellular and extracellular forces is needed if we are to conducted meaningful experiments on the relative contribution of cellular and extracellular thirst after varying durations of deprivation. What also needs to be inserted into this equation are dietary influences, which not only affect the movement of water between cellular and extracellular compartments but also modulate renal excretion of salt and water as well as digestive losses.

Salt Appetite—The Adrenal Mineralocorticoid Connection

The third problem that received much experimental attention prior to the recent explosion of thirst-related research was salt appetite. Richter's classic experiments of the 1930s and 1940s demonstrated that rats display an apparently innate preference for mildly sapid solutions that is greatly intensified by salt deficient diets, adrenalectomy, and large "pharmacological" doses of the adrenal mineralocorticoids. More recent investigations have added acute sodium depletion to the list of experimental treatments that elicit a true salt appetite.

The interaction of aldosterone with the renin–angiotensin system in the conservation of sodium by the kidney and the effects of extracellular thirst stimuli on salt appetite were not elucidated until 20 years later. The possibility that salt appetite itself might be due to a similar interaction between angiotensin and aldosterone in the brain has been discussed and put to experimental test only within the last decade.

The reasons for the delayed appearance and unusual persistence of salt appetite under many different experimental conditions are the subject of contemporary research and debate in many laboratories. Plausible explanations of the delayed appearance are available, including Stricker's suggestion that salt appetite cannot be expressed until the initial water drinking response to hypovolemia has resulted in osmotic dilution of plasma. When one adds to this the possibility that plasma may have access to salt reserves in interstitial tissue, a delayed response becomes plausible. Whether these explanations can account for delayed salt appetite in other situations remains to be established. The principal, unresolved problem is, however, the persistence of salt appetite, often for days, weeks, and in at least one instance apparently permanently. An explanation of this phenomenon would seem to be of interest far beyond the confines of salt appetite research.

The brain mechanisms responsible for salt appetite received experimental attention after Andersson and McCann's report in 1956 that electrical stimulation of the perifornical hypothalamus caused goats to avidly lick a block of salt. Wolf and colleagues demonstrated in the 1960s that lesions in the lateral hypothalamus abolished salt appetite in the rat without interfering with the preference for mildly sapid solutions. More recently, lesions in the the zona incerta and ventromedial thalamus have been shown to produce similar effects. The septum, nucleus medianus, and portions of the corticomedial amygdala appear to exert opposite, inhibitory effects. Damage to these areas increases the preference for isotonic and mildly hypertonic saline solutions, and electrical stimulation reduces it. The effect of these experimental procedures on true salt appetite remains to be elucidated. There is some evidence of an interaction between the septal and amygdaloid mechanisms but no information at all how the other brainstem regions, which appear to promote the expression of sodium appetite, are interrelated or what their relationship to thirst-related brain mechanisms might be.

Epstein and colleagues have shown that intracranial angiotensin elicits salt appetite in the rat particularly when administered in conjunction with systemic or central injections of aldosterone. It will be interesting to discover where in the brain angiotensin acts to affect sodium appetite and what the nature of the central interaction between aldosterone and renin may be.

The 1950s—A Time of Transition and the Seeds of Controversy

Although a good many questions were unresolved, it seemed to many investigators of the late 1940s and 1950s that the principal physiological basis for thirst, cellular dehydration, had been discovered. Sodium appetite appeared securely related to the adrenal gland, and it seemed but a matter of time until the apparent paradox that salt appetite could be elicited by adrenalectomy as well as large doses of its mineralocorticoid hormones deoxycorticosterone and aldosterone could be resolved.

All through the neurosciences, the decade was a time of exciting discoveries, made possible by the development of the stereotaxic instrument and detailed atlases of the brain that allowed investigators, for the first time, to directly study subcortical functions with a degree of precision not dreamed possible earlier.

In 1951, Anand and Brobeck published their classic paper on the devastating effects of lateral hypothalamic (LH) lesions on water and food intake in rats and cats. Their colleagues from the University of Pennsylvania, including Stellar, Epstein, and Teitelbaum, conducted what amounts to one of the first careful and integrated anatomical, physiological, and behavioral analyses of the effects of subcortical lesions. After many years of study, they concluded that rats do recover voluntary ingestive behavior after (LH) lesions if properly nursed and intubated with liquid food and water, often for weeks or months, but fail to drink in response to hypertonic salt loads and become adipsic or severely hypodipsic when food-deprived. This detailed description of the effects of hypothalamic lesions was complemented by reports from several other laboratories of drinking after electrical stimulation of the lateral hypothalamus of sated dogs, goats, and rats. These observations and the resulting conclusion that the lateral hypothalamus contains a major integrative mechanism for thirst became the subject of an enormous amount of research, debate, and controversy in later years.

As early as 1961, Morgane questioned what had become known as the "hypothalamocentric" theory on the basis of his observation that lesions in the globus pallidus, which is a major relay station in the extrapyramidal motor system, produced adipsia (and aphagia). He suggested that the effects of LH lesions might be due to an interruption of pallidofugal fiber systems. The hypothesis found few supporters, at least in part because the syndrome described by Morgane seemed quite different and far more generally debilitating than the effects of bilateral LH damage.

A more serious challenge was raised when Ungerstedt reported adipsia (as well as aphagia) combined with severe sensorimotor dysfunctions in rats with electrolytic or neurotoxin lesions in the substantia nigra that interrupted the dopaminergic nigrostriatal pathways. It was subsequently shown by Teitelbaum and associates that lesions in the LH itself produced apparently similar sensorimotor deficits, which tended to recovery in parallel with voluntary ingestive behavior. Stricker and colleagues next showed that intracerebroventricular injections of the neurotoxin 6-OHDA, in combination with a compound that protects noradrenergic cells, also results in sensorimotor and arousal dysfunctions, provided brain dopamine is depleted by 95% or more.

I have reviewed this series of events here because it is at the heart of a most important unresolved controversy. There is no doubt that LH lesions produce severely debilitating sensorimotor and arousal dysfunctions, which may well be responsible for the acute effects of the lesions. I do, however, question the validity of Stricker's hypothesis that the apparently permanent thirst deficits, including adipsia or severe hypodipsia during food deprivation and unresponsiveness to cellular as well as all extracellular dipsogens, reflect persisting "subclinical" arousal deficits that so severely impair the animal's ability to deal with the stress of the experiment as to render it incapable of the simple act of drinking.

(Why, for instance, should the gradual onset of thirst during food deprivation be such a traumatic stressor?)

It is true that 6-OHDA–treated rats do display some delayed drinking after certain dipsogens and respond more readily when tested during the dark, active phase of the day or after the administration of some stimulants. Although these observations are cited in support of the "arousal" hypothesis, I would think that a high baseline level of arousal, especially when it is due to an exogenous stimulant, would make it more difficult to deal with stressful situations rather than less. It is, in any, case true that significant effects on water intake are seen only after far more severe brain dopamine depletions than those typically seen in rats with large LH lesions, suggesting that the neurotoxin may produce quite different and more severe effects on catecholaminergic arousal functions.

Last, but not least, I would like to mention an extensive analysis of the effects of surgical knife cuts in and around the hypothalamus that I and my associates have conducted over the course of several years. The various knife cuts, which interrupted fibers of passage without local cellular damage, produced deficits in ingestive behavior as well as sensorimotor and arousal functions and striatal dopamine depletions but little or nothing in the way of significant correlations between the three variables. One might remember, in this context, that there are some early reports of apparently "pure" adipsia during the acute phase of some LH lesions. (In one of these experiments, some animals ate normally and drank milk but no water.) There are also reports of adipsia and hypodipsia and persistent impairments in responsiveness to hypertonic saline loads after kainic acid lesions in the LH that did not interfere with dopaminergic projections to the striatum and produced no evidence of sensorimotor or arousal impairments (indeed, the animals were hyperactive).

This is not the place for a listing of all the observations one can cite in support of the original view of the LH as a major integrative mechanism for thirst (or in defense of the sensorimotor/arousal alternative). It is, however, appropriate to point out that the scales are far more balanced than many contemporary writers have assumed. It seems appropriate to enter a plea for a more even-handed treatment of all available observations and, most importantly, for a renewed unbiased experimental attack on an important problem that has been shunted to the back burner because it has been controversial.

The 1960s—A Turn to New Directions

The 1960s gave birth to several fundamental discoveries that continue to be the subject of investigation and debate. Without doubt the most significant of these were the results of a series of experiments by Fitzsimons and colleagues at Cambridge University that demonstrated that experimental procedures that lowered blood volume and/or pressure, without disturbing the osmotic balance between cellular and extracellular fluid compartments, induce thirst in sated animals. These include hemorrhage, polyethylene glycol-induced intraperitoneal or subcutaneous edema, and lowered blood pressure produced by ligation of the abdominal or thoracic inferior vena cava or renal arteries. Other investigators showed that beta-adrenergic drugs, which result in a general lowering of blood pressure (Lehr *et al.*), or intraperitoneal glucose dialysis, which removes sodium from plasma and promotes the movement of water into cells (Falk), also elicits drinking. This "extracellular thirst" has been the subject of much recent experimentation and debate.

The 1960s also saw the rapid growth of a new discipline, neuropharmacology, spurred by the discovery that brain neurons seemed to rely on more than one chemical messenger. In order to address the vexing problems created by the fact that electrolytic lesions as well as electrical stimulation of the hypothalamus seemed to affect food as well as water intake, I decided to investigate the possibility that functionally distinct neural systems in areas of extensive anatomical overlap might use different neurotransmitters in order to prevent interference. In 1960, I succeeded in demonstrating that intrahypothalamic injections of acetylcholine, or its synthetic relative carbachol, produce only drinking in sated rats (feeding was, in fact, temporarily inhibited). Microinjections of norepinephrine through the same cannulae elicited feeding but not drinking. Control experiments indicated that the effects were pharmacologically specific since the appropriate receptor blockers selectively inhibited carbachol-induced drinking and norepinephrine-induced eating. Although the techniques used in these experiments were crude by today's standards, the results have been replicated in many subsequent investigations.

The initial reports stimulated a flurry of research that confirmed selective effects of carbachol and related receptor blockers, not only on ad libitum drinking, but also on deprivation-induced drinking, and drinking in response to systemic hypertonic saline. Interest in the phenomenon subsequently waned when it was shown that carbachol drinking was not confined to the hypothalamus, which at the time seemed to be the principal if not sole region of the brain concerned with thirst and sodium appetite. The potentially important implications of subsequent observations from Routtenberg's laboratory that icv as well as subfornical organ injections appeared to be effective at the lowest doses of carbachol (as well as intracranial angiotensin) should be investigated further, since they may hold the key to our understanding of the central action of angiotensin (discussed below). The inhibitory effects of intrahypothalamic norepinephrine (and similar effects of preoptic area injections) similarly deserve more attention than they have received in recent years. Like the LH lesions syndrome, carbachol drinking has been spurned in recent years because of the controversy surrounding it.

The 1970s & 1980s—Increasing Concern with Mechanisms of Action

Having established that extracellular as well as cellular water depletion could elicit thirst, the logical next question was how these general systemic changes are translated into the subjective sensation of thirst. Presumably, this required a peripheral or central sensory receptor mechanism in communication with brain mechanisms capable of transducing the information into conscious thirst sensations.

Osmoreceptors and Related Brain Mechanisms

In the case of cellular thirst, the classic work of Verney and subsequent electrophysiological investigations had firmly implicated cells in the preoptic region in the release of antidiuretic hormone in response to systemic salt load.

That similar "osmoreceptor" mechanisms in the region might also be responsible for cellular thirst has been suggest by experiments conducted by Epstein and others, which demonstrate that microinjections of hypertonic saline into the preoptic region or the adjacent tissues of the AV3V can elicit drinking whereas lesions in the area sometimes produce an apparently selective impairment in drinking response to systemic salt loads. The concept of a preoptic "osmoreceptor" mechanism has been widely accepted, although the evidence is not as unequivocal as one might wish. Not only do lesions in the area typically produce at least transient adipsia, but most seem to impair the drinking response to extracellular dipsogens as well. Lesions in other brain areas, such as the zona incerta and tissues rostral to the anterior pole of the third ventricle, also reduce or abolish drinking responses to systemic hypertonic saline and do so, often more selectively than preoptic lesions themselves.

It seems likely that further study of the problem will result in the discovery of a larger "osmosensitive" zone, which includes but is not confined to the preoptic region. In view of the fact that this larger area also seems to include mechanisms concerned with drinking responses to various extracellular stimuli, as well as angiotensin itself, the central interaction between cellular and extracellular influences will require further investigation.

The Renin–Angiotensin System and Extracellular Thirst

In the case of the extracellular thirst that was discovered during the 1960s, there was no historical evidence of brain receptors that might respond directly to vascular volume or pressure. However, evidence of two possible messenger systems soon became available.

In the late 1960s angiotensin II as well as its precursors angiotensin I and renin were shown to be potent dipsogens in numerous species. The following 20 years of intensive research will go down in the history of the field as the decades of the renin–angiotensin system.

Because all extracellular thirst stimuli release renin, Fitzsimons suggested that angiotensin might inform the brain of vascular hypovolemia and/or hypotension either directly by acting on brain tissue, or indirectly by modulating the sensitivity of stretch receptors in the low-pressure end of the circulatory system.The first of these suggestions was promptly supported by the observation that intracranial injections of renin, A-I, or A-II, in doses far too small to produce systemic effects, elicit drinking in a wide variety of species. The second remains to be evaluated (discussed below).

The discovery of the dipsogenic effects of systemic as well as central angiotensin is perhaps the greatest achievement of thirst research in recent decades but also presents us with unprecedented challenges. It is widely believed that a direct central action of angiotensin may play an important role in extracellular thirst, but there are numerous unresolved problems that have been the subject of an enormous amount of research and will require much additional consideration before we can hope to understand the role of the renin–angiotensin system in extracellular thirst. This is not the place for a review of the enormously complex experimental literature that has accumulated in recent years, but a brief summary of the critical issues and problems may help provide a grasp of the current state of the field.

We might begin by distinguishing between several issues: (a) Does angiotensin under normal circumstances play a significant role in transmitting information about blood volume and pressure to the brain and does this information act on mechanisms specifically related to extracellular thirst? (b) Is this an essential channel of information for some or all systemic extracellular thirst stimuli, at least under some conditions, or do neural afferents that originate from stretch receptors in the great veins and atria of the heart transmit duplicating information to the brain? (c) Does the release of renin modulate the sensitivity of the neural receptor system under some or all conditions of hypovolemia and hypotension? Most, though not all investigators in the field would accept the first proposition; few if any would agree with the second. All, I believe, would agree that we do not yet have sufficient evidence on the third to even venture an educated guess. Indeed, the essential challenge for the field for the 1990s is to separate the components of this puzzle.

With respect to the first question, there is no doubt that exogenous renin or angiotensin administered systemically can be dipsogenic. However, there has been controversy on whether the doses required are within the physiological range, and whether the quantities of water consumed in response to threshold doses are comparable to those drunk during experimentally induced hypovolemia. Fitzsimons, Mann, and others have argued that exogenous doses, well within the limits of plasma values seen after experimental treatments which result in hypovolemia, produce reliable drinking. Stricker has argued that the doses are too high and the total quantity of water consumed not significant. He suggests that endogenous renin plays only a permissive role in extracellular thirst by helping to raise blood pressure and thus to restore the behavioral competence required to seek and consume water. Robinson and Evered have turned this argument around and proposed that angiotensin may, in fact, have a true dipsogenic effect that is partially masked when A-II is administered to animals in normal water balance because the exogenous angiotensin results in hypertension that interferes with drinking. There are arguments (and data) as well as counterarguments (and data) on both sides of this important issue. A resolution of the problem would seem to be one of the most important, if also most difficult, tasks for the next decade.

The second issue has been addressed, in part, by examining the effects of nephrectomy, or pharmacological blockade of the renin–angiotensin system, on drinking responses to various extracellular dipsogens. If I may summarize and undoubtedly oversimplify a complex story, nephrectomy reduces but rarely abolishes drinking responses to some extracellular stimuli (such as caval ligation and, in some species, isoproterenol) but has little or no effect on others (such as polyethylene glycol or hemorrhage). The results of experiments on drug-induced blockade of various aspects of the renin–angiotensin system have also not been consistent. Intravenous as well as icv injections of antiserum to A-II have been reported to block drinking after PG as well as isoproterenol. On the other hand, drugs that block angiotensin receptors, or the conversion of the physiologically inactive A-I to the dipsogenic A-II, have been shown to block the dipsogenic effects of renin or angiotensin without affecting ad libitum drinking, deprivation-induced drinking, or the response to various extracellular dipsogens such as polyethylene glycol or isoproterenol in most experiments. Only very high doses of converting-enzyme inhibitors have been shown to have inhibitory effects; lower doses have been been reported to facilitate the response to extracellular dipsogens. There are plausible explanations for the apparent inconsistencies, but on balance the literature does not strongly support the conclusion that angiotensin is an essential messenger for all extracellular dipsogens. Indeed, even the weaker conclusion that it is an essential pathway for some extracellular thirst stimuli is supported only rather tenuously as yet. More conclusive experiments in this important area may have to await the development of more powerful and selective drugs or a better understanding to the nature (and location) of the central actions of A-II.

On the third issue raised above—the possible action of angiotensin on atrial stretch receptors—we have, as yet, deplorably little information. Fitzsimons suggested many years ago that angiotensin could influence extracellular thirst not only by a direct action on the brain but also by modulating the sensitivity of neural receptors in the great veins and atria of the heart. There is electrophysiological evidence for such stretch receptors in the walls of blood vessels and low-pressure chambers of the heart, but little direct information on their relation to thirst and essentially none concerning their sensitivity to circulating angiotensin.

Partial occlusion of the venous return to the heart elicits drinking, but the specific role of atrial stretch receptors in this effect is obscure because the effect is reduced or abolished by central as well as systemic injections of the angiotensin blocker saralasin. Inflation of balloons in the pulmonary vein near the left atrium of the heart, or in the junction of the superior vena cava and right atrium of the heart, has been reported to reduce ad libitum intake was well as drinking in response to several extracellular thirst stimuli. Because the procedure had little effect on plasma renin activity, and did not prevent a normal renin response to polyethylene glycol or isoproterenol, the observed inhibitory effects on drinking may reflect the results of a direct stimulation of neural receptors. None of these experiments have directly demonstrated a modulating action of angiotensin on the sensitivity of atrial stretch receptors, and there is some doubt whether the inflation of balloons can be compared with the pressure increases resulting from blood-pressure increases within the normal physiological range.

The last issue I would like to raise for a brief review and suggestions for further study in this context is the question of where angiotensin acts in the brain and how it gets there. Under normal circumstances, plasma angiotensin cannot cross the blood–brain barrier and also fails to enter cerebrospinal fluid. It is thus likely to act on cells in one of the fenestrated periventricular organs that are on the blood side of the barrier. There is good evidence that angiotensin acts on cells of the the subfornical organ, which projects to the AV3V and other regions of the brainstem that have been implicated in thirst. There is, however, also significant evidence for a direct A-II action on cells in the region of the OVLT and nucleus medianus, and there is some doubt that these structures are readily accessible from plasma. There is also evidence that icv injections of A-II retain dipsogenic properties when the SFO is destroyed or rendered inaccessible by cold-cream plugs. This suggests that angiotensin in CSF may gain access to other angiotensin-sensitive brain structures. The region of the OVLT and nucleus medianus has been proposed as a likely target because local lesions abolish the drinking response to systemic as well as icv angiotensin; neurons in the area are sensitive to angiotensin; and plausible mechanisms that could transport angiotensin from CSF to the region have been postulated. Yet there is little evidence for entry of blood-borne A-II into CSF, and the question needs to be addressed of how CSF angiotensin could be affected by changes in extracellular hydration.

There are also experimental data suggesting that injections of A-II into the preoptic region are dipsogenic. Epstein and others have argued that intraparenchymal injections of A-II and its precursors are dipsogenic only because of seepage into CSF and subsequent transport to SFO or, possibly, some other circumventricular site of action. Others have argued that the balance of the available experimental data instead favors the hypothesis that the preoptic area (and possibly other brain sites as well) may contain neurons sensitive to angiotensin, which could be produced by nerve cells and act as a neurotransmitter or neuromodulator. All components of the renin–angiotensin system are present in brain tissue, and there is rapidly increasing evidence that a variety of systemic peptides may indeed act in brain, apparently independently of their peripheral function. The possibility that preoptic A-II may have neurotransmitter or neuromodulator functions has not received the attention it deserves because the ventricular diffusion hypothesis seemed to have settled the matter. I believe further study is in order.

Other Centrally Acting Chemicals

The decade of the 1980s has seen a surge of interest in the action of various chemicals, including peripherally active peptides, on the brain. A group of peptides that has attracted the attention of thirst researches are compounds extracted from amphibian skin. One group, the tachykinins, inhibit, in a dose-dependent manner, drinking responses to icv angiotensin and carbachol. Most also inhibit water intake after cellular dehydration, but only at considerably higher doses. It is interesting, and possibly useful, that at least one of the tachykinins seems to affect cellular thirst selectively. The bombesins, a second group, selectively antagonize angiotensin-induced drinking when administered icv in very low doses. Higher doses also affect carbachol drinking.

These peptides appear to act only centrally. The possibility that intraparenchymal injections of them could be used to distinguish neural mechanisms that may be specifically related to cellular or extracellular thirst (or possibly even different types of extracellular thirst signals) has not been systematically explored.

A second class of chemicals that appear to have differential central effects on A-II–mediated drinking consists of members of the prostaglandin E (PGE) family. Very low icv doses of PGE reduce drinking responses to central as well as systemic A-II. At higher doses, icv PGE also attenuates the drinking response to polyethylene glycol. Cellular dehydration thirst and drinking in response to icv carbachol are not affected. There has been a good deal of research concerning the possibility that PGE may directly or indirectly counteract and terminate the action of A-II in the brain. The hypothesis received a significant amount of support from several studies but seems currently out of favor because icv injections of compounds that inhibit the biosynthesis of prostaglandins have had inconsistent effects on drinking after icv angiotensin. Further research on this interesting problem would seem to be warranted. The PGEs may also provide a potentially useful tool for isolating A-II–sensitive brain mechanisms and distinguishing between cellular and extracellular thirst pathways.

Bibliography

Abdelaal, A. E., Mercer, P. F., and Mogenson, G. J. (1974a). Drinking elicited by polyethylene glycol and isoproterenol reduced by antiserum to angiotensin-II. *Can. J. Physiol. Pharmacol.* **52**, 362–363.

Abedaal, A. E., Mercer, P. F., and Mogenson, G. J. (1976). Plasma angiotensin II levels and water intake following β-adrenergic stimulation, hypovolemia, cellular dehydration, and water deprivation. *Pharmacol. Biochem. Behav.* **4**, 317–321.

Abdelaal, A. E., Assaf, S. Y., Kucharczyk, J., and Mogenson, G. J. (1974b). Effect of ablation of the subfornical organ on water intake elicited by systemically administered angiotensin II. *Can. J. Physiol. Pharmacol.* **52**, 1217–1220.

Abraham, S. F., Baker, R. M., Blaine, E. H., Denton, D. A., and McKinley, M. J. (1975). Water drinking induced in sheep by angiotentin: A physiological or pharmacological effect? *J. Comp. Physiol. Psychol.* **88**, 503–518.

Abraham, S. F., Denton, D. A., McKinley, M. J., and Weisinger, R. S. (1976). Effect of an angiotensin antagonist, Sar [1]-Ala[8]-Angiotensin II on physiological thirst. *Pharmacol. Physiol. Behav.* **4**, 243–247.

Ackermann, U., and Irizawa, T. G. (1984). Synthesis and renal activity of rat atrial granules depend on extracellular volume. *Am. J. Physiol.* **247**, R750–752.

Adachi, A., Niijima, A., and H. L. Jacobs. (1976). An hepatic osmoreceptor mechanism in the rat: Electrophysiological and behavioral studies. *Am. J. Physiol.* **231**, 1043–1049.

Adolph, E. F. (1943). "Physiological Regulations." Jacques Cattell Press, Lancaster, Pa.

Adolph, E. F. (1947a). "Physiology of Man in the Desert." Interscience, New York.

Adolph, E. F. (1947b). Urges to eat and drink in rats. *Am. J. Physiol.* **151**, 110–125.

Adolph, E. F. (1947c). Water metabolism. *Annu. Rev. Physiol.* **9**, 381–408.

Adolph, E. F. (1948). Water ingestion and excretion in rats under some chemical influences. *Am. J. Physiol.* **155**, 309–316.

Adolph, E. F. (1950). Thirst and its inhibition in the stomach. *Am. J. Physiol.* **161**, 374–386.

Adolph, E. F. (1964). Regulation of body water content through water ingestion. *In* "Thirst: Proceedings of the First International Symposium on Thirst in the Regulation of Body Water" (M. J. Wayner, ed.), pp. 5–14. Pergamon Press, Oxford.

Adolph, E. F., Barker, J. P., and Hoy, P. A. (1954). Multiple factors in thirst. *Am. J. Physiol.* **178**, 538–562.

Ahren, G. L., Landin, M. L. and Wolf, G. (1978). Escape from deficits in sodium intake after thalamic lesions as a function of preoperative experience. *J. Comp. Physiol. Psychol.* **92**, 544–554.

Aiken, J. W., and Vane, R. J. (1973). Intrarenal prostaglandin release attenuates the renal vasoconstrictor activity of angiotensin. *J. Pharmacol. Exp. Ther.* **184**, 678–687.

Alheid, G. F., and Grossman, S. P. (1974). Aphagia and adipsia in rats produced by knife cuts ventral to the globus pallidus. *Neurosci. Abstr.* **3**, 115.

Alheid, G. F., Kelly, J., McDermott, L. J., Halaris, A., and Grossman, S. P. (1977a). Supersensitivity to norepinephrine or dopamine antagonists after knife cuts that produce aphagia and adipsia in rats. *Pharmacol. Biochem. Behav.* **6**, 647–657.

Alheid, G. F., McDermott, L. J., Kelly J., Halaris, A., and Grossman, S. P. (1977b). Deficits in food and water intake after knife cuts that deplete striatal DA or hypothalamic NE in rats. *Pharmacol. Biochem. Behav.* **6**, 273–287.

Almli, R. C. (1971). Hypovolemia at the polyethylene glycol induced onset of drinking. *Physiol. Behav.* **7**, 369–374.

Almli, R. C., and Weiss, C. S. (1974). Drinking behaviors: Effects of lateral preoptic and lateral hypothalamic destruction. *Physiol. Behav.* **13**, 527–538.

Almli, R. C., Weiss, C. S., and Tondat, L. M. (1975). Does hypovolemia plus cellular dehydration equal water deprivation? *Behav. Biol.* **13**, 445–456.

Almli, C. R., Golden, G. T., and McMullen, N. T. (1976). Ontogeny of drinking behavior of preweaning rats with lateral preoptic damage. *Brain Res. Bull.* **1**, 437–442.

Anand, B. K., and Brobeck, J. R. (1951). Hypothalamic control of food intake in rats and cats. *Yale J. Biol. Med.* **24**, 123–140.

Andersson, B. (1953). The effect of injections of hypertonic NaCl-solutions into different parts of the hypothalamus of goats. *Acta Physiol. Scand.* **28**, 188–201.

Andersson, B. (1955). Observations on the water and electrolyte metabolism in the goat. *Acta Physiol. Scand.* **33**, 50–65.

Andersson, B. (1971). Thirst-and brain control of water balance. *Am. Scientist* **59**, 408–415.

Andersson, B. (1973). Invited comments: Osmoreceptors versus sodium receptors. *In* "The Neuropsychology of Thirst" (A. N. Epstein, H. R. Kissileff, and E. Stellar, eds.), pp. 113–116. Wiley, New York.

Andersson, B. (1978). Regulation of water intake. *Physiol. Rev.* **58**, 582–603.

Andersson, B., and Eriksson, L. (1971). Conjoint action of sodium and angiotensin on brain mechanisms controlling water and salt balances. *Acta Physiol. Scand.* **81**, 18–29.

Andersson, B., and Larsson, S. (1956). Water and food intake and the inhibitory effect of amphetamine on drinking and eating before and after "prefrontal lobotomy" in dogs. *Acta Physiol. Scand.* **38**, 22–30.

Andersson, B., and Leksell, L. G. (1975). Effects on fluid balance of intraventricular infusions of prostaglandin E-1. *Acta Physiol. Scand.* **93**, 286–288.

Andersson, B., and McCann, S. M. (1955). A further study of polydipsia evoked by hypothalamic stimulation in the goat. *Acta Physiol. Scand.* **33**, 333–346.

Andersson, B., and McCann, S. M. (1956). Drinking, antidiuresis and milk ejection from electrical stimulation within the hypothalamus of the goat. *Acta Physiol. Scand.* **35**, 191–201.

Andersson, B., and Westbye, O. (1970). Synergistic action of sodium and angiotensin on brain mechanisms controlling fluid balance. *Life Sci.* **9**, 601–608.

Andersson, B., and Wyrwicka, W. (1957). Elicitation of a drinking motor conditioned reaction by electrical stimulation of the hypothalamic "drinking area" in the goat. *Acta Physiol. Scand.* **41**, 194–198.

Andersson, B., Dallman, M. F., and Olsson, K. (1969). Observations on central control of drinking and of the release of antidiuretic hormone (ADH). *Life Sci.* **8**, 425–432.

Andersson, B., Jobin, M., and Olsson K. (1967). A study of thirst and other effects of an increased sodium concentration in the 3rd brain ventricle. *Acta Physiol. Scand.* **69**, 29–36.

Andersson, B., Leksell, L. G., and Lishajko F. (1975). Perturbations in fluid balance induced by medially placed forebrain lesions. *Brain Res.* **99**, 261–275.

Andersson, B., Leksell, L. G., and Rundgren, M. (1982). Regulation of water intake. *Annu. Rev. Nutr.* **2**, 73–89.

Andersson, B., Eriksson, L., Fernandez, O., Kolmodin, G. G., and Oltner, R. (1972). Centrally mediated effects of sodium and angiotensin II on arterial blood pressure and fluid balance. *Acta Physiol. Scand.* **85**, 398–407.

Andersson, K., Fuxe, K., Agnati, L. F., Ganten, D. and Zim, I. (1982). Intraventricular injections of renin increase turnover in the tuberoinfundibular dopamine neurons and reduce the secretion of prolactin in male rats. *Acta Physiol. Scand.* **116**, 317–320.

Antelman, S. M., Rowland, N. E., and Fisher, A. E. (1976). Stress related recovery from lateral hypothalamic aphagia. *Brain Res.* **102**, 346–350.

Antelman, S. M., Rowland, N. E., and Fisher, A. E. (1977). Stimulation bound ingestive behavior: A view from the tail. *Physiol. Behav.* **17**, 743–748.

Arden, F. (1934). Experimental observations upon thirst and on potassium overdosage. *Austral. J. Exp. Biol. Med. Sci.* **12**, 121–122.

Arslan, Y., Burckhardt, R., Jawaharlal, K., Ornstein, K., and Peters, G. (1986). Effects of narcotic analgesics on water and food intake in normal rats. *In* "The Physiology of Thirst and Sodium Appetite" (G. deCaro, A. N. Epstein, and M. Massi, eds.), pp. 527–534. Plenum Press, New York.

Assaf, S. Y., and Mogenson, G. J. (1976). Evidence that angiotensin II acts on the preoptic region to elicit water intake. *Pharmacol. Biochem. Behav.* **5**, 679–699.

Asscher, A. W., and Anson, S. G. (1963). A vascular permeability factor of renal origin. *Nature* **198**, 1097–1099.

Atarashi, K., Mulrow, P. J., Franco-Saenz, R., Snajdar, R., and Rapp, J. (1984). Inhibition of aldosterone production by an atrial extract. *Science* **224**, 992–994.

Atkinson, J., Kaeserman, H. P., Lambelet, J., Peters, G., and Peters-Haefeli, L. (1979). The role of circulating renin in drinking in response to isoprenaline. *J. Physiol.* **291**, 61–73.

Avrith, D. B., and Fitzsimons, J. T. (1980). Increased sodium appetite in the rat induced by intracranial administration of components of the renin-angiotensin system. *J. Physiol.* **301**, 349–364.

Avrith, D. B., and Fitzsimons, J. T. (1983). Renin-induced sodium appetite: Effects on sodium balance and mediation by angiotensin in the rat. *J. Physiol.* **337**, 479–496, 1983.

Balagura, S., Wilcox, R. H., and Coscina, D. V. (1969). The effects of diencephalic lesions on food intake and motor activity. *Physiol. Behav.* **4**, 629–633.

Balment, R. J., Brimble, M. J., and Forsling, M. L. (1980). Release of oxytocin induced by salt loading and its influence on renal excretion in the male rat. *J. Physiol.* **308**, 439–449.

Barker, J. L. (1976). Peptides: roles in neuronal excitability. *Physiol. Rev.* **56**, 435–452.

Barney, C. C., Katovich, M. J., and Fregly, M. J. (1980). The effect of acute administration of an angiotensin converting enzyme inhibitor, captopril (SQ 14,225), on experimentally induced thirsts in rats. *J. Pharmacol. Exp. Ther.* **212**, 53–57.

Bealer, S. L., and Johnson, A. K. (1979). Sodium consumption following lesions surrounding the anteroventral third ventricle. *Brain Res. Bull.* **4**, 287–290.

Beilharz, S., Denton, D. A., and Sabine, J. R. (1962). The effect of concurrent deficiency of water and sodium on sodium appetite in sheep. *J. Physiol.* **163**, 378–390.

Bellin, S. I., Landas S., Bhatnagar R. K., and Johnson, A. K. (1984a). The role of catecholamines in discrete AV3V nuclei: Alterations in drinking and pressor responses to angiotensin following 6-hydroxydopamine. *Fed. Proc.* **43**, 1070.

Bellin, S. I., McRae-Deguerce, A., Landas, S., and Johnson, A. K. (1984b). Noradrenergic (NE) cell transplants into 6-HDA-denervated ventral lamina terminalis nuclei restore drinking responses to systemic angiotensin II (ANG II). *Soc. Neurosci. Abstr.* **10**, 1011.

Bellows, R. T. (1939). Time factors in water drinking in dogs. *Am. J. Physiol.* **125**, 87–97.

Bellows, R. T., and Van Wagenen, W. P. (1938). The relationship of polydipsia and polyuria in diabetes insipidus. A study of diabetes insipidus in dogs with and without esophageal fistulae. *J. Nerv. Mental Disorders* **88**, 417–473.

Bellows, R. T., and Van Wagenen, W. P. (1939). The effect of resection of the olfactory, gustatory and trigeminal nerves on water drinking in dogs without and with diabetes insipidus. *Am. J. Physiol.* **126**, 13–19.

Bernard, C. (1856). "Leçons de physiologie expérimentale appliquée à la médecine faites au Collège de France Cours du Semestre d'Ete, 1855," Vol. II, pp. 49–52. Bailliere, Paris.

Berridge, K. C., Flynn, F. W., Schulkin, J., and Grill, H. J. (1984). Sodium depletion enhances salt palatability in rats. *Behav. Neurosci.* **98**, 652–660.

Besch, N. F., and van Dyne, G. C. (1969). Effects of locus and size of septal lesions on consummatory behavior in the rat. *Physiol. Behav.* **4**, 953–958.

Black, S. L. (1976). Preoptic hypernatremia syndrome and the regulation of water balance in the rat. *Physiol. Behav.* **17**, 473–482.

Black, S. L., and Mogenson, G. J. (1973). The regulation of serum sodium in septal lesioned rats: A test of two hypotheses. *Physiol. Behav.* **10**, 379–384.

Black, S. L., Kucharczyk, J., and Mogenson, G. J. (1974). Disruption of drinking to intracranial angiotensin by a lateral hypothalamic lesion. *Pharmacol. Biochem. Behav.* **2**, 515–522.

Black, S. L., Mok, A. C. S., Cope, D. L., and Mogenson, G. J. (1973). Activation of lateral hypothalamic neurons by the injection of angiotensin into the preoptic area of the rat. *Fed. Proc.* **32**, Abstr. 930.

Blaine, E. H. (1986). Atrial natriuretic factor. *Fed. Proc.* **45**, 2360–2391

Blair-West, J. R., Coghlan, J. P., Cranon, D. A., Funder, J. W., and Scoggins, B. A. (1973). Increased aldosterone secretion during sodium depletion with inhibition of renin release. *Am. J. Physiol.* **224**, 1409–1414.

Blair-West, J. R., Coghlan, J. P., Denton, D. A., Funder, J. W., Scoggins, B. A., and Wright, R. D. (1971). Effects of the heptapeptide (2-8) and the hexapeptide (3-8) fragments of angiotensin II on aldosterone secretion. *J. Clin. Endocrin. Metabl.* **40**, 530–533.

Blank, D. L., and Wayner, M. J. (1975). Lateral preoptic single unit activity: Effects of various solutions. *Physiol. Behav.* **15**, 723–730.

Blass, E. M. (1974). Evidence for basal forebrain osmoreceptors in the rat. *Brain Res.* **82**, 69–76.

Blass, E. M., and Chapman, H. W. (1971). An evaluation of the contribution of cholinergic mechanism to thirst. *Physiol. Behav.* **7**, 679–686.

Blass, E. M., and Epstein, A. N. (1971). A lateral preoptic osmosensitive zone for thirst in the rat. *J. Comp. Physiol. Psychol.* **76**, 378–394.

Blass, E. M., and Fitzsimons, J. T. (1970). Additivity of effect and interaction of a cellular and extracellular stimulus of drinking. *J. Comp. Physiol. Psychol.* **70**, 200–205.

Blass, E. M., and Hall, W. G. (1976). Drinking termination: Interactions between hydrational, orogastric and behavioral controls in rats. *Psychol. Rev.* **183**, 356–374.

Blass E. M., and Hanson D. G. (1970). Primary hyperdipsia in the rat following septal lesions *J. Comp. Physiol. Psychol.* **70**, 87–93.

Blass, E. M., Nussbaum, A. I., and Hanson, D. G. (1974). Septal hyperdipsia: Specific enhancement of drinking to angiotensin in rats. *J. Comp. Physiol. Psychol.* **87**, 422–439.

Blass, E. M., Jobaris, R., and Hall, W. (1976). Oropharyngeal control of drinking in rats. *J. Comp. Physiol. Psychol.* **90**, 909–916.

Block, M. L., and Fisher, A. E. (1970). Anticholinergic central blockade of salt-aroused and deprivation-induced thirst. *Physiol. Behav.* **5**, 525–527.

Block, M. L., and Fisher, A. E. (1975). Cholinergic and dopaminergic blocking agents modulate water intake elicited by deprivation, hypovolemia, hypertonicity and isoproterenol. *Pharmacol. Biochem. Behav.* **3**, 251–261.

Block, M. L., Vallier, G. H., and Glickman, S. E. (1974). Elicitation of water ingestion in the mongolian gerbil (*Meriones Unguiculatus*) by intracranial injections of angiotensin II and l-norepinephrine. *Pharmacol. Biochem. Behav.* **2**, 235–242.

Blundell, J. E., and Herberg, L. J. (1973). Primary polyuria accompanies "hunger" elicited by intrahypothalamic injection of noradrenaline. *Neuropharmacologia* **12**, 597–599.

Booth, D. A. (1968). Mechanism of action of norepinephrine in eliciting an eating response on injection into the rat hypothalamus. *J. Pharmacol. Exp. Ther.* **160**, 336–348.

Booth, D. A., and Brookover, T. (1968). Hunger elicited in the rat by a single injection of bovine crystalline insulin. *Physiol. Behav.* **3**, 439–446.

Bott, E., Denton, D. A., and Weller, S. (1965). Water drinking in sheep with oesophageal fistulae. *J. Physiol.* **176**, 323–336.

Boyle, P. C., and Keesey, R. E. (1975). Chronically reduced levels of body weight in LH lesioned rats maintained upon diets and drinking solutions of varying palatability, *J. Comp. Physiol. Psychol.* **88**, 218–223.

Braun-Menéndez, E. (1952). Aumento del apetito especifico para la sal provocado por la desoxicorticosterona; sustancias que potencian o inhiben esta accion. *Rev. Soc. Argent. Biol.* **28**, 23–32.

Bridge, J. G., and Hatton, G. I. (1973). Septal unit activity in response to alterations in blood volume and osmotic pressure. *Physiol. Behav.* **10**, 769–774.

Brody, M. J., and Johnson, A. K. (1980). Role of the anteroventral third ventricle region in fluid and electrolyte balance, arterial pressure regulation, and hypertension. *In* "Frontiers in Neuroendocrinology," Vol. 6 (L. Martini and W. F. Ganong eds.), pp. 249–292. Raven Press, New York.

Brody, M. J., Fink, G. D., Buggy, J., Haywood, J. R., Gordon, F., and Johnson, A. K.

(1978). The role of the anteroventral third ventricle (3AV3V) region in experimental hypertension. *Circ. Res.* **43**, 2–13.

Brody, M. J., Haywood, J. R., and Touw, K. B. (1980). Neural mechanisms in hypertension. *Annu. Rev. Physiol.* **42**, 441–453.

Brophy, P. D., and Levitt, R. A. (1974). Dose-response analysis of angiotensin- and renin-induced drinking in the cat. *Pharmacol. Biochem. Behav.* **2**, 509–514.

Brown, B., and Grossman, S. P. (1980). Evidence that nerve cell bodies in the zona incerta influence ingestive behavior. *Brain Res. Bull.* **5**, 593–597.

Brown, D. R., and Holtzman, S. G. (1979). Suppression of deprivation-induced food and water intake in rats and mice by naloxone. *Pharmacol. Biochem. Behav.* **11**, 567–573.

Brownfield, M. S., Reid, I. A., Ganten, D., and Ganong, F. (1982). Differential distribution of immunoreactive angiotensin and angiotensin-converting enzyme in rat brain. *Neuroscience* **7**, 1759–1769.

Brunn, F. (1925). The sensation of thirst. *J. Am. Med. Assoc.* **85**, 234–235.

Bruno, J. P., Snyder, A. M., and Stricker, E. M. (1984). Effects of dopamine-depleting brain lesions on suckling and weaning in rats. *Behav. Neurosci.* **98**, 156–161.

Bruno, J. P., Zigmond, M. J., and Stricker, E. M. (1986). Rats given dopamine-depleting brain lesions as neonates do not respond to acute homeostatic imbalances as adults. *Behav. Neurosci.* **100**, 125–128.

Bryant, R. W., and Falk, J. L. (1973). Angiotensin I as a dipsogen: Efficacy in brain independent of conversion to angiotensin II. *Pharmacol. Biochem. Behav.* **1**, 469–475.

Bryant, R. W., Epstein, A. N., Fitzsimons, J. T., and Fluharty, S. J. (1980). Arousal of a specific and persistent sodium appetite in the rat with continuous intracerebroventricular infusion of angiotensin II. *J. Physiol.* **301**, 365–382.

Buerger, P. B., Levitt, R. A., and Irwin, D. A. (1973). Chemical stimulation of the brain: Relationship between neural activity and water ingestion in the rat. *J. Comp. Physiol. Psychol.* **12**, 278–285.

Buggy, J. (1977). Drinking elicited by angiotensin or hyperosmotic stimulation of the rat antero-ventral third ventricle: Single or separate neural substrates? *In* "Central Actions of Angiotensin and Related Hormones" (J. P. Buckley, C. M. Ferrario and M. F. Lokhandwala eds.). Pergamon Press, New York.

Buggy, J. (1978). Block of cholinergic-induced thirst after obstruction of anterior ventral third ventricle or periventricular preoptic ablation. *Neurosci. Abstr.* **4**, 172.

Buggy, J., and Fisher A. E. (1976). Anterolateral third ventricle site of action for angiotensin induced thirst. *Pharmacol. Biochem. Behav.* **4**, 651–660.

Buggy, J., and Johnson, A. K. (1977a). Anteroventral third ventricle periventricular ablation: Temporary adipsia and persisting thirst deficits. *Neurosci. Lett.* **5**, 177–182.

Buggy, J., and Johnson, A. K. (1977b). Preoptic-hypothalamic periventricular lesions: Thirst deficits and hypernatremia. *Am. J. Physiol.* **233**, R44–52.

Buggy, J., and Johnson, A. K. (1978). Angiotensin-induced thirst: Effects of third ventricle obstruction and periventricular ablation. *Brain Res.* **149**, 117–128.

Buggy, J., Fink, G. D., Haywood, J. R., Johnson, A. K., and Body, M. J. (1977a). Interruption of the maintenance phase of established hypertension by ablation of the anteroventral third ventricle (AV3V) in rats. *Clin. Exp. Hypertens.* **1**, 337–353.

Buggy, J., Fink, G. D., Johnson, A. K. and Brody, M. J. (1977b). Prevention of the development of renal hypertension by anteroventral third ventricular tissue lesions. *Circ. Res. (Suppl. 1)* **40**, I110-I117.

Buggy, J., Fisher, A. E., Hoffman, W. E., Johnson, A. K., and Phillips, M. I. (1975). Ventricular obstruction: Effect on drinking induced by intracranial injections of angiotensin. *Science* **190**, 72–74.

Buggy, J., Fisher, A. E., Hoffman, W. E., Johnson, A. K., and Phillips, M. I. (1978a). Reply to Simpson, J. B. and A. Routtenberg, Subfornical organ: A dipsogenic site of action of angiotensin II. *Science* **201**, 380–381.

Buggy, J., Haywood, J. R., Fink, G. D., Phillips, M. I., and Brody, M. J. (1978b). Central responses to angiotensin: No role for area postrema in rat. *Fed. Proc.* **37**, 3085.

Buggy, J., Hoffman, W. E., Phillips, M. I., Fisher, A. E., and Johnson, A. K. (1979). Osmosensitivity of rat third ventricle and interactions with angiotensin. *Am. J. Physiol.* **236**, R75–82.

Burckhardt, R., Peters-Haefeli, L., and Peters, G. (1975). The mechanism of thirst-induction by intrahypothalamic renin. *In* "Control Mechanisms of Drinking" (G. Peters, J. T. Fitzsimons, and L. Peters-Haefeli eds.), pp. 103–107. Springer Verlag, New York.

Burke, G. H., Mook, D. G., and Blass, E. M. (1972). Hyperreactivity to quinine associated with osmotic thirst in the rat. *J. Comp. Physiol. Psychol.* **78**, 32–39.

Cadnapaphornchai, P., Boykin, J., Harbottle, J. A., McDonald, K. M., and Schrier, R. W. (1975). Effect of angiotensin II on renal water excretion. *Am. J. Physiol.* **228**, 155–159.

Caggiula, A. R. (1969). Stability of behavior produced by electrical stimulation of the rat hypothalamus. *Brain, Behav. Evolut.* **2**, 343–358.

Cannon, W. B. (1919). The physiological basis of thirst. *Proc. R. Soc. (Lond.)* **90**, 283–301.

Cannon, W. B. (1934). Hunger and thirst. *In* "A Handbook of General Experimental Psychology" (Carl Murchison, ed.), pp. 247–263. Clark University Press, Worcester, Mass.

Cantalamessa, F., deCaro, G., Massi, M., and Micossi, L. G. (1982a). A study on behavioural alterations induced by intracerebroventricular administration of bombesin to rats. *Pharmacol. Res. Commun.* **14**, 163–173.

Cantalamessa, F., deCaro, G., Massi, M., and Micossi, L. G. (1982b). Stimulation of drinking behaviour and of renin release induced by intracerebroventricular injection of D-Ala²-D-Leu⁵-enkephalin to rats. *Pharmacol. Res. Commun.* **14**, 141–148.

Cantalamessa, F., deCaro, G., Massi, M., and Perfumi, M. (1984). Possible influence of tachykinins on body fluid homeostasis in the rat. *J. Physiol.* **79**, 524–530.

Carey, R. J. (1969). Contrasting effects of anterior and posterior septal injury on thirst motivated behavior. *Physiol. Behav.* **4**, 759–764.

Carey, R., and Procopia, G. (1974). Differential effects of septal, preoptic, and habenula ablations on thirst-motivated behaviors in rats. *J. Comp. Physiol. Psychol.* **86**, 1163–1172.

Chapman, W., and Epstein, A. N. (1970). Prandial drinking induced by atropine. *Physiol. Behav.* **5**, 549–554.

Chiaraviglio, E. (1969). Effects of lesions in the septal area and olfactory bulbs on sodium chloride intake. *Physiol. Behav.* **4**, 693–697.

Chiaraviglio, E. (1971). Amygdaloid modulation of sodium chloride and water intake in the rat. *J. Comp. Physiol. Psychol.* **76**, 401–407.

Chiaraviglio, E. (1972). Mesencephalic influences on the intake of sodium chloride and water in the rat. *Brain Res.* **44**, 73–82.

Chiaraviglio, E. (1976). Effect of renin-angiotensin system on sodium intake. *J. Physiol.* **255**, 57–66.

Chiaraviglio, E., and Pérez-Guaita, M. F. (1986). Effect of cerebroventricular infusion of hypertonic sodium solutions on sodium intake in rats. *In* "The Physiology of Thirst and Sodium Appetite" (G. de Caro, A. N. Epstein and M. Massie eds.), pp. 503–508. Plenum Press, New York.

Cizek, L. J., and Nocenti, M. R. (1965). Relationship between food and water ingestion in the rat. *Am. J. Physiol.* **208**, 615–620.

Cizek, L. J., Semple, R. E., Huang, K. C., and Gregersen, M. I. (1951). Effect of extracellular electrolyte depletion on water intake in dogs. *Am. J. Physiol.* **164**, 415–422.

Coburn, P. C., and Stricker, E. M. (1978). Osmoregulatory thirst in rats after lateral preoptic lesions. *J. Comp. Physiol. Psychol.* **92**, 350–361.

Cohen, M. L., and Kurz, K. D. (1982). Angiotensin converting enzyme inhibition in tissues from spontaneously hypertensive rats after treatment with captopril or MK–421. *J. Pharmacol. Exp. Ther.* **220**, 63–69.

Conrad, L. A., and Pfaff, D. W. (1976). Efferents from medial basal forebrain and hypothalamus in the rat. *J. Comp. Neurol.* **169**, 185–220.

Cooling, M. J., and Day, M. D. (1975). Angiotensin-induced drinking in the cat. *In* "Control Mechanisms of Drinking" (G. Peters, J. T. Fitzsimons, and L. Peters-Haefeli, eds.), pp. 132–135. Springer Verlag, New York.

Cooper, K. E. (1987). The neurobiology of fever: Thoughts on recent developments. *Ann. Rev. Neurosci.* **10**, 297–324.

Cooper, S. J. (1982a). Specific benzodiazepine antagonist Ro15–1788 and thirst-induced drinking in the rat. *Neuropharmacology* **21**, 775–780.

Cooper, S. J. (1982b). Effects of opiate antagonists and of morphine on chlordiazepoxide-induced hyperdipsia in the water-deprived rat. *Neuropharmacology* **21**, 1013–1017.

Cooper, S. J. (1982c). Enhancement of osmotic- and hypovolemic-induced drinking by chlordiazepoxide in rats is blocked by naltrexone. *Pharmacol. Biochem. Behav.* **17**, 921–925.

Cooper, S. J. (1983a). Benzodiazepines, barbiturates and drinking. *In* "Theory in Psychopharmacology," Vol. 2. (S. J. Cooper, ed.). Academic Press, London.

Cooper, S. J. (1983b). Effects of chlordiazepoxide on drinking compared in rats challenged with hypertonic saline, isoproterenol or polyethylene glycol. *Life Sci.* **32**, 2453–2459.

Cooper, S. J. (1986). Benzodiazepine and endorphinergic mechanisms in relation to salt and water intake. *In* "The Physiology of Thirst and Sodium Appetite" (G. deCaro, A. N. Epstein, and M. Massi, eds.), pp. 239–244. Plenum Press, New York.

Cooper, S. J., and Gilbert, D. B. (1984). Naloxone suppresses fluid consumption in tests of choice between sodium chloride solutions and water in male and female water-deprived rats. *Psychopharmacology* **84**, 362–367.

Cooper, S. J., and Gilbert, D. B. (1986). Dopaminergic modulation of choice in salt preference tests. *In* "The Physiology of Thirst and Sodium Appetite" (G. deCaro, A. N. Epstein, and M. Massi, eds.), pp. 453–458. Plenum Press, New York.

Cooper, S. J., and Turkish, S. (1983). Effects of naloxone and its quarternary analogue on fluid consumption in water-deprived rats. *Neuropharmacology* **22**, 797–800.

Corbit, J. D. (1965). Effect of intravenous sodium chloride on drinking in the rat. *J. Comp. Physiol. Psychol.* **60**, 397–406.

Corbit, J. D. (1967). Effects of hypervolemia on drinking in the rat. *J. Comp. Physiol. Psychol.* **64**, 250–255.

Corbit, J. D., and Tuchapsky, S. (1968). Gross hypervolemia: Stimulation of diuresis without effect upon drinking. *J. Comp. Physiol. Psychol.* **65**, 38–41.

Cort, J. H. (1952). The renal response to extrarenal depletion of the blood volume. *J. Physiol.* **116**, 307–319.

Coscina, D. V., Grant, L. D., Balagura, S., and Grossman, S. P. (1972). Hyperdipsia following serotonin-depleting midbrain lesions. *Nature* **235**, 63–64.

Costales, M., Fitzsimons, J. T., and Vijande, M. (1984). Increased sodium appetite and polydipsia induced by partial aortic occlusion in rats. *J. Physiol.* **352**, 467–481.

Costales, M., Vijande, M., Marìn, B., Brime, J. I., and Lopez-Sela, P. (1986). Renin-dependence of insulin-induced thirst. *In* "The Physiology of Thirst and Sodium Appetite" (G. deCaro, A. N. Epstein, and M. Massi, eds.), pp. 181–186. Plenum Press, New York.

Covian, M. R., Gentil, C. G., and Antunes-Rodrigues, J. (1972). Water and sodium chloride intake following microinjections of angiotensin-II into the septal area of the rat. *Physiol. Behav.* **9**, 373–377.

Cox, J. R., Cruz, C. E., and Ruger, J. (1978). Effects of total amygdalectomy upon regulation of salt intake in rats. *Brain Res. Bull.* **3**, 4431–435.

Cox, V. C., and Valenstein, E. S. (1969a). Distribution of hypothalamic sites yielding stimulus-bound behavior. *Brain Behav. Evolut.* **2**, 359–376.

Cox, V. C., and Valenstein, E. S. (1969b). Effects of stimulus intensity on behavior elicited by hypothalamic stimulation. *J. Comp. Physiol. Psychol.* **69**, 730–733.

Crone, C. (1965). The permeability of brain capillaries to nonelectrolytes. *Acta Physiol. Scand.* **64**, 407–4317.

Cross, B. A., and Green, J. D. (1959). Activity of single neurones in the hypothalamus: Effect of osmotic and other stimuli. *J. Physiol.* **148**, 554–569.

Currie, M. G., Geller, D. M., Cole, B. R., Boylan, J. G., YuSheng, W., Holmberg, S. W., and Needleman, P. (1983). Bioactive cardiac substances: Potent vasorelaxant activity in mammalian atria. *Science* **221**, 71–73.

Czech, D. A., Stein, E. A., and Blake, M. J. (1983). Naloxone-induced hypodipsia: A CNS mapping study. *Life Sci.* **33**, 797–803.

Dalhouse, A. D., Langford, H. G., Walsh, D., and Barnes, D. (1986). Angiotensin and salt appetite: Physiological amounts of angiotensin given peripherally increase salt appetite in the rat. *Behav. Neurosci.* **100**, 597–602.

Darrow, D. C., and Yannet, H. (1935). The changes in distribution of body water accompanying increase and decrease in extracellular electrolyte. *J. Clin. Invest.* **14**, 266–275.

DeBold, A. J. (1986). Atrial natriuretic factor (A.J. DeBold Chair). *Fed. Proc.* **45**, 2081–2132.

DeBold, A. J., Bornstein, H. B., Veress, A. T., and Sonnenberg H. (1981). A rapid and potent natriuretic response to intravenous injections of atrial myocardial extract in rats. *Life Sci.* **28**, 89–94.

DeCaro, G. (1986). Effects of peptides of the "gut-brain-skin triangle" on drinking behaviour of rats and birds. *In* "The Physiology of Thirst and Sodium Appetite" (G. deCaro, A. N. Epstein, and M. Massi, eds.), pp. 213–226. Plenum Press, New York.

DeCaro, G., and Micossi, L. G. (1986). Selective antidipsogenic effect of kassinin in Wistar rats. *In* "The Physiology of Thirst and Sodium Appetite" (G. deCaro, A. N. Epstein, and M. Massi, eds.), pp. 245–249. Plenum Press, New York.

DeCaro, G., Massi, M., and Micossi, L. G. (1978a). Antidipsogenic effect of intracranial injections of substance P to rats. *J. Physiol.* **279**, 133–140.

DeCaro, G., Massi, M., and Micossi, L. G. (1980a). Effect of bombesin on drinking induced by angiotensin II, carbachol and water deprivation in the rat. *Pharmacol. Res. Commun.* **12**, 657–666.

DeCaro, G., Massi, M., and Micossi, L. G. (1980b). Bombesin potently stimulates water intake in the pigeon. *Neuropharmacology* **19**, 867–870.

DeCaro, G., Massi, M., and Perfumi, M. (1978c). Potent dipsogenic effect of physalaemin in the pigeon. *Pharmacol. Res. Commun.* **10**, 861–870.

DeCaro, G., Micossi, L. G., and Piccinin, G. (1977). Antidipsogenic effect of intraventricular administration of eledoisin to rats. *Pharmacol. Res. Commun.* **9**, 489–500.

DeCaro, G., Mariotti, M., Massi, M., and Micossi, L. G. (1980b). Dipsogenic effect of angiotensin II, bombesin and tachykinins in the duck. *Pharmacol. Biochem. Behav.* **13**, 229–233.

DeCaro, G., Massi, M., Micossi, L. G., and Perfumi, M. (1982). Angiotensin II antagonists versus drinking induced by bombesin or eledoisin in pigeons. *Peptides* **3**, 631–636.

DeCaro, G., Massi, M., Micossi, G. L., and Perfumi, M. (1984a). Drinking and feeding inhibition by ICV pulse injection or infusion of bombesin, ranatensin and litorin to rats. *Peptides* **5**, 607–613.

DeCaro, G., Massi, M., Micossi, G. L., and Perfumi, M. (1984b).Effect of dermorphin and related peptides on drinking behaviour of the rat. *In* "Central and Peripheral Endorphins: Basic and Clinical Aspects" (E. E. Müller and A. R. Genazzani, eds.), pp. 145–149. Raven Press, New York.

DeCaro, G., Massi, M., Micossi, G. L., and Venturi, F. (1978b). Physalaemin, a new potent antidipsogen in the rat. *Neuropharmacology* **17**, 925–929.

DeCaro, G., Massi, M., Perfumi, M., and Venturi, F. (1983). Sensitivity of different nuclei of rat brain to the anti-dipsogenic effects of tachykinins. *Appetite* **4**, 198–204.

Denton, D. A. (1966). Some theoretical considerations in relation to innate appetite for salt. *Conditioned Reflex* **1**, 144–170.

Denton, D. (1982). "The Hunger for Salt." Springer Veralg, New York.

Devor, M., Wise, R. A., Milgram, N. W., and Hoebel, B. G. (1970). Physiological control of hypothalamically elicited feeding and drinking. *J. Comp. Physiol. Psychol.* **73**, 226–232.

DeWied, D. (1966). Effect of autonomic blocking agents and structurally related substances on the "salt arousal of drinking." *Physiol. Behav.* **1**, 193–197.

DiCara, L., and Wilson, L. M. (1974). Role of gustation in sodium appetite. *Physiol. Psychol.* **2**, 43–44.

Dicker, S. E., and Nunn, J. (1957). The role of antidiuretic hormone during water deprivation in rats. *J. Physiol.* **136**, 235–248.

Dickinson, C. J., and Ferrario, C. M. (1974). Central neurogenic effects of angiotensin. *In* "Angiotensin" (Handbook of Experimental Pharmacology, Vol. 37) (I. H. Page and F. M. Bumpus, eds.), pp. 408–416. Springer Verlag, Heidelberg.

Dumas, C. L. (1803). "Principes de Physiologie," Vol. IV. Deterville, Paris.

Dunn, F. L., Brennan, T. J., Nelson, A. E., and Robertson G. L. (1973). The role of blood osmolality and volume in regulating vasopressin secretion in the rat. *J. Clin. Invest.* **52**, 3212–3219.

Elattar, T. M. A. (1978). Prostaglandins: Physiology, biochemistry, pharmacology and clinical applications. *J. Oral Pathol.* **7**, 175–207.

Elfont, R. M., and Fitzsimons., J. T. (1981). Captopril induced drinking depends on and is enhanced by renin. *J. Physiol.* **319**, 71P–72P.

Elfont, R. M., and Fitzsimons, J. T. (1983). Renin-dependence of captopril-induced drinking after ureteric ligation in the rat. *J. Physiol.* **343**, 17–30.

Elfont, R. M., Epstein, A. N., and Findlay, A. L. (1980). The role of the subfornical organ in angiotensin-induced drinking in the North American opossum. *J. Physiol.* **301**, 49P.

Elfont, R. M., Epstein, A. N., and Fitzsimons, J. T. (1984). Involvement of the renin-angiotensin system in captopril-induced sodium appetite in the rat. *J. Physiol.* **354**, 11–27.

Elkinton, J. R., and Squires, R. D. (1951). The distribution of body fluids in congestive heart failure. I: Theoretic considerations. *Circulation* **4**, 679–696.

Elkinton, J. R., and Taffel, M. (1942). Prolonged water deprivation in the dog. *J. Clin. Invest.* **21**, 787–794.

Elliott, M. E., and Goodfriend, T. L. (1986). Inhibition of aldosterone synthesis by atrial natriuretic factor. *Fed. Proc.* **45**, 2376–2381.

Ellis, S., Axt, K., and Epstein, A. N. (1984). The arousal of ingestive behaviors by chemical injection into the brain of the suckling rat. *J. Neurosci.* **3**, 945–955.

Emmers, R. (1973). Interaction of neural systems which control body water. *Brain Res.* **49**, 323–347.

Eng, R., and Miselis,Z R. R. (1981). Polydipsia and abolition of angiotensin-induced drinking after transections of subfornical organ efferent projections in the rat. *Brain Res.* **225**, 200–206.

Epstein, A. N. (1960). Water intake without the act of drinking. *Science* **131**, 497–498.

Epstein, A. N. (1967). Oropharyngeal factors in feeding and drinking. *In* "Handbook of Physiology, Section 6, Alimentary Canal," Vol. I, "Control of Food and Water Intake" (C. F. Code, ed.), pp. 197–218. Williams & Wilkins, Baltimore.

Epstein, A. N. (1978). Consensus, controversies, and curiosities. *In* Angiotensin-Induced Thirst: Peripheral and Central Mechanisms (M. J. Fregly, ed.), *Fed. Proc.* **37**, 2711–2715.

Epstein, A. N. (1982). Mineralocorticoids and cerebral angiotensin may act together to produce sodium appetite. *Peptides* **3**, 493–494.

Epstein, A. N. (1983). The Neuropsychology of Drinking. *In* "Handbook of Behavioral Neurobiology," Vol. 6, "Motivation" (E. Satinoff and P. Teitelbaum, eds.), pp. 367–423. Plenum Press, New York.

Epstein, A. N. (1986). Hormonal synergy as the cause of salt appetite. *In* "The Physiology of Thirst and Sodium Appetite" (G. deCaro, A. N. Epstein, and M. Massi, eds.), pp. 395–404. Plenum Press, New York.

Epstein, A. N., and Hsiao, S. (1975). Angiotensin as dipsogen. *In* "Control Mechanisms of Drinking" (G. Peters, J. T. Fitzsimons, and L. Peters-Haefeli, eds.), pp.108–117. Springer Verlag, New York.

Epstein, A. N., and Milestone, R. (1968). Showering as a coolant for rats exposed to heat. *Science* **160**, 895–896.

Epstein, A. N., and Simpson, J. B. (1974). The dipsogenic action of angiotensin. *Acta Physiol. Latinoam.* **24**, 405–408.

Epstein, A. N., and Stellar, E. (1955). The control of salt preference in the adrenalectomized rat. *J. Comp. Physiol. Psychol.* **48**, 167–172

Epstein, A. N., and Teitelbaum, P. (1964). Severe and persistent deficits in thirst produced by lateral hypothalamic damage. *In* "Thirst in the Regulation of Body Water" (M. J. Wayner, ed.), pp. 395–406. Pergamon Press, Oxford.

Epstein, A. N., Fitzsimons, J. T., and Johnson, A. K. (1973). Prevention by angiotensin II antiserum of drinking induced by intracranial angiotensin. *J. Physiol.* **230**, 42–43.

Epstein, A. N., Fitzsimons, J. T., and Johnson, A. K. (1974). Peptide antagonists of the renin-angiotensin system and the elucidation of the receptors for angiotensin-induced drinking. *J. Physiol.* **238**, 34–35.

Epstein, A. N., Fitzsimons, J. T., and Rolls (nee Simons), B. J. (1970). Drinking induced by injection of angiotensin into the brain of the rat. *J. Physiol.* **210**, 457–474.

Epstein, A. N., Fitzsimons, J. T., and Simons, B. J. (1969). Drinking caused by the intracranial injection of angiotensin in the rat. *J. Physiol.* **200**, 98–100P.

Epstein, A. N., Spector, D., Samman, A., and Goldblum, C. (1964). Exaggerated prandial drinking in rats without salivary glands. *Nature* **201**, 1324–1325.

Epstein, A. N., Zhang, D-M., Schultz, J., Rosenberg, M., Kupsha, P., and Stellar, E. (1984). The failure of ventricular sodium to control sodium appetite in the rat. *Physiol. Behav.* **32**, 683–686.

Ericksson, L., Fernández, O., and Olsson, K. (1971). Differences in the antidiuretic response to intracarotid infusions of various hypertonic solutions in the conscious goat. *Acta Physiol. Scand.* **83**, 554–562.

Ernits, T., and Corbit, J. D. (1973). Taste as a dipsogenic stimulus. *J. Comp. Physiol. Psychol.* **83**, 27–31.

Evered, M. D., and Fitzsimons, J. T. (1976a). Drinking induced by angiotensin in the pigeon (*Columbia livia*). *J. Physiol.* **263**, 193–194P.

Evered, M. D., and Fitzsimons, J. T. (1976b). Peptide specificity of receptors for angiotensin-induced thirst in the pigeon (*Columbia livia*). *J. Physiol.* **263**, 252–253P.

Evered, M. D., and Mogenson, G. J. (1976). Regulatory and secondary water intake in rats with lesions of the zona incerta. *Am. J. Physiol.* **230**, 1049–1057.

Evered, M. D., and Mogenson, G. J. (1977). Impairment in fluid ingestion in rats with lesions of the zona incerta. *Am. J. Physiol.* **233**, R53–58.

Evered, M. D., Fitzsimons, J. T., and deCaro, G. (1977). Drinking behaviour induced by intracranial injections of eledoisin and substance P in the pigeon. *Nature* **268**, 332–333.

Evered, M. D., Robinson, M. M., and Richardson, M. A. (1980). Captopril, given intracerebroventricularly, subcutaneously or by gavage inhibits angiotensin-converting enzyme activity in the rat brain. *Eur. J. Pharmacol.* **68**, 443–449.

Falcon, J. II, Hoffman, W. E., and Phillips, M. I. (1976). The role of the sympathetic nervous system in the vasopressor and drinking response to angiotensin II. *Fed. Proc. Fed. Am. Socs. Exptl. Biol.* **35,** 651.

Falk, J. L. (1961). The behavioral regulation of water-electrolyte balance. *In* "Nebraska Symposium on Motivation" (M. R. Jones, ed.), pp. 1–33. University of Nebraska Press, Lincoln.

Falk, J. L. (1965a). Water intake and NaCl appetite in sodium depletion. *Psychol. Rep.* **16**, 315–325.

Falk, J. L. (1965b). Limitations to the specificity of NaCl appetite in sodium-depleted rats. *J. Comp. Physiol. Psychol.* **60**, 393–396.

Falk, J. L. (1966). Serial sodium depletion and NaCl solution intake. *Physiol. Behav.* **1**, 75–77.

Falk J. L., and Bryant R. W. (1973). Salivarectomy: Effect on drinking produced by isoproterenol, diazoxide and NaCl loads. *Pharmacol. Biochem. Behav.* **1**, 207–210.

Falk, J. L., and Lipton, J. M. (1967). Temporal factors in the genesis of NaCl appetite by intraperitoneal dialysis. *J. Comp. Physiol. Psychol.* **63**, 247–251.

Falk, J. L., and Tang, M. (1973). Nonuremic hyperosmolality produced by sodium depletion. *Physiol. Behav.* **10**, 793–799.

Falk, J. L., and Tang, M. (1980). Rapid sodium depletion and salt appetite induced by intraperitoneal dialysis. *In* "Biological and Behavioral Aspects of Salt Intake" (M. R. Kare, M. J. Fregly, and R. A. Bernard, eds.). pp. 205–220. Academic Press, New York.

Falk, J. L., Forman, S., and Tang, M. (1973). Dissociation of dipsogenic and depressor responses produced by hypotensive agents. *Pharmacol. Biochem. Behav.* **1**, 709–718.

Feldberg, W. (1975). Body temperature and fever: Changes in our views during the last decade. *Proc. R. Soc. Lond. Ser. B* **191**, 199–229.

Feldberg, W., and Saxena, P. N. (1971). Fever produced by prostaglandin E_1. *J. Physiol.* **217**, 547–556.

Feldberg, W., and Saxena, P. N. (1975). Prostaglandins, endotoxin and lipid A on body temperature in rats. *J. Physiol.* **249**, 601–615.

Felix, D. (1976). Peptide and acetylcholine interaction on neurones of the cat subfornical organ. *Arch. Pharmacol.* **292**, 15–20.

Felix, D., and Akert, K. (1974). The effect of angiotensin II on neurons of the cat subfornical organ. *Brain Res.* **76**, 350–353.

Felix, D., and Schlegel, W. (1978). Angiotensin receptive neurons in the subfornical organ. Structure-activity relations. *Brain Res.* **149**, 107–116.

Felix, D., Schelling, P., and Haas, H. L. (1982). Angiotensin in single neurons. *In* "Experimental Brain Research (Suppl. 4)" (D. Ganten, M. Printz, M. I. Phillips, and B. Schölkens, eds.), pp. 255–269. Springer Verlag, Heidelberg.

Felix, D., Gambino, M. C., Yong, Y., and Schelling, P. (1986). Angiotensin-sensitive sites in the central nervous system. *In* "The Physiology of Thirst and Sodium Appetite" (G. deCaro, A. N. Epstein, and M. Massi, eds.), pp. 135–140. Plenum Press, New York.

Ferrario, C. M., Gildenberg, P. L., and McCubbin, J. W. (1972). Cardiovascular effects of angiotensin mediated by the central nervous system. *Circ. Res.* **30**, 257–262.

Ferreyra, M. C., and Chiaraviglio, E. (1977). hanges in volemia and natremia and onset of sodium appetitie in sodium depleted rats. *Physiol. Behav.* **19**, 197–201.

Feuerstein, G., Krausz, M., and Gutman, Y. (1978). Effect of indomethacin on water intake of the rat. *Pharmacol. Biochem. Behav.* **9**, 893–894.

Fibiger, H. C., Phillips, A. G., and Clolston, R. A. (1973a). Regulatory deficits after unilateral electrolytic or 6-OHDA lesions of the substantia nigra. *Am. J. Physiol.* **225**, 1282–1287.

Fibiger, H. C., Zis, A. P., and McGeer, E. G. (1973b). Feeding and drinking deficits after 6-hydroxydopamine administration in the rat: Similarities to the lateral hypothalamic syndrome. *Brain Res.* **55**, 135–148.

Findlay, A. L. R., and Epstein, A. N. (1980). Increased sodium intake is somehow induced in rats by intravenous angiotensin II. *Hormones Behav.* **14**, 86–92.

Findlay, A. L. R., Elfont, R. M., and Epstein, A. N. (1980). The site of the dipsogenic action of angiotensin II in the North American opossum. *Brain Res.* **198**, 85–94.

Fisher, A. E. (1973). Relationship between cholinergic and other dipsogens in the central mediation of thirst. *In* "The Neuropsychology of Thirst: New Findings and Advances in Concepts" (A. N. Epstein, H. R. Kissileff, and E. Stellar, eds.), pp. 243–278. Wiley and Sons, New York.

Fisher, A. E., and Buggy, J. (1975). Central mediation of water and sodium intake: A dual role for angiotensin? *In* "Control Mechanisms of Drinking" (G. Peters, J. T. Fitzsimons, and L. Peters-Haefeli, eds.), pp. 138–147. Springer Verlag, New York.

Fisher, A. E., and Coury, J. (1962). Cholinergic tracing of a central neural circuit underlying the thirst drive. *Science* **138**, 691–693.

Fisher, A. E., and Levitt, R. A. (1967). Drinking induced by carbachol: Thirst circuit or ventricular modification? An answer to Routtenberg. *Science* **157**, 838–841.

Fitzsimons, J. T. (1957). Normal drinking in rats. *J. Physiol.* **138**, 39P.

Fitzsimons, J. T. (1961a). Drinking by nephrectomized rats injected with various substances. *J. Physiol.* **155**, 563–579.

Fitzsimons, J. T. (1961b). Drinking by rats depleted of body fluid without increase in osmotic pressure. *J. Physiol.* **159**, 297–309.

Fitzsimons, J. T. (1963). The effect of slow infusions of hypertonic solutions on drinking and drinking thresholds in rats. *J. Physiol.* **167**, 344–354.

Fitzsimons, J. T. (1964). Drinking caused by constriction of the inferior vena cava in the rat. *Nature* **204**, 479–480.

Fitzsimons, J. T. (1966). Hypovolemic drinking and renin. *J. Physiol.* **186**, 130–131.

Fitzsimons, J. T. (1967). The kidney as a thirst receptor. *J. Physiol.* **191**, 128–129.

Fitzsimons, J. T. (1969a). The role of renal thirst factor in drinking induced by extracellular stimuli. *J. Physiol.* **201**, 349–368.

Fitzsimons, J. T. (1969b). Effects of nephrectomy on the additivity of certain stimuli of drinking in the rat. *J. Comp. Physiol. Psychol.* **68**, 308–314.

Fitzsimons, J. T. (1970a). The renin-angiotensin system in the control of drinking. *In* "The Hypothalamus" (L. Martini, M. Motta, and F. Fraschini, eds.), pp. 195–212. Academic Press, New York.

Fitzsimons, J. T. (1970b). Interactions of intracranially administered renin or angiotensin and other thirst stimuli on drinking. *J. Physiol.* **210**, 152–153P.

Fitzsimons, J. T. (1971a). The effect on drinking of peptide precursors and of shorter chain peptide fragments of angiotensin II injected into the rat's diencephalon. *J. Physiol.* **214**, 295–303.

Fitzsimons, J. T. (1971b). The hormonal control of water and sodium intake. *In* "Frontiers in Neuroendocrinology" (L. Martini and W. F. Ganong, eds.), pp. 103–128. Oxford University Press, New York.

Fitzsimons, J. T. (1971c). The physiology of thirst: A review of the extraneural aspects of the mechanisms of drinking. *In* "Progress in Physiological Psychology," Vol. 4 (E. Stellar and J. M. Sprague, eds.), pp. 119–201. Academic Press, New York.

Fitzsimons, J. T. (1972). Thirst. *Physiol. Rev.* **52**, 468–561.

Fitzsimons, J. T. (1973). Angiotensin as a thirst regulating hormone. *In* "Endocrinology" (R. O. Scow, F. J. G. Ebling, and I. W. Henderson, eds.), pp. 711–716. Excerpta Medica, Amsterdam.

Fitzsimons, J. T. (1975). The renin-angiotensin system and drinking behavior. *In* Hormones, homeostasis and the brain (W. H. Gispen, T. B. van Wimersma Greidanus, B. Bohus, and D. de Wied, eds.). *Prog. Brain Res.* **42**, 215–233.

Fitzsimons, J. T. (1979). "The Physiology of Thirst and Sodium Appetite." Cambridge University Press, Cambridge.

Fitzsimons, J. T. (1986). Endogenous angiotensin and sodium appetite. *In* "The Physiology of Thirst and Sodium Appetite" (G. deCaro, A. N. Epstein, and M. Massi, eds.), pp. 383–394. Plenum Press, New York.

Fitzsimons, J. T. and Evered, M. D. (1977). Angiotensin and the regulation of water balance. In: "Endocrinology, Vol. I" (V. James ed.), pp. 57–61. Excerpta Medica, Amsterdam.

Fitzsimons, J. T., and Kaufman, S. (1977). Cellular and extracellular dehydration and angiotensin as stimuli to drinking in the common iguana. *J. Physiol.* **265**, 443–463.

Fitzsimons, J. T., and Kucharczyk, J. (1978). Drinking and haemodynamic changes induced in the dog by intracranial injection of components of the renin-angiotensin system. *J. Physiol.* **276**, 419–434.

Fitzsimons, J. T., and LeMagnen, J. (1969). Eating as a regulatory control of drinking in the rat. *J. Comp. Physiol. Psychol.* **67**, 273–283.

Fitzsimons, J. T., and Moore-Gillon, M. J. (1979). Short-latency, graded drinking response to reduction in venous return in the dog. *J. Physiol.* **295**, 76P.

Fitzsimons, J. T., and Moore-Gillon, M. J. (1980a). Pulmo-atrial junctional receptors and the inhibition of drinking. *J. Physiol.* **307**, 74–75P.

Fitzsimons, J. T., and Moore-Gillon, M. J. (1980b). Drinking and antidiuresis in response to reductions in venous return in the dog: Neural and endocrine mechanisms. *J. Physiol.* **308**, 403–416.

Fitzsimons, J. T., and Oatley, K. (1968). Additivity of stimuli for drinking in rats. *J. Comp. Physiol. Psychol.* **66**, 450–455.

Fitzsimons, J. T., and Setler, P. E. (1971). Catecholaminergic mechanisms in angiotensin-induced drinking. *J. Physiol.* **218**, 43–44P.

Fitzsimons, J. T., and Setler, P. E. (1975). The relative importance of central nervous catecholaminergic and cholinergic mechanisms in drinking response to angiotensin and other thirst stimuli. *J. Physiol.* **250**, 613–631.

Fitzsimons, J. T., and Simons, B. J. (1968). The effect of angiotensin on drinking in the rat. *J. Physiol.* **196**, 39–41P.

Fitzsimons, J. T., and Simons, B. J. (1969). The effect on drinking in the rat of intravenous infusions of angiotensin, given alone or in combination with other stimuli of thirst. *J. Physiol.* **203**, 45–57.

Fitzsimons, J. T., and Stricker, E. M. (1971). Sodium appetite and the renin-angiotensin system. *Nature* **231**, 58–60.

Fitzsimons, J. T., and Szczepanska-Sadowska E. (1974). Drinking and antidiuresis elicited by isoprenaline in the dog. *J. Physiol.* **239**, 251–267.

Fitzsimons, J. T., and Wirth, J. B. (1976). The neuroendocrinology of thirst and sodium appetite. *In* "Central Nervous Control of Na$^+$ Balance—Relations to the Renin-Angiotensin System" (W. Kaufman and D. K. Krause, eds.), pp. 80–93. Georg Thieme, Stuttgart.

Fitzsimons, J. T., and Wirth, J. B. (1978). The renin-angiotensin system and sodium appetite. *J. Physiol.* **274**, 63–80.

Fitzsimons, J. T., Epstein, A. N., and Johnson, A. K. (1978a). Peptide antagonists of the renin-angiotensin system in the characterization of the receptors for angiotensin-induced thirst. *Brain Res.* **153**, 319–331.

Fitzsimons, J. T., Kucharczyk, J., and Richards, G. (1978b). Systemic angiotensin-induced drinking in the dog: A physiological phenomenon. *J. Physiol.* **276**, 435–448.

Fitzsimons, J. T., Massi, M., and Thornton, S. N. (1981). Permissive effect of cerebrospinal fluid (Na) on drinking in response to cellular dehydration in the pigeon *Columbia livia*. *J. Physiol.* **315**, 14P.

Fluharty, S. J. (1981). Cerebral prostaglandin biosynthesis and angiotensin-induced drinking in rats. *J. Comp. Physiol. Psychol.* **95**, 915–923.

Fluharty, S. J., and Epstein, A. N. (1980). Effects of intracerebroventricular arachidonic acid and indomethacin on angiotensin-induced drinking. *In* "Advances in Prostaglandin and Thromboxin Research," Vol. 8 (B. Samuelson, P. W. Ramwell, and R. Paoletti, eds.), pp. 1231–1234. Raven Press, New York.

Fluharty, S. J., and Epstein, A. N. (1983). Sodium appetite elicited by intracerebroventricular infusion of angiotensin II in the rat: II. Synergistic interaction with systemic mineralocorticoids. *Behav. Neuroscience* **97**, 746–758.

Fluharty, S. J., and Manaker, S. (1983). Sodium appetite elicited by intracerebroventricular infusion of angiotensin II in the rat: I. Relationship to urinary sodium excretion. *Behav. Neurosci.* **97**, 738–745.

Franklin, K. B., and Quartermain, D. (1970). Comparison of the motivational properties of deprivation induced drinking elicited by central carbachol stimulation. *J. Comp. Physiol. Psychol.* **71**, 390–395.

Frankmann, S. P., Dorsa, D. M., Sakai, R. R., and Simpson, J. B. (1986). A single experience with hyperoncotic colloid dialysis persistently alters water and sodium intake. *In* "The Physiology of Thirst and Sodium Appetite" (G. deCaro, A. N. Epstein, and M. Massi, eds.), pp. 115–121. Plenum Press, New York.

Freeman, R. H., Davis, J. O., and Vari, R. C. (1985). Renal response to atrial natriuretic factor in conscious dogs with caval constriction. *Am. J. Physiol.* **248**, R495–500.

Fregly, M. J. (1980). Effect of the angiotensin converting enzyme inhibitor, captopril, on NaCl appetite of rats. *J. Pharmacol. Exp. Ther.* **215**, 407–412.

Fregley, M. J., and Kelleher, D. L. (1980). Antidipsogenic effect of clonidine on isoproterenol-induced water intake. *Appetite* **1**, 279–289.

Fregly, M. J., and Rowland, N. E. (1986). Role for alpha-$_2$-adrenoreceptors in experimentally-induced drinking in rats. *In* "The Physiology of Thirst and Sodium Appetite" (G. deCaro, A. N. Epstein, and M. Massi, eds.), pp. 509–519. Plenum Press, New York.

Fregly, M. J., and Waters, W. I. (1966a). Effect of mineralocorticoids on spontaneous sodium chloride appetite of adrenalectomized rats. *Physiol. Behav.* **1**, 65–74.

Fregly, M. J., and Waters, W. I. (1966b). Effect of desoxycorticosterone acetate on NaCl appetite of propylthiouracil-treated rats. *Physiol. Behav.* **1**, 133–138.

Fregly, M. J., Greenleaf, J. E., and Rowland, N. E. (1986). Effects of intraperitoneal and intragastric loading with water and isosmotic solutions of saline and glucose on water intake of dehydrated rats. *Brain Res. Bull.* **16**, 415–420.

Fregley, M. J., Rowland, N. E., and Greenleaf, J. E. (1983). Effects of yohimbine and tolazoline on isoproterenol- and angiotensin II-induced water intake in rats. *Brain Res. Bull.* **10**, 121–126.

Fuller, L. M., and Fitzsimons, J. T. (1986). Influence of sodium load on angiotensin-induced sodium appetite. *In* "The Physiology of Thirst and Sodium Appetite" (G. deCaro, A. N. Epstein, and M. Massi, eds.), pp. 419–424. Plenum Press, New York.

Gandelman, R. J., Panksepp, J., and Trowill, J. (1968). Preference behavior differences between water deprivation-induced and carbachol-induced drinkers. *Commun. Behav. Biol. A* **1**, 341–346.

Ganong, W. F. (1971). "Review of Medical Physiology," pp. 264–287. Lange Medical Publications, Los Altos, Calif.

Ganong, W. F. (1972). Sympathetic effects of renin secretion: Mechanism and physiological role. *In* "Control of Renin Secretion" (T. A. Assaykeen, ed.), Vol. 17: "Advances in Experimental Medicine and Biology," pp. 17–32. Plenum Press, New York.

Ganong, W. F. (1984). The brain renin-angiotensin system. *Annu. Rev. Physiol.* **46**, 17–31.

Ganten, D., Fuxe, K., Phillips, M. I., Mann, J. F. E., and Ganten, U. (1978). The brain isorenin-angiotensin system: Biochemistry, localization, and possible role in drinking and blood pressure regulation. *In* "Frontiers in Neuroendocrinology," Vol. 5 (W. F. Ganong and L. Martini, eds.), pp. 61–100. Raven Press, New York.

Ganten, D., Hutchinson, S., and Schelling, P. (1975). The intrinsic brain iso-renin angiotensin system: Its possible role in central mechanisms of blood pressure regulation. *Clin. Sci. Mol. Med.* **48**, 265s–268s.

Ganten, D., Hutchinson, J. S., Schelling, P., Ganten, U., and Fischer, H. (1976). The isorenin angiotensin systems in extrarenal tissue. *Clin. Exp. Pharmacol. Physiol.* **3**, 103–126.

Garay, K. F., and Leibowitz, S. F. (1974). Antidiuresis is produced by adrenergic receptor stimulation of the supraoptic nucleus. *Fed. Proc.* **33**, 563 (Abstr.).

Gardiner, T. W., and Stricker, E. M. (1985a). Hyperdipsia in rats after electrolytic lesions of nucleus medianus. *Am. J. Physiol.* **248**, R214–223.

Gardiner, T. W., and Stricker, E. M. (1985b). Impaired drinking responses of rats with lesions of nucleus medianus: Circadian dependence. *Am. J. Physiol.* **248**, R224–230.

Gardiner, T. W., Verbalis, J. G., and Stricker, E. M. (1985). Impaired secretion of vasopressin and oxytocin in rats after lesions of nucleus medianus. *Am. J. Physiol.* **249**, R681-R688.

Gardiner, T. W., Jolley, J. R., Vagnucci, A. H., and Stricker, E. M. (1986). Enhanced sodium appetite in rats with lesion centered upon nucleus medianus. *Behav. Neurosci.* **100**, 531–535.

Gehlert, D. R., Speth, R. C., and Wamsley, J. K. (1986). Distribution of [^{125}I]angiotensin binding sites in the rat brain: a quantitative autoradiographic study. *Neurosci.* **18**, 837–856.

Gellai, M., Allen, D. E., and Beeuwkes R. (1986). Contrasting views on the action of atrial peptides: lessons from studies of conscious animals. *Fed. Proc.* **45**, 2387–2391.

Gentil, C. G., Antunes-Rodrigues, J., Négro-Vilar, A., and Covian, M. R. (1968). Role of amygdaloid complex in sodium chloride and water intake in the rat. *Physiol. Behav.* **3**, 981–985.

Gentil, C. G., Mogenson, G. J., and Stevenson, J. A. F. (1971). Electrical stimulation of septum, hypothalamus, and amygdala and saline preference. *Am. J. Physiol.* **220**, 1172–1177.

Gerald, M. C., and Maikel, R. P. (1972). Studies on the possible role of brain histamine in behaviour. *Br. J. Pharmacol.* **44**, 462–471.

Giardina, A. R., and Fisher, A. E. (1971). Effect of atropine on drinking induced by carbachol, angiotensin and isoproterenol. *Physiol. Behav.* **7**, 653–655.

Gilman, A. (1937). The relation between blood osmotic pressure, fluid distribution, and voluntary water intake. *Am. J. Physiol.* **120**, 323–328.

Gold, R. M. (1967). Aphagia and adipsia following unilateral and bilaterally asymmetrical lesions in rats. *Physiol. Behav.* **2**, 211–220.

Goldstein, D. J., Marante-Perez, D. J., Gunst, J. P., and Jalperin, J. A. (1979). Prostaglandin E$_1$ inhibits acute cell dehydration thirst. *Pharmacol. Biochem. Behav.* **10**, 895–898.

Gordon, F. J., Haywood, J. R., Brody, M. J., and Johnson, A. K. (1982). Effect of ablation of an angiotensin and osmosensitive brain region on the development of hypertension in spontaneously hypertensive rats. *Hypertension* **4**, 387–393.

Grace, J. E. (1968). Central nervous system lesions and saline intake in the rat. *Physiol. Behav.* **3**, 387–393.

Greer, M. A. (1955). Suggestive evidence of a primary "drinking center" in hypothalamus of the rat. *Proc. Soc. Exp. Biol. Med.* **89**, 59–62.

Grill, H. J., Schulkin, J., and Flynn, F. W. (1986). Sodium homeostasis in chronic decerebrate rats. *Behav. Neurosci.* **100**, 536–543.

Gross, F., Brunner, H., and Ziegler, M. (1965). Renin-angiotensin system, aldosterone, and sodium balance. *Recent Prog. Horm. Res.* **21**, 119–127.

Gross, J. B., and Bartter, F. C. (1973). Effects of prostaglandins E_1, A_1, and F_2 on renal handling of salt and water. *Am. J. Physiol.* **225**, 218–225.

Grossman, S. P. (1960). Eating or drinking elicited by direct adrenergic or cholinergic stimulation of hypothalamus. *Science* **132**, 301–302.

Grossman, S. P. (1962a). Direct adrenergic and cholinergic stimulation of hypothalamic mechanisms. *Am. J. Physiol.* **202**, 872–882.

Grossman, S. P. (1962b). Effects of adrenergic and cholinergic blocking agents on hypothalamic mechanisms. *Am. J. Physiol.* **202**, 1230–1236.

Grossman, S. P. (1964). Effects of chemical stimulation of the septal area on motivation. *J. Comp. Physiol. Psychol.* **58**, 194–200.

Grossman, S. P. (1971). Changes in food and water intake associated with an interruption of the anterior or posterior fiber connections of the hypothalamus. *J. Comp. Physiol. Psychol.* **75**, 23–31.

Grossman, S. P. (1984). A reasessment of the brain mechanisms that control thirst. *Neurosci. Biobehav. Rev.* **8**, 95–104.

Grossman, S. P. (1986). The role of the zona incerta in water intake regulation. *In* "The Physiology of Thirst and Sodium Appetite" (G. de Caro, A. N. Epstein, and M. Massi, eds.), pp. 355–360. Plenum Press, New York.

Grossman, S. P., and Grossman, L. (1971). Food and water intake in rats with parasagittal knife cuts medial and lateral to the lateral hypothalamus. *J. Comp. Physiol. Psychol.* **74**, 148–156.

Grossman, S. P., and Grossman, L. (1973). Persisting deficits in rats "recovered" from transections of the fibers which enter or leave the hypothalamus laterally. *J. Comp. Physiol. Psychol.* **85**, 515–527.

Grossman, S. P., and Grossman, L. (1977). Food and water intake in rats after transections of fibers en passage in the tementum. *Physiol. Behav.* **18**, 647–658.

Grossman, S. P., and Grossman, L. (1978). Parametric study of the regulatory capabilities of rats with rostromedial zona incerta lesions: Responsiveness to hypertonic saline and polyethylene glycol. *Physiol. Behav.* **21**, 432–440.

Grossman, S. P., and Grossman, L. (1982). Iontophoretic injections of kainic acid into the rat lateral hypothalamus: Effects on ingestive behavior. *Physiol. Behav.* **29**, 553–559.

Grossman, S. P., and Hennessy, J. W. (1976). Differential effects of coronal cuts through the posterior hypothalamus on food intake and body weight in male and female rats. *Physiol. Behav.* **17**, 89–102.

Grossman, S. P., Grossman, L., and Halaris, A. E. (1977). Effects on hypothalamic and telencephalic NE and 5-HT of tegmental knife cuts that produce hyperphagia and hyperdipsia in the rat. *Pharmacol. Biochem. Behav.* **6**, 101–106.

Grossman, S. P., Dacey, D., Hallaris, A. E., Collier, T., and Routtenberg, A. (1978). Aphagia and adipsia after preferential destruction of nerve cell bodies in the hypothalamus. *Science* **202**, 557–559.

Gutman, Y., Benzakein, F., and Livneh, F. (1971). Polydipsia induced by isoprenaline and by lithium: Relations to kidney and renin. *Eur. J. Pharmacol.* **16**, 380–384.

Gutman, Y., and Krausz, M. (1973). Drinking induced by dextran and histamine: Relation to kidneys and renin. *Eur. J. Pharmacol.* **23**, 256–263.

Guyton, A. C. (1987). "Human Physiology and Mechanisms of Disease," 4th Ed. W. B. Saunders, Philadelphia.

Haber, E. (1976). The role of renin in normal and pathological cardiovascular homeostasis. *Circulation* **54**, 849–861.

Haberich, J. J. (1968). Osmoreception in the portal system. *Fed. Proc.* **27**, 1137–1141.

Hainsworth, F. R. (1967). Saliva spreading, activity and body temperature regulation in the rat. *Am. J. Physiol.* **212**, 1288–1292.

Hall, W. G. (1973). A remote stomach clamp to evaluate oral and gastric controls of drinking in the rat. *Physiol. Behav.* **11**, 897–901.

Hall, W. G., and Blass, E. M. (1975). Orogastric, hydrational and behavioral controls of drinking following water deprivation in rats. *J. Comp. Physiol. Psychol.* **89**, 939–954.

Hall, W. G., and Blass, E. M. (1977). Orogastric determinants of drinking in rats: Interaction between absorptive and peripheral controls. *J. Comp. Physiol. Psychol.* **91**, 365–373.

Hall, W., Blass, E. M., and Russell, J. (1976). Oropharyngeal control of drinking in rats. *J. Comp. Physiol. Psychol.* **9**, 909–916.

Haller, A. (1764). Fames et sitis. *In* "Elementa Physiologiae Corporis Humanis," Vol. 6, pp. 164–187. Sumptibus Societatis Typographicae, Berne.

Hartle, D. K., Haywood, J. R., Johnson, A. K., and Brody, M. J. (1979). The effect of anteroventral third ventricle (AV3V) lesions of plasma renin activity in the Grollman model of renal hypertension. *Fed. Proc.* **38**, 1233.

Hartzell, A. K., Paulus, R. A., and Schulkin, J. (1985). Brief preoperative exposure to saline protects rats against behavioral impairments in salt appetite following central gustatory damage. *Behav. Brain Res.* **15**, 9–13.

Harvey, J. A., and Hunt, H. F. (1965). Effects of septal lesions on thirst in the rat as indicated by water consumption and operant responding for water reward. *J. Comp. Physiol. Psychol.* **59**, 49–56.

Hatton, G. I. (1976). Nucleus circularis: is it an osmoreceptor in the brain? *Brain Res. Bull.* **1**, 123–131.

Hatton, G. I., and Bennett, C. T. (1970). Satiation of thirst and termination of drinking: Roles of plasma osmolality and absorption. *Physiol. Behav.* **5**, 479–487.

Hayward, J. N., and Vincent, J. D. (1970). Osmosensitive single neurons in the hypothalamus of unanesthetized monkeys. *J. Physiol.* **210**, 947–992.

Haywood, J. R., Fink, G. D., Buggy, J., Boutelle, S., Johnson, A. K., and Brody, M. J. (1983). Prevention of two-kidney one-clip renal hypertension in the rat by ablation of anteroventral third ventricle (AV3V) tissue. *Am. J. Physiol.* **245**, H683-H689.

Healy, D. P., and Printz, M. P. (1984). Distribution of immunoreactive angiotensin II, angiotensin I, angiotensinogen and renin in the CNS of intact and nephrectomized rats. *Hypertension* **6**, 1–130.

Hendler, N. H., and Blake, W. D. (1969). Hypothalamic implants of angiotensin II, carbachol, and norepinephrine on water and NaCl solution intake in rats. *Commun. Behav. Biol.* **4**, 41–48.

Hendry, D. P., and Rasche, R. H. (1961). Analysis of a new non-nutritive positive reinforcer based on thirst. *J. Comp. Physiol. Psychol.* **54**, 477–483.

Hennessy, J. W., and Grossman, S. P. (1976). Overeating and obesity produced by interruption of the caudal connections of the hypothalamus: Evidence of hormonal and metabolic disruption. *Physiol. Behav.* **17**, 103–110.

Hennessy, J. W., Grossman, S. P., and Kanner, M. A. (1977). A study of the etiology of the hyperdipsia produced by coronal knife cuts in the posterior hypothalamus. *Physiol. Behav.* **18**, 73–80.

Hernández-Peon, R., Chavez-Ibarra, G., Morgane, P. J., and Timo-Iaria, C. (1962). Cholinergic pathways for sleep, alertness and rage in the limbic midbrain circuit. *Acta Neurol. Latinoam.* **8**, 93–96.

Hill, D. L., and Almli, C. R. (1983). Parabrachial nuclei damage in infant rats produces residual deficits in gustatory preferences/aversions and sodium appetite. *Dev. Psychobiol.* **16**, 519–533.

Hirano, T., Takei, Y., and Kobayashi, H. (1978). Angiotensin and drinking in the eel and frog. *In* "Osmotic and Volume Regulation" (C. Barker Jorgenson and E. Skadhaupe, eds.), pp. 123–128. Munksgaard, Copenhagen.

Hoffman, W. E., and Phillips, M. I. (1976a). Evidence for Sar[1]-Ala[8]-Angiotensin crossing the blood cerebrospinal fluid barrier to antagonize central effects of angiotensin II. *Brain Res.* **109**, 541–552.

Hoffman, W. E., and Phillips, M. I. (1976b). Regional study of cerebral ventricle sensitive sites to angiotensin II. *Brain Res.* **110**, 541–552.

Hoffman, W. E., and Phillips, M. I. (1976c). The effect of subfornical organ lesions and ventricular blockade on drinking induced by angiotensin II. *Brain Res.* **108**, 59–73.

Hoffman, W. E., and Phillips, M. I. (1976d). A pressor response to intraventricular injections of carbachol. *Brain Res.* **108**, 59–73.

Hoffman, W. E., and Phillips, M. I. (1977). The role of ADH in the pressor response to intra-ventricular angiotensin II. *In* "Central Actions of Angiotensin" (J. P. Buckley and C. Ferrario, eds.), Pergamon Press, New York.

Hoffman, W. E., and Schmid, P. G. (1979). Cardiovascular and antidiuretic effects of central prostaglandin E_2. *J. Physiol.* **288**, 159–169.

Hoffman, W. E., Ganten, U., Phillips, M. I., Schmid, P. G., Schelling, P., and Ganten, D. (1978). Inhibition of drinking in water-deprived rats by combined central angiotensin II and cholinergic receptor blockade. *Am. J. Physiol.* **234**, F41-F47.

Hoffman, W. E., Schmid, P. G., Phillips, M. I., Falcon, J., and Weet, J. F. (1977). Release of pressor amounts of antidiuretic hormone by intraventricular injections of angiotensin II and carbachol. *Neuropharmacology* **16**, 463–472.

Holman, G. (1969). Intragastric reinforcement effect. *J. Comp. Physiol. Psychol.* **69**, 432–441.

Holmes, J. H., and Cizek, L. J. (1951). Observations on sodium chloride depletion in the dog. *Am. J. Physiol.* **164**, 407–414.

Holmes, J. H., and Gregersen, M. I. (1947). Relation of the salivary flow to the thirst produced in man by intravenous injection of hypotonic salt solution. *Am. J. Physiol.* **151**, 252–257.

Holmes, J. H., and Gregersen, M. I. (1950). Observations on drinking induced by hypertonic solutions. *Am. J. Physiol.* **162**, 326–337.

Holmes, J. H., and Montgomery, A. V. (1951). Observations on relation of hemorrhage to thirst. *Am. J. Physiol.* **167**, 796 (Abstr.).

Holmes, J. H., and Montgomery, A. V. (1953). Thirst as a symptom. *Am. J. Med. Sci.* **225**, 281–286.

Horovitz, Z. P. (1981). "Angiotensin Converting Enzyme Inhibitors." Urban and Schwarzenberg, Baltimore.

Hosutt, J. A., Rowland, N., and Stricker, E. M. (1978). Hypotension and thirst in rats after isoproterenol treatment. *Physiol. Behav.* **21**, 593–598.

Hosutt, J. A., Rowland, N., and Stricker, E. M. (1981). Impaired drinking responses of rats with lesions of the subfornical organ. *J. Comp. Physiol. Psychol.* **95**, 104–113.

Houpt, K. A., and Epstein, A. N. (1971). The complete dependence of beta-adrenergic drinking on the renal dipsogen. *Physiol. Behav.* **7**, 897–902.

Hsiao, S., Epstein, A. N., and Camardo, J. S. (1977). The dipsogenic potency of intravenous angiotensin. *Horm. Behav.* **8**, 129–140.

Huang, K. C. (1955). Effect of salt depletion and fasting on water exchange in the rabbit. *Am. J. Physiol.* **181**, 609–615.

Huang, Y., and Mogenson, G. (1972). Neural pathways mediating drinking and feeding in rats. *Exp. Neurol.* **37**, 269–286.

Hunt, J. N. (1956). Some properties of an alimentary osmoreceptor mechanism. *J. Physiol.* **132**, 267–288.

Hunt, J. N., and Stubbs, D. F. (1975). The volume and energy content of meals as determinants of gastric emptying. *J. Physiol.* **245**, 209–225.

Hutchinson, R. R., and Renfrew, J. W. (1967). Modification of eating and drinking: Interactions between chemical agent, deprivation state, and site of stimulation. *J. Comp. Physiol. Psychol.* **63**, 408–416.

Ishibashi, S., Oomura, Y., Gueguen, B., and Nicolaidis, S. (1985). Neuronal responses in subfornical organ and other regions to angiotensin II applied by various routes. *Brain Res. Bull.* **14**, 307–314.

Iovino, M., and Steardo, L. (1986). The role of the septal area in the regulation of drinking behavior and plasma ADH secretion. *In* "The Physiology of Thirst and Sodium Appetite" (G. deCaro, A. N. Epstein, and M. Massi, eds.), pp. 367–374. Plenum Press, New York.

Iovino, M., Poenaru, S., and Annunziato, L. (1983). Basal and thirst-evoked vasopressin secretion in rats with electrolytic lesions of the medio-ventral septal area. *Brain Res.* **258**, 123–126.

Jacquin, M. F. (1983). Gustation and ingestive behavior in the rat. *Behav. Neurosci.* **97**, 98–109.

Jacquin, M. F., and Zeigler, H. P. (1983). Trigeminal orosensation and ingestive behavior in the rat. *Behav. Neurosci.* **97**, 62–97.

Jalowiec, J. E., and Stricker, E. M. (1970a). Restoration of body fluid balance following acute sodium deficiency in rats. *J. Comp. Physiol. Psychol.* **70**, 238–244.

Jalowiec, J. E., and Stricker, E. M. (1970b).Sodium appetite in rats after apparent recovery from acute sodium deficiency. *J. Comp. Physiol. Psychol.* **73**, 238–244.

Jalowiec, J. E., Crapanzano, J. E., and Stricker, E. M. (1966). Specificity of salt appetite by hypovolemia. *Psychonom. Sci.* **6**, 331–332.

Janssen, S. (1936). Pharmacologische Beinflussung des Durstes. *Arch. Exp. Pathol. Pharmakol.* **181**, 126–127.

Jerome, C., and Smith, G. P. (1982a). Gastric vagotomy inhibits drinking after hypertonic saline. *Physiol. Behav.* **28**, 371–374.

Jerome, C., and Smith, G. P. (1982b). Gastric or coeliac vagotomy decreases drinking after peripheral angiotensin II. *Physiol. Behav.* **29**, 533–536.

Jerome, C., and Smith, G. P. (1984). Development of the drinking deficit to hypertonic saline in rats after abdominal vagotomy. *Physiol. Behav.* **32**, 819–821.

Jeulin, A. C., and Nicolaidis, S. (1986). Integrative rostromedial diencephalic neurons are comodulated by vasopressin and angiotensin. *In* "The Physiology of Thirst and

Sodium Appetite" (G. deCaro, A. N. Epstein, and M. Massi, eds.), pp. 43–57. Plenum Press, New York.

Johnson, A. K. (1975). The role of the cerebral ventricular system in angiotensin-induced thirst. *In* "Control Mechanisms of Drinking" (G. Peters, J. T. Fitzsimons, and L. Peters-Haefeli, eds.), pp. 117–122. Springer Verlag, New York.

Johnson, A. K. (1979). Role of the periventricular tissue of the anteroventral third ventricle in body fluid homeostasis. *In* "Nervous System and Hypertension" (P. Meyer and H. Schmitt, eds.), pp. 106–114. John Wiley and Sons, New York.

Johnson, A. K. (1983). Periventricular structures of the lamina terminalis: their role in angiotensin-induced thirst. *In* "Abstracts of the Evian Symposium on Body Fluid Homeostasis" (S. Nicolaidis and J. T. Fitzsimons, eds.), p. 23. Acad. Sci., Paris.

Johnson, A. K. (1985). The periventricular anterolateral third ventricle (AV3V): Its relationship with the subfornical organ and neural systems involved in maintaining body fluid homeostasis. *Brain Res. Bull.* **15**, 595–601.

Johnson, A. K., and Buggy, J. (1977). A critical analysis of the site of action for the dipsogenic effect of angiotensin II. *In* "Central Actions of Angiotensin and Related Hormones" (J. P. Buckley and C. M. Ferrario, eds.), pp. 357–386. Pergamon Press, New York.

Johnson, A. K., and Buggy, J. (1978). Periventricular preoptic-hypothalamus is vital for thirst and normal water economy. *Am. J. Physiol.* **234**, R122–127.

Johnson, A. K., and Epstein, A. N. (1975). The cerebral ventricles as the avenue for the dipsogenic action of intracranial angiotensin. *Brain Res.* **86**, 399–418.

Johnson, A. K., and Schwob, J. E. (1975). Cephalic angiotensin receptors mediating drinking to systemic angiotensin II. *Pharmacol. Biochem. Behav.* **3**, 1077–1084.

Johnson, A. K., Hoffman, W. E., and Buggy, J. (1978). Attenuated pressor responses to intracranially injected stimuli and altered antidiuretic activity following preoptic-hypothalamic periventricular ablation. *Brain Res.* **157**, 161–166.

Johnson, A. K., Bealer, S. L., McNeil, J. R., Schoun, J., and Möhring, J. (1980). The influence of the periventricular tissue of the anteroventral third ventricle (AV3V) on the release of vasopressin (VP). *Soc. Neurosci. Abstr.* **6**, 696.

Johnson, A. K., Buggy, J., Fink, G. D., and Brody, M. J. J. (1981a). Prevention of renal hypertension and of the central pressor effect of angiotensin by ventromedial hypothalamic ablation. *Brain Res.* **205**, 225–264.

Johnson, A. K., Mann, J. F. E., Rascher, W., Johnson, J. K., and Ganten, D. (1981b). Plasma angiotensin II concentrations and experimentally induced thirst. *Am. J. Physiol.* **240**, R229–R234.

Johnson, A. K., Robinson, M. M., and Mann, J. F. E. (1986). The role of the renal renin-angiotensin system in thirst. In "The Physiology of Thirst and Sodium Appetite" (G. deCaro, A. N. Epstein, and M. Massi eds.), pp. 161–180. Plenum Press, New York.

Kakolewski, J., Deaux, E., Christensen, J., and Chase, B. (1971). Diurnal patterns in water and food intake and body weight changes in rats with lateral hypothalamic lesions. *Am. J. Physiol.* **221**, 711–718.

Kanter, G. S. (1953). Excretion and drinking after salt loading in dogs. *Am. J. Physiol.* **174**, 89–94.

Kapatos, G., and Gold, R. M. (1972a). Tongue cooling during drinking: A regulator of water intake in rats. *Science* **176**, 658–686

Kapatos, G., and Gold, R.M. (1972b). Rats drink less cool water: A change in the taste of water? *Science* **178**, 1121.

Katovich, M. J., Barney, C. C., Fregley, M., and McCaa, R. (1979). Effect of an angiotensin converting enzyme inhibitor (SQ 14,225) on β-adrenergic and angiotensin-induced thirsts. *Eur. J. Pharmacol.* **56**, 123–130.

Kaufman, S. (1984). Role of right atrial receptors in the control of drinking in the rat. *J. Physiol.* **349**, 389–396.

Kaufman, S. (1986a). Control mechanisms of salt appetite. *In* "The Physiology of Thirst and Sodium Appetite" (G. deCaro, A. N. Epstein, and M. Massi, eds.), pp. 459–463. Plenum Press, New York.

Kaufman, S. (1986b). Relationship between right atrial stretch and plasma renin activity. *In* "The Physiology of Thirst and Sodium Appetite" (G. deCaro, A. N. Epstein, and M. Massi, eds.), pp.109–114. Plenum Press, New York.

Keil, L. C., Summy-Long, J., and Severs, W. B. (1975). Release of vasopressin by angiotensin II. *Endocrinology* **96**, 1063–1064.

Kenney, N. J. (1980). A case study of the neuroendocrine control of goal-directed behavior: the interaction between angiotensin II and prostaglandin E_1 in the control of water intake. *In* "Neural Mechanisms of Goal-Directed Behavior and Learning" (R. F. Thompson, L. H. Hicks, and V. B. Shvyrkov, eds.), pp. 437–446. Academic Press, New York.

Kenney, N. J. (1986). Suppression of water intake by the E prostaglandins. *In* "The Physiology of Thirst and Sodium Appetite" (G. deCaro, A. N. Epstein, and M. Massi, eds.), pp. 227–238. Plenum Press, New York.

Kenney, N. J., and Epstein, A. N. (1978). The antidipsogenic role of the E-prostaglandins. *J. Comp. Physiol. Psychol.* **92**, 204–219.

Kenney, N. J., and Moe, K. E. (1981). The role of endogenous prostaglandin E in angiotensin-II induced drinking. *J. Comp. Physiol. Psychol.* **95**, 383–390.

Kenney, N. J., and Moe, K. E. (1982). Cellular dehydration and hypovolemia: Effect of acetylsalicylic acid on drinking. *Pharmacol. Biochem. Behav.* **17**, 73–76.

Kenney, N. J., and Perara, E. (1980). Pressor action of centrally administered prostaglandin E_1. *In* "Advances in Prostaglandin and Thromboxane Research," Vol. 8 (B. Samuelson, P. W. Ramwell, and R. Paoletti, eds.), Raven Press, New York.

Kenney, N. J., Moe, K. E., and Skoog, K. M. (1981). The antidipsogenic action of peripheral prostaglandin E$_2$. *Pharmacol. Biochem. Behav.* **15**, 263–269.

King, B. M., and Grossman, S. P. (1977). Response to glucoprivic and hydrational challenges by normal and hypothalamic hyperphagic rats. *Physiol. Behav.* **18**, 463–473.

Kissileff, H. R. (1969a). Food associated drinking in the rat. *J. Comp. Physiol. Psychol.* **67**, 284–300.

Kissileff, H. R. (1969b). Oropharyngeal control of prandial drinking. *J. Comp. Physiol. Psychol.* **67**, 309–319.

Kissileff, H. R. (1971). Acquisition of prandial drinking in weanling rats recovering from lateral hypothalamic lesions. *J. Comp. Physiol. Psychol.* **77**, 97–109.

Kissileff, H. R. (1973). Nonhomeostatic controls of drinking. *In* "The Neuropsychology of Thirst" (A. N. Epstein, H. R. Kissileff, and E. Stellar, eds.), pp.163–198. Wiley and Sons, New York.

Kissileff, H. R., and Epstein, A. N. (1969). Exaggerated prandial drinking in the "recovered lateral" rat without saliva. *J. Comp. Physiol. Psychol.* **67**, 301–308.

Kissileff, H. R., and Hoeffer, R. (1975). Reduction of saline intake in adrenalectomized rats during chronic intragastric infusions of saline. *In* "Control Mechanisms of Drinking" (G. Peters, J. T. Fitzsimons, and L. Peters-Heafeli, eds.), pp. 22–24. Springer Verlag, Heidelberg.

Kleeman, C. F., Dawson, H., and Levin, E. (1962). Urea transport in the central nervous system. *Am. J. Physiol.* **203**, 739–747.

Knepel, W., Nutto, D., and Meyer, D. K. (1982). Effect of transection of subfornical organ efferent projections on vasopressin release induced by angiotensin or isoprenaline in the rat. *Brain Res.* **248**, 180–184.

Kozlowski, S., and Drzewiecki, K. (1973). The role of osmoreceptors in portal circulation in control of water intake in dogs. *Acta Physiol. Polon.* **24**, 325–330.

Kozlowski, S., and Szcsepanska-Sadowska, E. (1975). Mechanisms of hypervolaemic thirst and interactions between hypovolaemia, hyperosmolality and the antidiuretic system. *In* "Control Mechanisms of Drinking" (G. Peters, J. T. Fitzsimons, and L. Peters-Haefeli, eds.), pp. 25–35. Springer Verlag, Berlin.

Kozlowski, S., Drzewiecki, K., and Zurawski, W. (1972). Relationship between osmotic reactivity of the thirst mechanism and the angiotensin and aldosterone level in the blood of dogs. *Acta Physiol. Polon.* **23**, 417–425.

Kraly, F. S. (1978). Abdominal vagotomy inhibits osmotically induced drinking in the rat. *J. Comp. Physiol. Psychol.* **92**, 999–1013.

Kraly, F. S. (1983). A probe for the histaminergic component of drinking in the rat. *Physiol. Behav.* **31**, 229–232.

Kraly, F. S. (1986). Histamine plays a role in drinking elicited by eating in the rat. *In*

"The Physiology of Thirst and Sodium Appetite" (G. deCaro, A. N. Epstein, and M. Massi, eds.), pp. 295–299. Plenum Press, New York.

Kraly, F. S., and Specht, S. M. (1984). Histamine plays a major role for drinking elicited by spontaneous eating in rats. *Physiol. Behav.* **33**, 611–614.

Kraly, F. S., Gibbs, J., and Smith, G. P. (1975). Disordered drinking after abdominal vagotomy in rats. *Nature* **258**, 226–228.

Kraly, F. S., Miller, L. A., and Hecht, E. S. (1983). Histaminergic mechanisms for drinking elicited by insulin in the rat. *Physiol. Behav.* **31**, 233–236.

Kriekhaus, E. E., and Wolf, G. (1968). Acquisition of sodium by rats: Interaction of innate mechanisms and learning. *J. Comp. Physiol. Psychol.* **65**, 197–201.

Kucharczyk, J., and Mogenson, G. J. (1975). Separate lateral hypothalamic pathways for extracellular and intracellular thirst. *Am. J. Physiol.* **228**, 295–301.

Kucharczyk, J., and Mogenson, G. J. (1976). Specific deficits in regulatory drinking following electrolytic lesions of the lateral hypothalamus. *Exp. Neurol.* **53**, 371–385.

Kucharczyk, J., Assaf, S. Y., and Mogenson, G. J. (1976). Differential effects of brain lesions on thirst induced by the administration of angiotensin II to the preoptic region, subfornical organ and anterior third ventricle. *Brain Res.* **108**, 327–337.

Kudo, T., and Baird, A. (1984). Inhibition of aldosterone production in the adrenal glomerulosa by atrial natriuretic factor. *Nature* **312**, 756–757.

Kühn, E. R. (1974). Cholinergic and adrenergic release mechanisms for vasopressin in the male rat: A study with injections of neurotransmitters and blocking agents into the third ventricle. *Neuroendocrinology* **16**, 255–264.

Landas, S., Phillips, M. I., Stamler, J. F., and Raizada, M. K. (1980). Visualization of specific angiotensin II binding sites in the brain by fluorescent microscopy. *Science* **210**, 791–793.

Lang, R. E., Tholken, A., Ganten, D., Luft, F. C., Rushmkoaho, H., and Unger, T. H. (1985). Atrial natriuretic factor—A circulating hormone stimulated by volume loading. *Nature* **314**, 264–266.

Laragh, J. H., and Sealy, J. E. (1973). The renin-angiotensin-aldosterone hormonal system and regulation of sodium, potassium, and blood pressure homeostasis. *In* "Handbook of Physiology Section 8, Renal Physiology" (J. Orloff and R. W. Berliner, eds.), pp. 831–908. Williams and Wilkins, Baltimore.

Laubie, M., and Schmitt, M. (1977). Sites of action of clonidine: Centrally mediated increase in vagal tone, centrally mediated hypotensive and sympatho-inhibitory effects. *Prog. Brain Res.* **47**, 337–348.

Leander, J. D., and Hynes, M. D. (1983). Opioid antagonists and drinking: Evidence of kappa receptor involvement. *Eur. J. Pharmacol.* **87**, 481–484.

Lee, M. C., Thrasher, T. N., and Ramsay, D. J. (1981). Is angiotensin essential in drinking induced by water deprivation and caval ligation? *Am. J. Physiol.* **240**, R75–80.

Leenen, F. H., and McDonald, R. H., Jr. (1974). Effect of isoproterenol on blood pressure, plasma renin activity and water intake in rats. *Eur. J. Pharmacol.* **26**, 129–135.

Leenen, F. H., and Stricker, E. M. (1974). Plasma renin activity and thirst following hypovolemia or caval ligation in rats. *Am. J. Physiol.* **226**, 1238–1242.

Leenen, F. H., Stricker, E. M., McDonald, R. H., Jr., and DeJong, W. (1975). Relationship between increase in plasma renin activity and drinking following different types of dipsogenic stimuli. *In* "Control Mechanisms of Drinking" (G. Peters, J. T. Fitzsimons, and L. Peters-Haefeli, eds.), pp. 84–88. Springer Verlag, New York.

Lehr, D. (1973). Invited Comment: Comments to papers on "Thirst" by Drs. Fisher, Harvey and Setler. In "The Neuropsychology of Thirst: New Findings and Advances in Concepts" (A. N. Epstein, H. R. Kissileff, and E. Stellar eds.), pp. 307–314. V. H. Winston & Sons, Washington.

Lehr, D., and Goldman, H. W. (1973). Continued pharmacological analysis of consummatory behavior in the albino rat. *Eur. J. Pharmacol.* **23**, 197–210.

Lehr, D., Goldman, H. W., and Casner, P. (1973). Renin-angiotensin role in thirst: Paradoxical enhancement of drinking by angiotensin converting enzyme inhibition. *Science* **182**, 1031–1034.

Lehr, D., Goldman, H. W., and Casner, P. (1975). Evidence against the postulated role of the renin-angiotensin system in putative renin-dependent drinking responses. *In* "Control Mechanisms of Drinking" (G. Peters, J. T. Fitzsimons, and L. Peters-Haefeli, eds.), pp. 79–83. Springer Verlag, New York.

Lehr, D., Mallow, J., and Kurkowski, M. (1967). Copious drinking and simultaneous inhibition of urine flow elicited by beta-adrenergic stimulation and contrary effect of alpha-adrenergic stimulation. *J. Pharmacol. Exp. Ther.* **158**, 150–163.

Leibowitz, S. F. (1970). Reciprocal hunger-regulating circuits involving alpha- and beta-adrenergic receptors located, respectively, in the ventromedial and lateral hypothalamus. *Proc. Natl. Acad. Sci. USA* **67**, 1063–1070.

Leibowitz, S. F. (1971a). Hypothalamic alpha- and beta-adrenergic systems regulate both thirst and hunger in the rat. *Proc. Natl. Acad. Sci. USA* **68**, 332–334.

Leibowitz, S. F. (1971b). Hypothalamic beta-adrenergic "thirst" system mediates drinking induced by carbachol and transiently by norepinephrine. *Fed. Proc.* **30**, 481.

Leibowitz, S. F. (1972). Central adrenergic receptors and the regulation of hunger and thirst. *In* "Neurotransmitters" (I. J. Kopin, ed.), "Research Publication of the Association for Research on Nervous and Mental Diseases," Vol. 50, pp. 327–358. Williams and Wilkins, Baltimore.

Leibowitz, S. F. (1973a). Histamine: A stimulatory effect on drinking in the rat. *Brain Res.* **63**, 440–444.

Leibowitz, S. F. (1973b). Brain norepinephrine and ingestive behavior. *In* "Frontiers in

Catecholamine Research" (E. Usdin and S. Snyder, eds.), pp. 711–713. Pergamon Press, Oxford.

Leibowitz, S. F. (1973c). Alpha-adrenergic receptors mediate suppression of drinking induced by hypothalamic amphetamine injection. *Fed. Proc.* **32**, 754 (Abstract).

Leibowitz, S. F. (1979). Histamine: Modifications of behavioral and physiological components of body fluid homeostasis. *In* "Histamine Receptors" (T. O. Yellin, ed.), pp. 219–253. Spectrum Press, New York.

Leibowitz, S. F. (1980). Neurochemical systems of the hypothalamus. *In* "Handbook of the Hypothalamus," Vol. 3, "Behavioral Studies of the Hypothalamus" (P. J. Morgane and J. Panksepp, eds.), pp. 299–437. Marcel Dekker, New York.

Leibowitz, S. F., and Rossakis. C. (1979a). Mapping study of brain dopamine- and epinephrine-sensitive sites which cause feeding suppression in the rat. *Brain Res.* **172**, 101–113.

Leibowitz, S. F., and Rossakis, C. (1979b). Pharmacological characterization of perifornical hypothalamic dopamine receptors mediating feeding inhibition in the rat. *Brain Res.* **172**, 115–130.

Leksell, L. G. (1976). Influence of prostaglandin E–1 on cerebral mechanisms involved in the control of fluid balance. *Acta Physiol. Scand.* **98**, 85–93.

Leksell, L. G., Congiu, M., Denton, D. A., Fei, T. D. W., McKinley, M. J., Tarjan, E., and Weisinger, R. S. (1981). Influence of mannitol-induced reduction in CSF sodium on nervous and endocrine mechanisms involved in control of fluid balance. *Acta Physiol. Scand.* **112**, 33–40.

LeMagnen, J., and Tallon, S. (1966). La periodicité spontanée de la prise d'aliments ad libitum du rat blanc. *J. Physiol.* **58**, 323–349.

LeMagnen, J., and Tallon, S. A. (1967). Les déterminants quantitatifs de la prise hydrique dans ses relations avec la prise d'aliments chez le rat. *C. R. Soc. Biol.* **161** 1243–1246.

Leschke, E. (1918). Über die Durstempfindung. *Arch. Psych. Nervenkr.* **59**, 773–781.

Levitt, D. R., and Teitelbaum, P. (1975). Somnolence, akinesia, and sensory activation of motivated behavior in the lateral hypothalamic syndrome. *Proc. Natl. Acad. Sci. USA* **72**, 2819–2823.

Levitt, R. A. (1971). Cholinergic substrate for drinking in the rat. *Psychol. Rep.* **29**, 431–448.

Levitt, R. A., and Fisher, A. E. (1966). Anticholinergic blockade of centrally induced thirst. *Science* **154**, 520–522.

Levy, C. J., and McCutcheon, B. (1974). Importance of postingestional factors in the satiation of sodium appetite in rats. *Physiol. Behav.* **13**, 621–625.

Lewis, M. E., Avrith, D. B., and Fitzsimons, J. T. (1979). Short-latency drinking and increased Na appetite after intracerebral microinjections of NGF in rats. *Nature* **279**, 440–442.

Lightman, S. L., Todd, K., and B. J. Everitt. (1984). Ascending noradrenergic projections from brainstem: Evidence for a major role in the regulation of blood pressure and vasopressin secretion. *Exp. Brain Res.* **55**, 145–151.

Liljestrand, G., and Zotterman, Y. (1954). The water taste in mammals. *Acta Physiol. Scand.* **32**, 291–303.

Lind, R. W., and Johnson A. K. (1981). Periventricular preoptic-hypothalamic lesions: Effects on isoproterenol-induced thirst. *Pharmacol. Biochem. Behav.* **15**, 563–565.

Lind, R. W., and Johnson, A. K. (1982a). On the separation of functions mediated by the AV3V region. *Peptides* **3**, 495–499.

Lind, R. W., and Johnson, A. K. (1982b). Subfornical organ-median preoptic connections and drinking and pressor responses to angiotensin II. *J. Neurosci.* **2**, 1043–1051.

Lind, R. W., and Johnson, A. K. (1982c). Central and peripheral mechanisms mediating angiotensin induced thirst. *In* "Experimental Brain Research" (Suppl. 4) (D. Ganten, M. Prinz, M. I. Phillips, and B. Schölkens, eds.), pp. 353–364. Springer Verlag, New York.

Lind, R. W., Ohman, L. E., Lansing, M. B., and Johnson, A. K. (1983). Transection of subfornical organ neural connections diminishes the pressor response to intravenously infused angiotensin II. *Brain Res.* **178**, 225–254.

Lind, R. W., Thunhorst, R. L., and Johnson, A. K. (1984). The subfornical organ and the integration of multiple factors in thirst. *Physiol. Behav.* **32**, 69–74.

Lind, R. W., Van Hoesen, G. W., and Johnson, A. K. (1982). An HRP study of the connections of the subfornical organ of the rat. *J. Comp. Neurol.* **210**, 265–277.

Linden, R. J., and Kappagoda, C. T. (1982). "Atrial Receptors." Cambridge University Press, Cambridge.

Lipton, J. M., Welch, J. P., and Clark, W. G. (1973). Changes in body temperature produced by injecting prostaglandin E_1, EGTA and bacterial endotoxin into the PO/AH region and the medulla oblongata of the rat. *Experientia* **29**, 806–808.

Longet, F. A. (1868). "Traité de Physiologie," Vol. I, pp. 21–38. Bailliere, Paris.

Lorens, S. A., Sorenson, J. P., and Yunger, L. M. (1971). Behavioral and neurochemical effects of lesions in the raphé system of the rat. *J. Comp. Physiol. Psychol.* **77**, 48–52.

Lotter, E. C., McKay, L. D., Mangiapane, M. L., Simpson, J. B., Vogel, K. E., Porte, D., Jr., and Woods, S. C. (1980). Intraventricular angiotensin elicits drinking in the baboon. *Proc. Soc. Exp. Biol. Med.* **163**, 48–51.

Lovett, D., and Singer, G. (1971). Ventricular modification of drinking and eating behavior. *Physiol. Behav.* **6**, 23–26.

Lubar, J. F., Boyce, B. A., and Schaefer, C. F. (1968). Etiology of polydipsia and polyuria in rats with septal lesions. *Physiol. Behav.* **3**, 289–292.

Lubar, J. F., Schaefer, C. F., and Wells, D. G. (1969). The role of the septal area in the regulation of water intake and associated motivational behavior. *Ann. N.Y. Acad. Sci.* **157**, 875–893.

MacPhail, E. M., and Miller, N. E. (1968). Cholinergic brain stimulation in cats, failure to obtain sleep. *J. Comp. Physiol. Psychol.* **65**, 499–503.

Maddison, S., Rolls, B. J., Rolls, E. T., and Wood, R. J. (1977). Analysis of drinking in the chronically cannulated monkey. *J. Physiol.* **272**, 4–5P.

Maddison, S., Rolls, B. J., Rolls, E. T., and Wood, R. J. (1980a). The role of gastric factors in drinking termination in the monkey. *J. Physiol.* **305**, 55–56P.

Maddison, S., Wood, R. J., Rolls, E. T., Rolls, B. J., and Gibbs, J. (1980b). Drinking in the rhesus monkey: Peripheral factors. *J. Comp. Physiol. Psychol.* **94**, 365–374.

Maebashi, M., and Yoshinaga, K. (1967). Effect of dehydration on plasma renin activity. *Jpn. Circ. J.* **31**, 609–613.

Magendie, F. (1822). "A Summary of Physiology," Transl. John Revere. Coale, Baltimore.

Malmo, R. B., and Mundl, W. J. (1975). Osmosensitive neurons in the rat's preoptic area: Medial-lateral comparison. *J. Comp. Physiol. Psychol.* **88**, 161–175.

Malmo, R. B., and Malmo, H. P. (1979). Responses of lateral preoptic neurons in the rat to hypertonic sucrose and NaCl. *Electroencephalogr. Clin. Neurophysiol.* **45**, 401–408.

Malmo, R. B., and Malmo, H. P. (1981). Responses of lateral preoptic neurons and behavioral reactions to angiotensin II and hypertonic NaCl and sucrose administered into the rat cerebral ventricle. *Electroencephalogr. Clin. Neurophysiol.* **52**, 72–80.

Malvin, R. L., Mouw, D., and Vander, A. J. (1977). Angiotensin: Physiological role in water-deprivation-induced thirst of rats. *Science* **197**, 171–173.

Malvin, R. L., Schiff, D., and Eiger, S. (1980). Angiotensin and drinking rates in the euryhaline killifish. *Am. J. Physiol.* **239**, R31–34.

Mangiapane, M. L., and Simpson, J. B. (1980a). Subfornical organ: Forebrain site of pressor and dipsogenic action of antiotensin II. *Am. J. Physiol.* **239**, R382–389.

Mangiapane, M. L., and Simpson, J. B. (1980b). Subfornical organ lesions reduce the pressor effect of systemic angiotensin II. *Neuroendocrinology* **31**, 380–384.

Mangiapane, M. L., and Simpson, J. B. (1983). Drinking and pressor responses after acetylcholine injections into subfornical organ. *Am. J. Physiol.* **244**, R508–513.

Mangiapane, M. L., Thrasher, T. N., Keil, L. C., Simpson, J. B., and Ganong, W. F. (1983). Deficits in drinking and vasopressin secretion after lesions of the nucleus medianus. *Neuroendocrinology* **37**, 73–77.

Mann, J. F. E., Johnson, A. K., and Ganten, D. (1980). Plasma angiotensin II: dipsogenic levels and angiotensin-generating capacity of renin. *Am. J. Physiol.* **238**, 372–377.

Mann, J. F. E., Eisele, S., Ganten, D., Johnson, A. K., Rettig, R., Ritz, E., and Unger T. (1986). Angiotensin dependent thirst following polyethylene glycol treatment in the rat. *In* "The Physiology of Thirst and Sodium Appetite" (G. deCaro, A. N. Epstein, and M. Massi, eds.), pp.199–203. Plenum Press, New York.

Mann, J. F. E., Johnson, A. K., Rascher, W., Genest, J., and Ganten, D. (1981). Thirst in the rat after ligation of the inferior vena cava: Role of angiotensin II. *Pharmacol. Biochem. Behav.* **15**, 337–341.

Mann, J. F. E., Phillips, I. Dietz, R., Haebara, H., and Ganten, D. (1978). Effects of central and peripheral angiotensin blockade in hypertensive rats. *Am. J. Physiol.* **234**, H626–637.

Manning, P. T., Schwartz, D., Katsube, N. C., Holmberg, S. W., and Needleman, P. (1985). Vasopressin-stimulated release of atriopeptin: Endocrine antagonists in fluid homeostasis. *Science* **229**, 395–397.

Margarinos, A. M., Coirini, H., DeNicola, H. F., and McEwen, B. S. (1986). Mineralocorticoid regulation of salt intake is preserved in hippocampectomized rats. *Neuroendocrinology* **44**, 494–497.

Marshall, J. F., and Teitelbaum, P. (1974). Further analysis of sensory inattention following lateral hypothalamic damage in rats. *J. Comp. Physiol. Psychol.* **86**, 375–395.

Marshall, J. F., Levitan, D., and Stricker, E. M. (1976). Activation-induced restoration of sensorimotor functions in rats with dopamine-depleting brain lesions. *J. Comp. Physiol. Psychol.* **90**, 536–546.

Marshall, J. F., Richardson, J. S., and Teitelbaum, P. (1974). Nigrostriatal bundle damage and the lateral hypothalamic syndrome. *J. Comp. Physiol. Psychol.* **87**, 808–830.

Marshall, J. F., Turner, B. H., and Teitelbaum, P. (1971). Sensory neglect produced by lateral hypothalamic damage. *Science* **174**, 523–525.

Massi, M., DeCaro, G., and Epstein, A. N. (1986a). Effect of tachykinins on sodium appetite in sodium depleted rats. *In* "Modulation of Central and Peripheral Transmitter Function" (G. Biggio, P. F. Spano, G. Toffano, and G. L. Gessa, eds.), pp. 545–548. Liviana Press, Padova, Italy.

Massi, M., DeCaro, G., Epstein, A. N., and Mazzarella, L. (1986b). Sensitivity to dipsogenic peptides of pigeons bearing lesions directed to the subfornical organ (SFO). *In* "The Physiology of Thirst and Sodium Appetite" (G. deCaro, A. N. Epstein, and M. Massi, eds.), pp. 251–256. Plenum Press, New York.

Massi, M., DeCaro, G., Perfumi, M., and Venturi, F. (1988). Mapping of brain sites sensitive to the antidipsogenic effect of tachykinins. *Peptides* **9**, 347–356.

Massi, M., Micossi, L. G., DeCaro, G., and Epstein, A. N. (1986c). Suppression of drinking but not feeding by central eledoisin and physalaemin in the rat. *Appetite* **7**, 63–70.

Mayer, A. (1900). Variations de la tension osmotique de sang chez les animaux privés de liquides. *C. R. Soc. Biol. Fil.* **53**, 153–155.

Mayer, A. (1901). "Essai sur la Soif. Ses causes et son méchanisme." Travail du laboratoire de pathologie expérimentale et comparée de la Faculté de Médecine de Paris. Félix Alcan, Paris.

McCaa, R. E., McCaa, C. S., and Guyton, A. C. (1975). Role of angiotensin II and potassium in the long term regulation of aldosterone secretion in intact conscious dogs. *Circ. Res. (Suppl.)* **36**, 57–67.

McCance, R. A. (1936).Experimental sodium chloride deficiency in man. *Proc. R. Soc. Lond.* **119b**, 245–268.

McCutcheon, B., and Levy, C. (1972). The relationship between NaCl reinforced bar-pressing and duration of sodium deficiency in rats. *Physiol. Behav.* **8**, 621–623.

McDermott, L. J., and Grossman, S. P. (1979). Regulation of caloric intake in rats with rostral zona incerta lesions: Effects of caloric density or palatability of the diet. *Physiol. Behav.* **23**, 1135–1140.

McDermott, L. J., and Grossman, S. P. (1980a). Circadian rhythms in ingestive behavior and responsiveness to glucoprivic and osmotic challenges in rats with rostral zona incerta lesions. *Physiol. Behav.* **24**, 575–584.

McDermott, L. J., and Grossman, S. P. (1980b). Responsiveness to 2-deoxy-D-glucose and insulin in rats with rostral zona incerta lesions. *Physiol. Behav.* **24**, 585–592.

McDermott, L. J., Alheid, G. F., Halaris, A., and Grossman, S. P. (1977a). A correlational analysis of the effects of surgical transections of three components of the MFB on ingestive behavior and hypothalamic, striatal and telencephalic amine concentrations. *Pharmacol. Biochem. Behav.* **6**, 203–214.

McDermott, L. J., Alheid, G. F., Kelly, J., Halaris, A., and Grossman, S. P. (1977b). Regulatory deficits after surgical transections of three components of the MFB: Correlation with regional amine depletions. *Pharmacol. Biochem. Behav.* **6**, 397–407.

McFarland, D. J., and Rolls, B. J. (1972). Suppression of feeding by intracranial injections of angiotensin. *Nature* **236**, 172–173.

McGiff, J. C., Terragno, N. A., Malik, K. U., and Lonigro, A. J. (1972). Release of prostaglandin A-like substances from canine kidney by bradykinin: Comparison with eledoisin. *Circ. Res.* **31**, 36–43.

McGowan, M. K., Brown, B., and Grossman, S. P. (1988a). Lesions of the MPO or AV3V: Influences on fluid intake. *Physiol. Behav.* **42**, 331–342.

McGowan, M. K., Brown, B., and Grossman, S. P. (1988b). Depletion of neurons from lateral preoptic area impairs drinking to various dipsogens. *Physiol. Behav.* **43**, 815–822.

McKenzie, J. S., and Denton, D. A. (1974). Salt ingestion responses to diencephalic electrical stimulation in the unrestrained conscious sheep. *Brain Res.* **70**, 449–466.

McKinley M. J., Blaine, E. H., and Denton, D. A. (1974). Brain osmoreceptors, cerebrospinal fluid electrolyte composition and thirst. *Brain Res.* **70**, 532–537.

McKinley, M. J., Denton, D. A., and Weisinger, R. S. (1978). Sensors for antidiuresis and thirst—osmoreceptors or CSF sodium detectors? *Brain Res.* **141**, 89–103.

McKinley, M. J., Denton, D. A., Leksell, L., Tarjan, E., and Weisinger, R. S. (1980). Evidence for cerebral sodium receptors involved in water drinking in sheep. *Physiol. Behav.* **25**, 501–504.

McKinley, M. J., Denton, D. A., Leksell, L. G., Mouw, D. R., Scoggins, B. A., Smith, M. H., Weisinger, R. S., and Wright, R. D. (1982). Osmoregulatory thirst in sheep is disrupted by ablation of the anterior wall of the optic recess. *Brain Res.* **236**, 210–215.

McKinley, M. J., Denton, D. A., Park, R. G., and Weisinger, R. S. (1983). Cerebral involvement in dehydration-induced natriuresis. *Brain Res.* **263**, 340–347.

McKinley, M. J., Denton, D. A., Leventer, M., Miselis, R. R., Park, R. G., Tarjan, E., Simpson, J. B., and Weisinger, R. S. (1986). Adipsia in sheep caused by cerebral lesions. *In* "The Physiology of Thirst and Sodium Appetite" (G. deCaro, A. N. Epstein, and M. Massi, eds.), pp. 321–326. Plenum Press, New York.

Mendelsohn, F. A. O., Quirion, R., Saavedra, J. M., Aguilera, G., and Catt, K. J. (1984). Autoradiographic localization of angiotensin II receptors in rat brain. *Proc. Natl. Acad. Sci., USA* **81**, 1575–1579.

Mendelson, J. (1970). Feedback control of hypothalamic drinking. *Physiol. Behav.* **5**, 779–781.

Mercer, P. F., Mogenson, G. J., and Paquette, S. Y. M. (1978). Sodium intake following destruction of the anterior hypothalamus in the rat. *Can. J. Physiol. Pharmacol.* **56**, 252–259.

Meyer, D. K., and Hertting, G. (1973). Influence of neuronal uptake-blocking agents on the increase in water intake and in plasma concentrations of renin and angiotensin I induced by phentolamine and isoprenaline. *Naunyn-Schmiedebergs Arch. Exp. Pathol. Pharmakol.* **280**, 191–200.

Meyer, D. K., and Hertting, G. (1975). Drinking induced by direct or indirect stimulation of beta-receptors: Evidence for involvement of the renin-angiotensin system. *In* "Control Mechanisms of Drinking" (G. Peters, J. T. Fitzsimons, and L. Peters-Haefeli, eds.), pp. 89–92. Springer Verlag, New York.

Meyer, D. K., Peskar, B., and Hertting, G. (1971a). Hemmung des durch blutdrucksenkende Pharmaka bei Ratten ausgelösten Trinkens durch Nephrektomie. *Experientia* **27**, 65–66.

Meyer, D. K., Peskar, B., Tauchmann, U., and Hertting, G. (1971b). Potentiation and abolition of the increase in plasma renin activity seen after hypotensive drugs in rats. *Eur. J. Pharmacol.* **16**, 278–282.

Meyer, D. K., Raucher, W., Peskar, B., and Hertting, G. (1973). The mechanisms of the drinking response to some hypotensive drugs: Activation of the renin-angiotensin system by direct or reflex-mediated stimulation of β-receptors. *Naunyn-Schmiedebergs Arch. Pharmakol.* **276**, 13–24.

Milgram, N. W., Devor, M., and Server, A. C. (1971). Spontaneous changes in waves induced by electrical stimulation of the lateral hypothalamus in rats. *J. Comp. Physiol. Psychol.* **75**, 491–499.

Miller, N. E. (1957). Experiments on motivation. Studies combining psychological, physiological, and pharmacological techniques. *Science* **126**, 1271–1278.

Miller, N. E. (1960). Motivational effects of brainstimulation and drugs. *Fed. Proc.* **19**, 846–853.

Miller, N. E. (1965). Chemical coding of behavior in the brain. *Science* **148**, 328–338.

Miller, N. E., Sampliner, R. I., and Woodrow, P. (1957). Thirst reducing effects of water by stomach fistula versus water by mouth, measured by both a consummatory and an instrumental response. *J. Comp. Physiol. Psychol.* **50**, 1–5.

Misantone, L. J., Ellis, S., and Epstein, A. N. (1980). Development of angiotensin-induced drinking in the rat. *Brain Res.* **186**, 195–202.

Miselis, R. R. (1981). The efferent projections of the subfornical organ of the rat: A circumventricular organ within a neural network subserving water balance. *Brain Res.* **230**, 1–23.

Miselis, R. R. (1986). The visceral neuraxis in thirst and renal functions. *In* "The Physiology of Thirst and Sodium Appetite" (G. deCaro, A. N. Epstein, and M. Massi, eds.), pp. 345–354. Plenum Press, New York.

Miselis, R. R., Shapiro, R. E., and Hand, P. J. (1979). Subfornical organ efferents to neural systems for control of body water. *Science* **205**, 1022–1023.

Mitchell, L. D., Wilkin, L. D., and Johnson, A. K. (1984). Angiotensin II afferents from circumventricular organs to the supraoptic nucleus. *Soc. Neurosci. Abstr.* **10**, 480.

Moe, K. E., and Epstein, A. N. (1986). Sodium appetite during captopril blockade of endogenous angiotensin formation. *In* "The Physiology of Thirst and Sodium Appetite" (G. deCaro, A. N. Epstein, and M. Massi, eds.), pp. 431–439. Plenum Press, New York.

Moe, K. E., Weiss, M. L., and Epstein, A. N. (1984) Sodium appetite during captopril blockade of endogenous angiotensin II formation. *Am. J. Physiol.* **247**, R356-R365.

Mogenson, G. J. (1971).Stability and modification of consummatory behavior elicited by electrical stimulation of the hypothalamus. *Physiol. Behav.* **6**, 255–260.

Mogenson, G. J. (1973). Hypothalamic limbic mechanisms in the control of water intake. *In* "The Neuropsychology of Thirst" (A. E. Epstein, H. R. Kissileff, and E. Stellar, eds.), pp. 119–142. V. H. Winston and Sons, Washington, D.C.

Mogenson, G. J., and Kucharczyk, J. (1975). Evidence that the lateral hypothalamus and midbrain participate in the drinking response elicited by intracranial angiotensin. *In* "Control Mechanisms of Drinking" (G. Peters, J. T. Fitzsimons, and L. Peters-Haefeli, eds.), pp. 127–131. Springer Verlag, New York.

Mogenson, G. J., and Kucharczyk, J. (1978). Central neural pathways for angiotensin-induced thirst. *Fed. Proc.* **37**, 2683–2688.

Mogenson, G. J., and Morgan, C.W. (1967). Effects of induced drinking on self-stimulation of the lateral hypothalamus. *Exp. Brain Res.* **3**, 111–116.

Mogenson, G. J., and Stevenson, J. A. F. (1966). Drinking and self-stimulation with electrical stimulation of the lateral hypothalamus. *Physiol. Behav.* **1**, 251–254.

Mogenson, G. J., and Stevenson, J. A. F. (1967). Drinking induced by electrical stimulation of the lateral hypothalamus. *Exp. Neurol.* **17**,119–127.

Mogenson, G. J., Gentil, C. G., and Stevenson, J. A. F. (1971). Feeding and drinking elicited by low and high frequencies of hypothalamic stimulation. *Brain Res.* **33**, 127–133.

Mogenson, G. J., Kucharczyk, J., and Assaf, S. (1977). Evidence for multiple receptors and neural pathways which subserve water intake initiated by antiotensin II. *In* "International Symposium on the Central Actions of Angiotensin and Related Hormones" (P. J. Buckley and C. Ferrario, eds.), pp. 493–502. Pergamon Press, New York.

Montemurro, D. G., and Stevenson, J. A. F. (1957). Adipsia produced by hypothalmic lesions. *Can. J. Biochem.* **35**, 31–37.

Montegomery, A. V., and Holmes, J. H. (1955). Gastric inhibition of the drinking response. *Am. J. Physiol.* **182**, 227–231.

Montgomery. M. F. (1931). The role of the salivary glands in the thirst mechanism. *Am. J. Physiol.* **96**, 221–227.

Mook, D. (1969). Some determinants of preference and aversion in the rat. *Ann. N.Y. Acad. Sci.* **157**, 1158–1170.

Moore-Gillon, M. J. (1980). Effects of vagotomy on drinking in the rat. *J. Physiol.* **308**, 417–726.

Moran, J. S., and Blass, E. M. (1976). Inhibition of drinking by septal stimulation in rats. *Physiol. Behav.* **17,** 23–27.

Morgane P. J. (1961). Alterations in feeding and drinking behavior of rats with lesions in globi pallidi. *Am. J. Physiol.* **201**, 420–428.

Morris, M., McCann, S. M., and Orias, R. (1976). Evidence for hormonal participation in the natriuretic and kaliuretic responses to intraventricular saline and norepinephrine. *Proc. Soc. Exp. Biol. Med.* **152**, 95–98.

Morris, M., McCann, S. M., and Orias, R. (1977). Role of transmitters in mediating hypothalamic control of electrolyte excretion. *Can. J. Physiol. Pharmacol.* **55**, 1143–1154.

Mouw, D., Bonjour, J. P., Malvin, R. L., and Vander, A. J. (1971). A central action of angiotensin in stimulating ADH release. *Am. J. Physiol.* **220**, 239–242.

Murphy, H. M., and Brown, T. S. (1970). Effects of hippocampal lesions on simple and preferential consummatory behavior in the rat. *J. Comp. Physiol. Psychol.* **72**, 404–415.

Myers, R. D. (1964). Emotional and autonomic responses following hypothalamic chemical stimulation. *Can. J. Psychol.* **18**, 6–14.

Myers, R. D. (1969). Chemical mechanisms in the hypothalamus mediating eating and drinking in the monkey. *Ann. N.Y. Acad. Sci.* **157**, 918–932.

Myers, R. D., and Sharpe, L. G. (1968). Chemical activation of ingestive and other hypothalamic regulatory mechanisms. *Physiol. Behav.* **3**, 987–995.

Myers, R. D., Hall, G. D., and Rudy, T. A. (1973). Drinking in the monkey evoked by nicotine or angiotensin II microinjected in hypothalamic and mesencephalic sites. *Pharmacol. Biochem. Behav.* **1**, 15–22.

Nachman, M. (1962). Taste preferences for sodium salts by adrenalectomized rats. *J. Comp. Physiol. Psychol.* **55**, 1124–1129.

Nachman, M. (1963). Taste preference for lithium chloride by adrenalectomized rats. *Am. J. Physiol.* **205**, 219–221.

Nachman, M., and Ashe, J. H. (1974). Effects of basolateral amygdala lesions on neophobia, learned taste aversions, and sodium appetite in rats. *J. Comp. Physiol. Psychol.* **87**, 622–643.

Nachman, M., and Valentino, D. A. (1966). Roles of taste and postingestional factors in the satiation of sodium appetite in rats. *J. Comp. Physiol. Psychol.* **62**, 280–283.

Nagel, J. A., and Satinoff, E. (1980). Mild cold exposure increases survival in rats with medial preoptic lesions. *Science* **208**, 301–303.

Nairn, R. C., Masson, G. M. C., and Corcoran, A. C. (1956). The production of serous effusions in nephrectomized animals by the administration of renal extracts and renin. *J. Pathol. Bacteriol.* **71**, 155–163.

Négro-Vilar, A., Gentil, C. G., and Covian, M. R. (1967). Alterations in sodium chloride and water intake after septal lesions in the rat. *Physiol. Behav.* **2**, 167–170.

Neill, D. B., and Linn, C. L. (1975). Deficits in consummatory responses to regulatory challenges following basal ganglia lesions in rats. *Physiol. Behav.* **14**, 617–624.

Nicolaidis, S. (1968). Neurophysiologie sensorielle. Résponses des unités osmosensible hypothalamique aux stimulation salines et aqueuses de la langue. *C. R. Acad. Sci. Ser. D* **267**, 2352–2355.

Nicolaidis, S. (1969a). Early systemic responses to orogastric stimulation in the regulation of food and water balance: functional and electrophysiological data. *Ann. N.Y. Acad. Sci.* **151**, 1176–1203.

Nicolaidis, S. (1969b). Discriminatory responses of hypothalamic osmosensitive units to gustatory stimulation in cats. *In* "Olfaction and Taste," Vol. 3 (C. Pfaffmann, ed.), pp. 569–573. Rockefeller University Press, New York.

Nicolaidis, S. (1970a). Mise en évidence de neurones barosensibles hypothalamiques antérieur et médian chez le chat. *J. Physiol.* **62**, 199–200.

Nicolaidis, S. (1970b). Résponse unitaire dans les aires antérieur et médianes de l'hypothalamus antérieur associées à des variations de pression artérielle et de volémie. *C. R. Acad. Sci.* **270**, 839–842

Nicolaidis, S., and Fitzsimons, J. T. (1975). La dééendance de la prise d'eau induite par l'angiotensine II envers la fonction vasomotrice cérébrale locale chez le rat. *C. R. Acad. Sci.* **281**, 1417–1420.

Nicolaidis, S., and Jeulin, A. C. (1984). Converging projections of hydromineral imbalances. *J. Physiol.* **79**, 406–415.

Nicolaidis, S., and Rowland, N. (1974). Long term self-intravenous drinking in the rat. *J. Comp. Physiol. Psychol.* **87**, 1–15.

Nicolaidis, S., and Rowland, N. (1975a). Regulatory drinking in rats with permanent access to a bitter fluid source. *Physiol. Behav.* **14**, 819–824.

Nicolaidis, S., and Rowland, N. (1975b). Systemic versus oral and gastro-intestinal metering of fluid intake. *In* "Control Mechanisms of Drinking" (G. Peters, J. T. Fitzsimons, and L. Peters-Haefeli, eds.), pp. 14–21. Springer Verlag, New York.

Nicolaidis, S., Ishibashi, S., Gueguen, B., Thornton, S. N., and de Beaurepaire, R. (1983). Iontophoretic investigation of identified SFO angiotensin responsive neurons firing in relation to blood pressure changes. *Brain Res. Bull.* **10**, 357–363.

Nicolaidis, S., Le Poncin-Lafitte, M., Danguir, J., Grosdemouge, C., and Rapin, J. R. (1981). Specific behaviors bound brain cartography of the glucose uptake in the rat. *Eur. Neurol.* **20**, 180–182.

Nicoll, R. A., and Barker, J. L. (1971). Excitation of supraoptic neurosecretory cells by angiotensin II. *Nature* **233**, 172–174.

Nováková, A., and Cort, J. H. (1966). Hypothalamic regulation of spontaneous salt intake in the rat. *Am. J. Physiol.* **211**, 919–925.

Novin, D. (1964). The effects of insulin on water intake in the rat. *In* "Thirst in the Regulation of Body Water" (M. J. Wayner, ed.), pp. 177–182. Pergamon Press, New York.

Novin, D., and Durham, R. (1969). Unit and D-C potential studies of the supraoptic nucleus. *Ann. N.Y. Acad. Sci.* **157**, 740–754.

Oakley, B., and Pfaffmann, C. (1962). Electrophysiologically monitored lesions in the gustatory thalamic relay of the albino rat. *J. Comp. Physiol. Psychol.* **55**, 155–160.

Oatley, K. (1964). Changes of blood volume and osmotic pressure in the production of thirst. *Nature* **202**, 1341–1342.

Oatley, K., and Dickinson, A. (1970). Air drinking and the measurement of thirst. *Anim. Behav.* **18**, 259–265.

Oehme, C. (1922). Die Enstehung der Durstempfindung und die Regulation der Wasserzufuhr. *Dtsch. Med. Wochensch.* **48**, 277.

O'Kelly, L. I., Falk, L. J., and Flint, D. (1954). The effects of preloads of water and sodium chloride on voluntary water intake of thirsty rats. *J. Comp. Physiol. Psychol.* **47**, 7–13.

Olds, J., Allen, W., and Briese, E. (1971). Differentiation of hypothalamic drive and reward centers. *Am. J. Physiol.* **221**, 368–375.

Olsson, K. (1969). Studies on central regulation of secretion of antidiuretic hormone (ADH) in the goat. *Acta Physiol. Scand.* **77**, 465–474.

Olsson, K. (1972). Dipsogenic effects of intracarotid infusions of various hyperosmolal solutions. *Acta Physiol. Scand.* **85**, 517–522.

Olsson, K. (1973). Further evidence for the importance of CSF Na$^+$ concentration in central control of fluid balance. *Acta Physiol. Scand.* **88**, 183–188.

Olsson, K. (1975). Attenuation of dehydrative thirst by lowering of the CSF (Na$^+$). *Acta Physiol. Scand.* **94**, 536–538.

Olsson, K., and Kolmodin, R. (1974). Accentuation by angiotensin II of the antidiuretic and dipsogenic responses to intracarotid infusions of NaCl and fructose. *Acta Endocrinol.* **75**, 333–341.

Olsson, K., and Rundgren, ;M. (1975). Inefficiency of isoprenaline to induce drinking in the goat. *Acta Physiol. Scand.* **93**, 553–559.

Olsson, K., Larsson, B., and Liljekvist, E. (1976). Intracerebroventricular glycerol: A potent inhibitor of ADH-release and thirst. *Acta Physiol. Scand.* **98**, 470–477.

Oomura, Y., Ono, T., Ooyama, H., and Wayner, M. J. (1969). Glucose and osmosensitive neurons in the rat hypothalamus. *Nature* **222**, 3282–284.

Osborne, M. J., Pooters, N., Angles d'Auriac, G., Epstein, A. N., Worcel, M., and Meyer, P. (1971). Metabolism of tritiated angiotensin II in anaesthetized rats. *Pflügers Arch. Gesammte Physiol.* **326**, 101–114.

Osborne, P. G., Weisinger, R. S., and Denton, D. A. (1983). Changes in cerebrospinal fluid [Na] and its effects on Na and water homeostasis in the Na-replete rat. *Appetite* **4**, 215–216.

Osborne, P. G., Denton, D. A., and Weisinger, R. S. (1987). Effect of variation of the composition of CSF in the rat upon drinking of water and hypertonic NaCl solutions. *J. Comp. Physiol. Psychol.* **101**, 371–377.

Osumi, Y., Oishi, R., Fujiwara, H., and Takatori, S. (1975). Hyperdipsia induced by bilateral destruction of the locus coeruleus in rats. *Brain Res.* **86**, 419–427.

Palovcik, R. A., and Phillips, M. I. (1984). Saralasin increases activity of hippocampal neurons inhibited by angiotensin II. *Brain Res.* **323**, 345–348.

Peart, W. S. (1969). A history and review of the renin-angiotensin system. *Proc. R. S. Lond.* **173B**, 317–325.

Peck, J. W. (1973). Discussion: Thirst(s) resulting from bodily water imbalances. *In* "The Neuropsychology of Thirst" (A. N. Epstein, H. R. Kissileff, and E. Stellar, eds.), pp. 99–112. Wiley and Sons, New York.

Peck, J. W., and Blass, E. M. (1975). Localization of thirst and antidiuretic osmoreceptors by intracranial injections in rats. *Am. J. Physiol.* **228**, 1501–1509.

Peck, J. W., and Novin, D. (1971). Evidence that osmoreceptors mediating drinking in rabbits are in the lateral preoptic area. *J. Comp. Physiol. Psychol.* **74**, 134–14

Peres, V. L., Gentil, D. G., Graeff, F. G., and Covian, M. R. (1974). Antagonism of the dipsogenic action of intraseptal angiotensin II in the rat. *Pharmacol. Biochem. Behav.* **2**, 597–602.

Perez-Guaita, M. F., and Chiaraviglio E. (1980). Effect of prostaglandin E_1 and its biosynthesis inhibitor indomethacin on drinking in the rat. *Pharmacol. Biochem. Behav.* **13**, 787–792.

Perfumi, M., deCaro, G., Massi, M., and Venturi, F. (1986). Inhibition of ang II-induced drinking by dermorphin given into the SFO or into the lateral ventricle of intact or of SFO lesioned rats. *In* "The Physiology of Thirst and Sodium Appetite" (G. deCaro, A. N. Epstein, and M. Massi, eds.), pp. 257–263. Plenum Press, New York.

Peskar, B., Meyer, D. K., Tauchman, U., and Hertting, G. (1970). Influence of isoproterenol, hydralazine and phentolamine on the renin activity of plasma and renal cortex of rats. *Eur. J. Pharmacol.* **9**, 394–396.

Pettersson, A., Ricksten, S. E., Towle, A. C., Hedner, J., and Hedner, T. (1985). Effect of blood volume expansion and sympathetic denervation on plasma levels of atrial natriuretic factor (ANF) in the rat. *Acta Physiol. Scand.* **124**, 309–311.

Pettinger, W. A., Keeton, T. K., Campbell, W. B., and Harper, D. C. (1976). Evidence for a renal alpha-adrenergic receptor inhibiting renin release. *Circ. Res.* **38**, 338–346.

Pettinger, W. A., Marchelle, M., and Augusto, L. (1971). Renin suppression by DOCA and NaCl in the rat. *Am. J. Physiol.* **204,** 1071–1074.

Phillips, M. I. (1978). Angiotensin in the brain. *Neuroendocrinology* **25**, 354–377.

Phillips, M. I. (1987). Functions of angiotensin in the central nervous system. *Annu. Rev. Physiol.* **49**, 413–435.

Phillips, M. I., and Felix, D. (1976). Specific angiotensin II receptive neurons in the cat subfornical organ. *Brain Res.* **109**, 531–540.

Phillips, M. I., and Hoffman, W. E. (1977). Sensitive sites in the brain for the blood pressure and drinking responses to angiotensin II. *In* "Central Actions of Angiotensin and Related Hormones" (J. P. Buckley and C. S. Ferrario, eds.), pp. 325–356. Pergamon Press, New York.

Phillips, M. I., Deshmukh, P., and Larsen, W. (1978). Morphological comparisons of the ventricular wall of subfornical organ and organum vasculosum of the lamina terminalis. *Scanning Electron Microsc.* **2**, 349–356.

Phillips, M. I., Felix, D., Hoffman, W. E., and Ganten, D. (1977a). Angiotensin-sensitive sites in the brain ventricular system. *In* "Society for Neuroscience Symposia" (W. M. Cowan and J. A. Ferrrendelli, eds.), pp. 308–339. Society for Neuroscience, Bethesda, Md.

Phillips, M. I., Leavitt, M., and Hoffman, W. E. (1974). Experiments on angiotensin II and the subfornical organ in the control of thirst. *Fed. Proc.* **33**, 1985 (Abstr.).

Phillips, M. I., Mann, H., Dietz, R., Hoffman, W. E., and Ganten, D. (1977b). Lowering of hypertension by central saralasin in the absence of plasma renin. *Nature* **270**, 445–447.

Phillips, M. I., Phipps, J., Hoffman, W. E., and Leavitt, M. (1975) Reduction of blood pressure by intracranial injection of angiotensin blocker (P113) in spontaneously hypertensive rats (SHR). *Physiologist* **18**, 350 (Abstract).

Powley, T. L., and Keesey, R. E. (1970). Relationship of body weight to the lateral hypothalamic feeding syndrome. *J. Comp. Physiol. Psychol.* **70**, 25–36.

Quartermain, D., Miller, N. E., and Wolf, G. (1967). Role of experience in relationship between sodium deficiency and rate of bar pressing for salt. *J. Comp. Physiol. Psychol.* **63**, 417–420.

Quartermain, D., Wolf, G., and Keselica J. (1969). Relation between medial hypothalamic damage and impairments in regulation of sodium intake. *Physiol. Behav.* **4**, 101–103.

Radford, E. P. (1959). Factors modifying water metabolism in rats fed dry diets. *Am. J. Physiol.* **196**, 1098–1108.

Radio, G. J., Summy-Long, J., Daniels-Severs, A. D., and Severs, W. B. (1972). Hydration changes produced by central infusion of angiotensin II. *Am. J. Physiol.* **223**, 1221–1226.

Raizada, M. K., Yang, J. W., Phillips, M. I., and Fellows, R. E. (1981). Rat brain cells in primary culture: Characterization of angiotensin II binding sites. *Brain Res.* **207**, 343–355.

Ramsay, D. J. (1978). Beta-adrenergic thirst and its relation to the renin-angiotensin system. *Fed. Proc.* **37**, 2689–2693.

Ramsay, D. J., and Ganong, W. F. (1980). CNS regulation of salt intake. *In Neuroendocrinology* (D. T. Krieger and J. C. Hughes, eds.), pp. 123–129. Sinauer, Sunderland, Mass.

Ramsay, D. J., and Reid, I. A. (1975). Some central mechanisms of thirst in the dog. *J. Physiol.* **253**, 517–525.

Ramsay, D. J., and Thrasher, T. N. (1986). Hyperosmotic and hypervolemic thirst. *In* "The Physiology of Thirst and Sodium Appetite" (G. deCaro, A. N. Epstein, and M. Massi, eds.), pp. 83–96. Plenum Press, New York.

Ramsay, D. J., Rolls, B. J., and Wood, R. J. (1975). The relationship between elevated water intake and oedema associated with congestive heart failure in the dog. *J. Physiol.* **244**, 303–312.

Ramsay, D. J., Rolls, B. J., and Wood, R. J. (1977a). Thirst following water deprivation in dogs. *J. Physiol.* **232**, 93–100.

Ramsay, D. J., Rolls, B. J., and Wood, R. J. (1977b). Body fluid changes which influence drinking in the water deprived rat. *J. Physiol.* **266**, 453–569.

Reed, D. J., and Woodbury, D. M. (1962). Effect of hypertonic urea on cerebrospinal fluid pressure and brain volume. *J. Physiol.* **164**, 252–264.

Reid, I. A., and Ramsay, D. J. (1975). The effects of intracerebroventricular administration of renin on drinking and blood pressure. *Endocrinology* **97**, 536–542.

Rettig, R., Ganten, D., and Johnson, A. K. (1981). Isoproterenol-induced thirst: Renal and extrarenal mechanisms. *Am. J. Physiol.* **241**, 152–157.

Rice, K. K., and Richter, C. P. (1943). Increased sodium chloride and water intake of normal rats treated with desoxycorticosterone acetate. *Endocrinology* **33**, 106–115.

Richardson, D. B., and Mogenson, G. J. (1981). Water intake elicited by injections of angiotensin II into the preoptic area of rats. *Am. J. Physiol.* **240**, R70–74.

Richter, C. P. (1936). Increased salt appetite in adrenalectomized rats. *Am. J. Physiol.* **115**, 155–161.

Richter, C. P. (1941). Sodium chloride and dextrose appetite of untreated and treated adrenalectomized rats. *Endocrinology* **29**, 115–125.

Richter, C. P. (1956). Salt appetite of mammals: Its dependence on instinct and metabolism. *In* "L'Instinct dans le Comportement des Animaux et de l'Homme," pp. 577–629. Masson, Paris.

Roberts, W. W. (1969). Are hypothalamic motivational mechanisms functionally and anatomically specific? *Brain, Behav. Evolut.* **2**, 317–342.

Robertson, G. L., and Athar, S. (1976). The interaction of blood osmolality and blood volume in regulating vasopressin secretion in man. *J. Clin. Endocrinol. Metab.* **42**, 613–620.

Robertson, G. L., Shelton, R. L., and Athar, S. (1976). The osmoregulation of vasopressin. *Kidney Int.* **10**, 25–37.

Robinson, M. M., and Evered, M. D. (1986). Angiotensin II and arterial pressure in the control of thirst. *In* "The Physiology of Thirst and Sodium Appetite" (G. deCaro, A. N. Epstein, and M. Massi, eds.), pp. 193–198. Plenum Press, New York.

Rogers, R. C., and Novin, D. (1983). The neurological aspects of hepatic osmoregulation. *In* "The Kidney in Liver Disease" (2nd ed.) (M. Epstein, ed.), pp. 337–350. Elsevier, New York.

Rojo-Ortega, J. M., and Genest, J. (1968). A method for production of experimental hypertension in rats. *Can. J. Physiol. Pharmacol.* **46**, 883–885.

Rolls, B. J. (1970). Drinking by rats after irritative lesions in the hypothalamus. *Physiol. Behav.* **5**, 1385–1393.

Rolls, B. J., and McFarland, D. J. (1973). Hydration releases inhibition of feeding produced by intracranial angiotensin. *Physiol. Behav.* **11**, 881–884.

Rolls, B. J., and Ramsay, D. J. (1975). The elvation of endogenous angiotensin and thirst in the dog. *In* "Control Mechanisms of Drinking" (G. Peters, J. T. Fitzsimons, and L. Peters-Haefeli, eds.), pp. 74–78. Springer Verlag, New York.

Rolls, B. J., and Rolls, E. T. (1982). "Thirst." Cambridge University Press, Cambridge.

Rolls, B. J., and Wood, R. J. (1977). Role of angiotensin in thirst. *Pharmacol. Biochem. Behav.* **6**, 245–250.

Rolls, B. J., and Wood, R. J. (1979). Homeostatic control of drinking: A surviving concept. *Behav. Brain Sci.* **2**, 116–117.

Rolls, B. J., Jones, B. P., and Fallows, D. J. (1972). A comparison of the motivational properties induced by intracranial angiotensin and water deprivation. *Physiol. Behav.* **9**, 777–782.

Rolls, B. J., Wood, R. J., and Rolls, E. T. (1980a). Thirst: The initiation, maintenance, and termination of drinking. *In* "Progress in Psychobiology and Physiological Psychology," Vol. 9 (J. M. Sprague and A. N. Epstein, eds.), pp. 263–321. Academic Press, New York.

Rolls, B. J., Wood, R. J., and Stevens R. M. (1978). Effects of palatability on body fluid homeostasis. *Physiol. Behav.* **20**, 15–19.

Rolls, B. J., Wood, R., Rolls, E. T., Lind, H., Lind, R., and Ledingham, J. G. (1980b). Thirst following water deprivation in humans. *Am. J. Physiol.* **239**, R476–482.

Rolls, B. J., Phillips, P. A., Ledingham, J. G. G., Forsling, M. L., Morton, J. J., and Crowe, M. J. (1986). Human thirst: The controls of water intake in healthy men. *In* "The Physiology of Thirst and Sodium Appetite" (G. deCaro, A. N. Epstein, and M. Massi, eds.), pp. 521–526. Plenum Press, New York.

Routtenberg, A. (1967). Drinking induced by carbachol: Thirst circuit or ventricular modification? *Science* **157**, 838–839.

Routtenberg, A. (1972). Intracranial chemical injections and behavior: A critical review. *Behav. Biol.* **7**, 601–641.

Routtenberg, A., and Simpson, J. B. (1971). Carbachol induced drinking at ventricular and subfornical organ sites of application. *Life Sci.* **10**, 481–490.

Rowland, N. (1976a). Circadian rhythms and partial recovery of regulatory drinking in rats recovered from lateral hypothalamic lesions. *J. Comp. Physiol. Psychol.* **90**, 382–393.

Rowland, N. (1976b). Endogenous circadian rhythms in rats recovered from lateral hypothalamic lesions. *Physiol. Behav.* **16**, 257–266.

Rowland, N. (1976c). Regulatory drinking following lateral hypothalamic lesions: Effects of chronic NaCl and water administrations. *Exp. Neurol.* **53**, 488–507.

Rowland, N. (1977). Regulatory drinking: Do physiological substrates have an ecological niche? *Biobehav. Rev.* **1**, 261–272.

Rowland, N. (1980). Impaired drinking to angiotensin II after subdiaphragmatic vagotomy in rats. *Physiol. Behav.* **24**, 1177–1180.

Rowland, N. (1982). Comparison of the suppression by naloxone of water intake induced in rats by hyperosmolality, hypovolemia and angiotensin. *Pharmacol. Biochem. Behav.* **16**, 87–91.

Rowland, N., and Engle, D. J. (1977). Feeding and drinking interactions after acute butyrophenon administration. *Pharmacol. Biochem. Behav.* **7**, 295–301.

Rowland, N., and Flamm C. (1977). Quinine drinking: more regulatory puzzles. *Physiol. Behav.* **18**, 1165–1170.

Rowland, N., and Nicolaidis, S. (1974). Periprandial self-intravenous "drinking" in the rat. *J. Comp. Physiol. Psychol.* **87**, 16–25.

Rowland, N., and Nicolaidis, S. (1976). Metering of fluid intake and determinants of ad libitum drinking in rats. *Am. J. Physiol.* **231**, 1–8.

Rowland, N., Grossman, L., and Grossman, S. P. (1979). Zona incerta lesions: Regulatory drinking deficits to intravenous NaCl, angiotensin but not to salt in the food. *Physiol. Behav.* **23**, 745–750.

Ruger, J., and Schulkin, J. (1980). Preoperative sodium appetite experience and hypothalamic lesions in rats. *J. Comp. Physiol. Psychol.* **94**, 914–920.

Rullier, J. (1821). Soif. *In* "Dictionaire des Sciences Médicinales par une Société de Médecins et de Chirurgiens," Vol. 55, pp. 448–490. Panckoucke, Paris.

Russell, P. J. D., Abdelaal, A. E., and Mogenson, G. J. (1975). Graded levels of hemorrhage, thirst and angiotensin II in the rat. *Physiol. Behav.* **15**, 117–119.

Ruwe, W. D., Naylor, A. M., and Veale, W. L. (1985). Perfusion of vasopressin within the rat brain suppresses prostaglandin E-hyperthermia. *Brain Res.* **338**, 219–224.

Saad, W. A., Antunes-Rodrigues, J., Gentil, C. G., and Covian, M. R. (1972). Interaction between hypothalamus, amygdala and septal area in the control of sodium chloride intake. *Physiol. Behav.* **9**, 629–636.

Sakai, K. K., Marsk, B. H., George, J., and Koester, A. (1974). Specific angiotensin II receptors in the organ culture canine supraoptic nuclus cells. *Life Sci.* **14**, 1337–1344.

Sakai, R. R. (1986). The hormones of renal sodium conservation act synergistically to arouse a sodium appetite in the rat. *In* "The Physiology of Thirst and Sodium Appetite" (G. deCaro, A. N. Epstein, and M. Massi, eds.), pp. 425–430. Plenum Press, New York.

Samson, W. K. (1985). Atrial natriuretic factor inhibits dehydration and hemorrhage-induced vasopressin release. *Neuroendocrinology* **40**, 277–279.

Sanger, D. J. (1983). Opiates and ingestive behavior. *In* "Theory in Psychopharmacology," Vol. 2 (S. J. Cooper, ed.). Academic Press, London.

Saper, C. B., and Levisohn, D. (1983). Afferent connections of the median preoptic nucleus in the rat: Anatomical evidence for a cardiovascular integrative mechanism in the anteroventral third ventricular (AV3V) region. *Brain Res.* **288**, 21–31

Saper, C. B., and Loewy, A. D. (1980). Efferent connections of the parabrachial nucleus in the rat. *Brain Res.* **197**, 291–317.

Saper, C. B., Reis, D. J., and Jon, T. (1983). Medullary catecholamine inputs to the anteroventral third ventricular cardiovascular regulatory region in the rat. *Neurosci. Lett.* **42**, 285–291.

Satinoff, E., Liran, J., and Clapman, R. (1982). Aberrations of circadian body temperature rhythms in rats with medial preoptic lesions. *Am. J. Physiol.* **242**, R352-R357.

Schelling, P., Hutchinson, J. S., Sponer, G., Ganten, U., Haebara, H., and Ganten, D. (1976). Permeability of the blood-cerebrospinal fluid (CSF) barrier for angiotensin II in rats. *Naunyn-Schmiedeberg's Arch. Pharmacol.* (*Suppl. 293*) **R36** (Abstr.).

Schiff, M. (1867). "Leçons sur la Physiologie de la Digestion. Faites au Muséum d'Histoire Naturelle de Florence" Vol. I (Emile Levier, ed.), pp. 41–42. Loescher, Florence.

Schiffrin, E. L., Gutkowska, J., and Genest, G. (1981). Mechanism of captopril-induced renin release in conscious rats. *Proc. Soc. Exp. Biol. Med.* **167**, 327–332.

Schmitt, M. (1973). Influences of hepatic portal receptors on hypothalamic feeding and satiety centers. *Am. J. Physiol.* **225**, 1089–1095.

Schmidt-Nielsen, B., Schmidt-Nielsen, K., Haupt, T. R., and Jarnum, S. A. (1956). Water balance of the camel. *Am. J. Physiol.* **185**, 185–194.

Schoelkens, B. A., Jung, W., and Steinbach, R. (1976). Blood pressure response to central and peripheral injection of angiotensin II and 8-C-phenylglycine analogue of angiotensin II in rats with experimental hypertension. *Clin. Sci. Mol. Med.* **51**, 403s–406s.

Schulkin, J. (1978). Mineralocorticoids, dietary conditions, and sodium appetite. *Behav. Biol.* **23**, 197–205.

Schulkin, J. (1982). Behavior of sodium deficient rats: The search for a salty taste. *J. Comp. Physiol. Psychol.* **96**, 628–634.

Schulkin, J., and Fluharty, S. J. (1985). Further studies on salt appetite following lateral hypothalamic lesions: Effects of preoperative alimentary experience. *Behav. Neurosci.* **99**, 929–935.

Schulkin, J., Arnell, P., and Stellar, E. (1985). Running to the taste of salt in mineralocorticoid-treated rats. *Hormones Behav.* **19**, 413–425.

Schulkin, J., Marini J., and Epstein, A. N. (1989). A role for the medial region of the amygdala in mineralocorticoid induced salt hunger. *Behav. Neurosci.,* **103**, 178–185.

Schulkin, J., Eng, R., and Miselis, R. R. (1983). The effects of disconnecting the subfornical organ on behavioral and physiological responses to alterations of body sodium. *Brain Res.* **263**, 351–355.

Schulkin, J., Flynn, F. W., Grill, H. J., and Norgren, R. (1985). Central gustatory lesions: III. Effects on salt appetite and taste aversion learning. *Neurosci. Abstr.* **11**, 1259.

Schwob, J. E., and Johnson A. K. (1975). Evidence for the involvement of the renin-angiotensin system in isoproterenol dipsogenesis. *Neurosci. Abstr.* **1**, 467

Sclafani, A., Berner, C. N., and Maul, G. (1973). Feeding and drinking pathways between medial and lateral hypothalamus in the rat. *J. Comp. Physiol. Psychol.* **85**, 29–51.

Sessler, M., and Salhi, M. D. (1981). Interaction of hypertonic NaCl and neural stimuli on lateral preoptic neurons. *Neurosci. Lett.* **26**, 319–324.

Setler, P. E. (1971). Drinking induced by injection of angiotensin II into the hypothalamus of the rhesus monkey. *J. Physiol.* **217**, 59–60P.

Setler, P. E. (1973). The role of catecholamines in thirst. *In* "The Neuropsychology of

Thirst" (A. N. Epstein, H. R. Kissileff, and E. Stellar, eds.), pp. 279–290. V. H. Winston and Sons, Washington, D.C.

Setler, P. E. (1975). Noradrenergic and dopaminergic influences on thirst. *In* "Control Mechanisms of Drinking" (G. Peters, J. T. Fitzsimons, and L. Peters-Haefeli, eds.), pp.62–73. Springer Verlag, New York.

Setler, P. E. (1977). The neuroanatomy and neuropharmacology of drinking. *In* "Handbook of Psychopharmacology," Vol.8, "Drugs, Neurotransmitters and Behavior" (L. L. Iversen, S. D. Iversen, and S. H. Snyder, eds.), pp. 131–158. Plenum Press, New York.

Severs, W. B., and Daniels-Severs, A. E. (1973). Effects of angiotensin on the central nervous system. *Pharmacol. Rev.* **25**, 415–449.

Severs, W. B., Summy-Long, J., and Daniels-Severs, A. E. (1973). Effect of a converting enzyme inhibitory (SQ 20881) on angiotensin-induced drinking. *Proc. Soc. Exp. Biol. Med.* **142**, 203–204.

Severs, W. B., Summy-Long, J., and Daniels-Severs, A. E. (1974). Angiotensin interaction with thirst mechanisms. *Am. J. Physiol.* **226**, 340–344.

Severs, W. B., Changaris, D. G., Keil, L. C., Summy-Long, J. Y., Klase, P. A., and Kapsha, J. M. (1978). Pharmacology of angiotensin-induced drinking behavior. *Fed. Proc.* **13**, 2699–2703.

Severs, W. B., Daniels, A. E., Smookler, H. H., Kinnard, W. J., and Buckley, J. P. (1966). Inter-relationship between angiotensin II and the sympathetic nervous system. *J. Pharmacol. Exp. Ther.* **153**, 530–537.

Severs, W. B., Daniels-Severs, A. E., Summy-Long, J., and Radio, G. J. (1971a). Effects of centrally administered angiotensin II on salt and water excretion. *Pharmacology* **6**, 242–252.

Severs, W. B., Kapsha, J. M., Klase, P. A., and Keil, L. C. (1977). Drinking behavior in water deprived rats after angiotensin receptor blockade. *Pharmacology* **15**, 254–258.

Severs, W. B., Summy-Long, J., Daniels-Severs, A. E., and Connor, J. D. (1971b). Influence of adrenergic blocking drugs on central angiotensin effects. *Pharmacology* **5**, 205–214.

Severs, W. B., Summy-Long, J., Taylor, J. S., and Connor, J. D. (1970). A central effect of angiotensin: Release of pituitary pressor material. *J. Pharmacol. Exp. Ther.* **74**, 27–34.

Shade, R. E., and Share, L. (1975). Vasopressin release during nonhypotensive hemorrhage and angiotensin infusion. *Am. J. Physiol.* **228**, 149–154.

Shapiro, R. E., and Miselis, R. R. (1978). Confirmation of the subfornical organ projection to the supraoptic nucleus in the rat. *Anat. Rec.* **190**, 538.

Sharpe, L. G., and Swanson, L. W. (1974). Drinking induced by injections of angiotensin into forebrain and mid-brain sites of the monkey. *J. Physiol.* **239**, 595–622.

Shrager, E. E., and Johnson, A. K. (1980). Anteroventral third ventricle (AV3V) region ablation: Chronic elevations of plasma renin concentration. *Brain Res.* **190**, 554–558.

Shrager, E. E., Osborne, M. J., Johnson, A. K., and Epstein, A. N. (1975). Entry of angiotensin into cerebral ventricles and circumventricular structures. *In* "Central Action of Drugs in Blood Pressure Regulation" (D. S. Davies and J. L. Reid, eds.). University Park Press, Baltimore.

Sibole, W., Miller, J. J., and Mogenson, G. J. (1971). Effects of septal stimulation on drinking elicited by electrical stimulation of the lateral hypothalamus. *Exp. Neurol.* **32**, 466–477.

Siegel, P. S., and Stuckey, H. L. (1947). The diurnal course of water and food intake in the normal mature rat. *J. Comp. Physiol. Psychol.* **40**, 365–370.

Silverman, A. J., Hoffman, D. L., and Zimmerman, E. A. (1981). The descending afferent connections of the paraventricular nucleus of the hypothalamus (PVN). *Brain Res. Bull.* **6**, 47–61.

Simansky, K. J., and Smith, G. P. (1983). Acute abdominal vagotomy reduces drinking to peripheral but not central angiotensin II. *Peptides* **4**, 159–163.

Simpson, J. B. (1975). Subfornical organ involvement in angiotensin-induced drinking. *In* "Control Mechanisms of Drinking" (G. Peters, J. T. Fitzsimons, and L. Peters-Haefeli, eds.), pp. 123–126. Springer Verlag, New York.

Simpson, J. B., and Routtenberg, A. (1972). The subfornical organ and carbachol induced drinking. *Brain Res.* **45**, 135–152.

Simpson, J. B., and Routtenberg, A. (1973). Subfornical organ: Site of drinking elicitation by angiotensin-II. *Science* **181**, 1172–1175.

Simpson, J. B., and Routtenberg, A. (1974). Subfornical organ: Acetylcholine application elicits drinking. *Brain Res.* **79**, 157–154.

Simpson, J. B., and Routtenberg, A. (1975). Subfornical organ lesions reduce intravenous angiotensin-induced drinking. *Brain Res.* **88**,154–161.

Simpson, J. B., and Routtenberg, A. (1978). Subfornical organ: A dipsogenic site of action of angiotensin II. *Science* **201**, 379–380.

Simpson, J. B., Epstein, A. N., and Camardo, J. S. (1978a). Localization of receptors for dipsogenic action of angiotensin II in the subfornical organ of rat. *J. Comp. Physiol. Psychol.* **92**, 581–608.

Simpson, J. B., Mangiapane, M. L., and Dellmann H. D. (1978b). Central receptor sites for angiotensin-induced drinking; A critical review. *Fed. Proc.* **37**, 2676–2682.

Simpson, J. B., Reed, M., Keil, L. C., Thrasher, T. N., and Ramsay, D. J. (1979). Forebrain analysis of vasopressin secretion and water intake induced by angiotensin II. *Fed. Proc.* **38**, 2969

Simpson, J. B., Reid, I. A., Ramsay, D. J., and Kipen, H. (1978c). Mechanism of the dipsogenic action of tetradecapeptide renin substrate. *Brain Res.* **157**, 63–72.

Simpson, J. B., Saad, W. A., and Epstein, A. N. (1976). The subfornical organ, the cerebrospinal fluid and the dipsogenic action of angiotensin. *In* "Regulation of Blood Pressure by the Central Nervous System" (G. Onesti, K. E. Kim, and M. Fernandes, eds.), pp. 191–202. Grune & Stratton, New York.

Singer, G., and Kelly, J. (1972). Cholinergic and adrenergic interaction in the hypothalamic control of drinking and eating behaviour. *Physiol. Behav.* **8**, 885–890.

Sirett, N. E., McLean, A. S., Bray, J. J., and Hubbard, J. I. (1977). Distribution of angiotensin II receptors in rat brain. *Brain Res.* **122**, 299–312.

Slangen, J. L., and Miller, N. E. (1969). Pharmacological tests for the function of hypothalamic norepinephrine in eating behavior. *Physiol. Behav.* **4**, 543–552.

Smith, G. P., and Jerome, C. (1983). Effects of total and selective abdominal vagotomies on water intake in rats. *J. Auton. Nerv. Sys.* **9**, 259–271.

Smith, R. W., and McCann, S. M. (1962). Alterations in food and water intake after hypothalamic lesions in the rat. *Am. J. Physiol.* **203**, 366–370.

Smith, R. W., and McCann, S. M. (1964). Increased and decreased water intake in the rat with hypothalamic lesions. *In* "Thirst" (M. J. Wayner, ed.), pp. 382–392. Pergamon Press, New York.

Snapir, N., Robinson, B., and Godschalk, M. (1976). The drinking response of the chicken to peripheral and central administration of angiotensin II. *Pharmacol. Biochem. Behav.* **5**, 5–10.

Snyder, J. J., and Levitt, R. A. (1975). Neural activity changes correlated with central anticholinergic blockade of cholinergically-induced drinking. *Pharmacol. Biochem. Behav.* **3**, 75–79.

Snyder, S. H., Axelrod, J., and Bauter, H. (1964). The fate of C^{14}-histamine in animal tissues. *J. Pharmacol. Exp. Ther.* **144**, 373–378.

Sommer, S. R., Novin, D., and LeVine, M. (1967). Food and water intake after intrahypothalamic injections of carbachol in the rabbit. *Science* **156**, 983–984.

Sorenson, J. P., and Harvey, J. A. (1971). Decreased brain acetylcholine after septal lesions in rats: Correlation with thirst. *Physiol. Behav.* **6**, 723–725.

Spielman, W. S., and Davis, J. O. (1974). The renin-angiotensin system and aldosterone secretion during sodium depletion in the rat. *Circ. Res.* **35**, 615–624.

Spitz, R. (1974). Induction of drinking by insulin in the rat. *Eur. J. Pharmacol.* **31**, 110–114.

Spoerri, V. (1963). Uber die Gefässversorgung des Subfornikal-organs der Ratte. *Acta Anat. (Basel)* **54**, 333–348.

Steggerda, F. R. (1941). Observations on the water intake in an adult man with dysfunctioning salivary glands. *Am. J. Physiol.* **132**,517–521.

Stein, L., and Seifter, J. (1962). Muscarinic synapses in the hypothalamus. *Am. J. Physiol.* **202**, 751–756.

Stellar, E., Hyman, R., and Samet, S. (1954). Gastric factors controlling water- and salt-solution drinking. *J. Comp. Physiol. Psychol.* **47**, 220–226.

Stitt, J. T. (1986). Prostaglandin E as the neural mediator of the febrile response. *Yale J. Biol. Med.* **59**, 137–149.

Strauss, M. B. (1957). "Body Water in Man: The Acquisition and Maintenance of Body Fluids." Little & Brown, Boston.

Stricker, E. M. (1966). Extracellular fluid volume and thirst. *Am. J. Physiol.* **211**, 232–238.

Stricker, E. M. (1968). Some physiological and motivational properties of the hypovolemic stimulus for thirst. *Physiol. Behav.* **3**,379–385.

Stricker E. M. (1969). Osmoregulation and volume regulation in rats: Inhibition of hypovolemic thirst by water. *Am. J. Physiol.* **217**, 98–105.

Stricker, E. M. (1971a). Inhibition of thirst in rats following hypovolemia and/or caval ligation. *Physiol. Behav.* **6**, 293–298.

Stricker, E. M. (1971b). Effects of hypovolemia and/or caval ligation on water and NaCl solution drinking by rats. *Physiol. Behav.* **6**, 299–305.

Stricker, E. M. (1973). Thirst, sodium appetite, and complementary physiological contributions to the regulation of intravascular fluid volume. *In* "The Neuropsychology of Thirst" (A. N. Epstein, H. R. Kissileff, and E. Stellar, eds.), pp. 73–98. Wiley and Sons, New York.

Stricker, E. M. (1976). Drinking by rats after lateral hypothalamic lesions: A new look at the lateral hypothalamic syndrome. *J. Comp. Physiol. Psychol.* **90**, 127–143.

Stricker, E. M. (1977). The renin-angiotensin system and thirst: A re-evaluation. II: Drinking elicited in rats by caval ligation or isoproterenol. *J. Comp. Physiol. Psychol.* **91**, 1220–1231.

Stricker, E. M. (1978a). The renin-angiotensin system and thirst: Some unanswered questions. *Fed. Proc.* **37**, 2704–2710.

Stricker, E. M. (1978b). Excessive drinking by rats with septal lesions during hypovolemia induced by subcutaneous colloid treatment. *Physiol. Behav.* **21**, 905–907.

Stricker, E. M. (1980). The physiological basis of sodium appetite: a new look at the "depletion-repletion"model. *In* "Biological and Behavioral Aspects of Salt Intake" (M. R. Kare, M. J. Fregly, and R. A. Bernard, eds.), pp. 185–204. Academic Press, New York.

Stricker, E. M. (1981). Thirst and sodium appetite after colloid treatment in rats. *J. Comp. Physiol. Psychol.* **95**, 1–25.

Stricker, E. M. (1983). Thirst and sodium appetite after colloid treatment in rats: Role of the renin-angiotensin-aldosterone system. *Behav. Neurosci.* **97**, 725–737.

Stricker, E. M. (1984). Thirst and sodium appetite after colloid treatment in rats with septal lesions. *J. Comp. Physiol. Psychol.* **98**, 356–360.

Stricker, E. M., Bradshaw, W. G., and McDonald, R. H, Jr. (1976). The renin-angiotensin system and thirst: A reevaluation. *Science* **194**, 1169–1171.

Stricker, E. M., and Jalowiec, J. E. (1970). Restoration of intravascular fluid volume following acute hypovolemia in rats. *Am. J. Physiol.* **218**, 191–196.

Stricker, E. M., and MacArthur, J. P. (1974). Physiological bases for different effects of extravascular colloid treatments on water and NaCl solution drinking by rats. *Physiol. Behav.* **13**, 389–394.

Stricker, E. M., and Verbalis, J. G. (1986). Interaction of osmotic and volume stimuli in regulation of neurohypophyseal secretion in rats. *Am. J. Physiol.* **250**, R267–275.

Stricker, E. M., and Verbalis, J. G. (1987). Central inhibitory control of sodium appetite in rats: Correlation with pituitary oxytocin secretion. *J. Comp. Physiol. Psychol.* **101**, 560–567.

Stricker, E. M., and Wolf, G. (1966). Blood volume and tonicity in relation to sodium appetite. *J. Comp. Physiol. Psychol.* **62**, 275–279.

Stricker, E. M., and Wolf, G. (1967). The effect of hypovolemia in rats with lateral hypothalamic damage. *Proc. Soc. Exp. Biol. Med.* **124**, 816–820.

Stricker, E. M., and Zigmond, M. J. (1974). Effects on homeostasis of intraventricular injections of 6-hydroxydopamine in rats. *J. Comp. Physiol. Psychol.* **86**, 973–994.

Stricker, E. M., and Zigmond, M. J. (1975). Brain catecholamines and thirst. *In* "Control Mechanisms of Drinking" (G. Peters, J. T. Fitzsimons, and L. Peters-Haefeli, eds.), pp. 55–61. Springer Verlag, New York.

Stricker, E. M., and Zigmond, M. J. (1976). Recovery of function following damage to central catecholamine-containing neurons: A neuro-chemical model for the lateral hypothalamic syndrome. *In* "Progress in Psychobiology and Physiological Psychology," Vol. 6 (J. M. Sprague and A. N. Epstein, eds.), pp. 121–188. Academic Press, New York.

Stricker, E. M., Swerdloff, A. F., and Zigmond, M. J. (1978). Intrahypothalamic injections of kainic acid produce feeding and drinking deficits in rats. *Brain Res.* **158**, 470–473.

Stricker, E. M., Vagnucci, A. H., and McDonald, R. H., Jr. (1979). Renin and aldosterone secretions during hypovolemia in rats: Relation to NaCl intake. *Am. J. Physiol.* **237**, R45–51.

Strominger, J. L. (1947). The relation between water intake and food intake in normal rats, and in rats with hypothalamic hyperphagia. *Yale J. Biol. Med.* **9**, 279–188.

Sturgeon, R. D., Brophy, P. D., and Levitt, R. A. (1973). Drinking elicited by intracranial microinjection of angiotensin in the cat. *Pharmacol. Biochem. Behav.* **1**, 353–355.

Summy-Long, J., and Severs, W. B. (1974). Angiotensin and thirst: Studies with a converting enzyme inhibitor and a receptor antagonist. *Life Sci.* **15**, 569–582.

Swanson, L. W., and Sharpe, L. G. (1973). Centrally induced drinking: Comparison of angiotensin II- and carbachol-sensitive sites in rats. *Am. J. Physiol.* **225**, 566–573.

Swanson, L. W., Kucharczyk, J., and Mogenson, G. J. (1978). Autoradiographic evidence for pathways from the medial preoptic area to the midbrain involved in the drinking response to angiotensin II. *J. Comp. Neurol.* **178**, 645–660.

Swanson, L. W., Sharpe, L. G., and Griffin, D. (1973a). Drinking to intracerebral angiotensin II and carbachol: Dose-response relationships and ionic involvement. *Physiol. Behav.* **10**, 595–600.

Swanson, L. W., Marshall, G. R., Needleman, P. A., and Sharpe, L. G. (1973b). Characterization of central angiotensin II receptors involved in the elicitation of drinking in the rat. *Brain Res.* **49**, 441–446.

Swanson, P. P., Timson, G. H., and Frazier, E. (1935). Some observations of the physiological adjustment of the albino rat to a diet poor in salts when edestin is the source of dietary protein. *J. Biol. Chem.* **109**, 729–737.

Sweet, C. S., Columbo, J. M., Gaul, S. L., Weitz, D., and Wenger, H. C. (1977). Inhibitors of the renin-angiotensin system in rats with malignant and spontaneous hypertension: Comparative antihypertensive effects of central vs. peripheral administration. *In* "Central Action of Angiotensin and Related Hormones" (J. P. Buckley and C. S. Ferrario, eds.), pp. 283–292. Pergamon Press, New York.

Szczepanska-Sadowska, E. (1973). Plasma ADH level and body water balance in dogs after moderate haemorrhage. *Bull. Acad. Pol. Sci.* **21**, 89–90.

Szczepanska-Sadowska, E., and Fitzsimons, J. T. (1975). The effects of angiotensin II, renin and isoprenaline on drinking in the dog. *In* "Control Mechanisms of Drinking" (G. Peters, J. T. Fitzsimons, and L. Peters-Haefeli, eds.), pp. 69–73. Springer Verlag, New York.

Szczepanska-Sadowska, E., Sobocinska, J., and Sadoswki, B. (1982). Central dipsogenic effect of vasopressin. *Am. J. Physiol.* **242**, R372–379.

Szczepanska-Sadowska, E., Gray, D., and Simon-Opperman, C. (1983). Vasopressin in blood and third ventricle CSF during dehydration, thirst and hemorrhage. *Am. J. Physiol.* **245**, R549–555.

Szczepanska-Sadowska, E., Simon-Opperman, C., Gray, D., and Simon, E. (1984). Plasma and cerebrospinal fluid vasopressin and osmolality in relation to thirst. *Pflügers Arch. Gesammte Physiol.* **400**, 294–299.

Szczepanska-Sadowska, E., Sobocinska, J., and Kozlowski, S. (1986). Osmotic thirst suppression after central administration of vasopressin antagonists. *In* "The Physiology of Thirst and Sodium Appetite" (G. deCaro, A. N. Epstein, and M. Massi, eds.), pp. 97–102. Plenum Press, New York.

Takayanagi, R., Tanaka, I., Maki, M., and Inagami, T. (1985). Effects of changes in water-sodium balance on levels of atrial natriuretic factor messenger RNA and peptide in rats. *Life Sci.* **36**, 1843–1848.

Takei, Y. (1977). Angiotensin and water intake in the Japanese quail (*Coturnix coturnix japonica*). *Gen. Comp. Endocrinol.* **31**, 364–372.

Tang, M. (1976). Dependence of polyethylene-glycol-induced dipsogenesis on intravascular fluid depletion. *Physiol. Behav.* **17**, 811–816.

Tang, M., and Falk, J. L. (1974). Sar-Ala angiotensin II blocks renin-angiotensin but not beta-adrenergic dipsogens. *Pharmacol. Biochem. Behav.* **2**, 401–408.

Tang, M., and Falk, J. L. (1979). Temporary peritoneal sequestration of NaCl and persistent NaCl appetite. *Physiol. Behav.* **22**, 595–597.

Teicher, M. H., and Blass, E. M. (1976). Lateral preoptic lesions in rats separate urge to drink from amount of water drunk. *Science* **191**, 1187–1189.

Teitelbaum, P. (1973). On the use of electrical stimulation to study hypothalamic structure and function (Discussion). *In* "The Neuropsychology of Thirst" (A. N. Epstein, H. R. Kissileff, and E. Stellar, eds.), pp. 143–154. John Wiley and Sons, New York.

Teitelbaum, P., and Epstein, A. N. (1962). The lateral hypothalamic syndrome: Recovery of feeding and drinking after lateral hypothalamic lesions. *Psychol. Rev.* **69**, 74–90.

Teitelbaum, P., and Stellar, E. (1954). Recovery from the failure to eat produced by hypothalamic lesions. *Science* **120**, 894–895.

Teitelbaum, P., and Wolgin, D. L. (1975). Neurotransmitters and the regulation of food intake. *Prog. Brain Res.* **42**, 235–249.

Teitelbaum, P., Schallert, T., and Wishaw, I. Q. (1983). Sources of spontaneity in motivated behavior. *In* "Handbook of Behavioral Neurobiology," Vol. 6, "Motivation" (E. Satinoff and P. Teitelbaum, eds.), pp. 23–66. Plenum Press, New York.

Teitelbaum, P., Schallert, T., deRyck, M., Wishaw, I. Q., and Golani, I. (1980). Motor subsystems in motivated behavior. *In* "Neural Mechanisms of Goal-Directed Behavior" (R. F. Thompson, L. H. Hicks, and V. B. Shvyrkov, eds.), pp. 127–144. Academic Press, New York.

Thornton, S. N. (1984). Drinking and renal responses to peripherally administered osmotic stimuli in the pigeon (*Columbia livia*). *J. Physiol.* **351**, 501–515.

Thornton, S. N., Jeulin, A. C., de Beaurepaire, R., and Nicolaidis, S. (1985). Iontophoretic application of angiotensin II, vasopressin and oxytocin in the region of the anterior hypothalamus in the rat. *Brain Res. Bull.* **14**, 211–215.

Thrasher, T. N., and Ramsay, D. J. (1986). The organum vasculosum laminae terminalis. *In* "The Physiology of Thirst and Sodium Appetite" (G. deCaro, A. N. Epstein, and M. Massi, eds.), pp. 327–332. Plenum Press, New York.

Thrasher, T. N., Keil, L. C., and Ramsay D. J. (1982c). Hemodynamic, hormonal and drinking responses to reduced venous return in the dog. *Am. J. Physiol.* **243**, R354–362.

Thrasher, T. N., Keil, L. C., and Ramsay, D. J. (1982b). Lesions of the organum vasculosum of the lamina terminalis (OVLT) attenuate osmotically-induced drinking and vasopressin secretion in the dog. *Endocrinology* **110**, 1837–1839.

Thrasher, T. N., Simpson, J. B., and Ramsay, D. J. (1982a). Lesions of the subformical organ block angiotensin-induced drinking in the dog. *Neuroendocrinology* **35**, 68–72.

Thrasher, T. N., Brown, C. J., Keil, L. C., and Ramsay, D. J. (1980a). Thirst and vasopressin release in the dog: An osmoreceptor or sodium receptor mechanism? *Am. J. Physiol.* **238**, R333–339.

Thrasher, T. N., Jones, R. G., Keil, L. C., Brown, C. J., and Ramsay, D. J. (1980b).

Drinking and vasopressin release during ventricular infusions of hypertonic solutions. *Am. J. Physiol.* **238**, R340–345.

Thrasher, T. N., Moore-Gillon, M., Wade, C. E., Keil, L. C., and Ramsay, D. J. (1983). Inappropriate drinking and secretion of vasopressin after caval constriction in dogs. *Am. J. Physiol.* **244**, R850–856.

Tondat, L. M., and Almli, C. R. (1975). Hyperdipsia produced by severing ventral septal fiber systems. *Physiol. Behav.* **15**, 701–706.

Tordoff, M. G., and Novin, D. (1982). Coeliac vagotomy attenuates the ingestive responses to epinephrine and hypertonic saline but not insulin, 2-deoxy-D-glucose or polyethylene glycol. *Physiol. Behav.* **29**, 605–613.

Tordoff, M. G., Schulkin, J., and Friedman, M. I. (1986). Hepatic contribution to satiation of salt appetite in rats. *Am. J. Physiol.* **251**, R1095-R1102.

Tordoff, M. G., Schulkin, J., and Friedman, M. I. (1987).Further evidence for hepatic control of salt intake in rats. *Am. J. Physiol.* **253,** R444–449.

Towbin, E. J. (1949). Gastric distention as a factor in the satiation of thirst in esophagostomized dogs. *Am. J. Physiol.* **159**, 533–541.

Towbin, E. J. (1955). Thirst and hunger behavior in dogs and the effects of vagotomy and sympathectomy. *Am. J. Physiol.* **182**, 377–382.

Tripodo, N. C., McCaa, R. E., and Guyton, A. C. (1976). Effect of prolonged angiotensin II infusion on thirst. *Am. J. Physiol.* **230**, 1063–1066.

Türker, R. K. (1986). A general review of the effects of angiotensin-peptides and 8-substituted analogs of angiotensin II. *In* "The Physiology of Thirst and Sodium Appetite" (G. deCaro, A. N. Epstein, and M. Massi, eds.), pp. 205–212. Plenum Press, New York.

Ueda, H., Katayama, S., and Kato, R. (1972). Area postrema angiotensin sensitive site in brain. *Adv. Exp. Biol. Med.* **17**, 109–116.

Unger, T., Ganten, D., Ludvig, G., and Lang, R. E. (1986). The brain-renin-angiotensin system: Update. *In* "The Physiology of Thirst and Sodium Appetite" (G. deCaro, A. N. Epstein, and M. Massi, eds.), pp. 123–133. Plenum Press, New York.

Ungerstedt, U. (1971). Adipsia and aphagia after 6-hydroxydopamine induced degeneration of the nigro-striatal dopamine system. *Acta Physiol. Scand. (Suppl.)* **367**, 95–122.

Urano, A., and Kobayashi, H. (1978). Effects of noradrenaline and dopamine injected into the supraoptic nucleus on urine flow rate in hydrated rats. *Exp. Neurol.* **60**, 140–150.

Valenstein, E. S. (1969). Behavior elicited by hypothalamic stimulation: A prepotency hypothesis. *Brain, Behav. Evolut.* **2**, 295–316.

Valenstein, E. S. (1970). Stability and plasticity of motivational systems. *In* "The Neurosciences: Second Study Program" (F. O. Schmitt, ed.), pp. 207–217. Rockefeller University Press, New York.

Valenstein, E. S. (1973). Invited comment: Electrical stimulation and hypothalamic function: historical perspective. *In* "The Neuropsychology of Thirst" (A. N. Epstein, H. R. Kissileff, and E. Stellar, eds.), pp. 155–161. John Wiley and Sons, New York.

Valenstein, E. S. (1976). The interpretation of behavior evoked by brain stimulation. *In* "Brain Stimulation Reward" (A. Wauquier and E. T. Rolls, eds.), pp. 65–88. North Holland, Amsterdam.

Valenstein, E. S., Cox, V. C., and Kakolewski, J. W. (1968). Modification of motivated behavior by electrical stimulation of the hypothalamus. *Science* **159**, 1119–1121.

Vance, W. B. (1970). The effects of vagotomy on the water intake of the white rat. *Psychon. Sci.* **20**, 21–22.

Van Houten, M., Posner, B. I., Kopriwa, B. M., and Brawer, J. R. (1979). Insulin-binding sites in the rat brain: In vivo localization to the circumventricular organs by quantitative radioautography. *Endocrinology* **105**, 666–673.

Van Houten, M., Schiffrin, E. L., Mann, J. E. F., Posner, B. I., and Boucher, R. (1980). Radioautographic localization of specific binding sites for blood-borne angiotensin II in the rat brain. *Brain Res.* **186**, 480–485.

Vaughn, E. D., Jr., Gavras, H., Laragh, J. H., and Koss, M. N. (1973). Vascular permeability factor: Dissociation from the angiotensin II induced pressor and drinking responses. *Nature* **242**, 334–335.

Veress, A. T., and Sonnenberg, H. (1984). Right atrial appendectomy reduces the renal response to acute hypervolemia in the rat. *Am. J. Physiol.* **247**, R610–613.

Verney, E. B. (1947). The antidiuretic hormone and factors which determine its release. *Proc. R. Soc. Lond. Ser. B* **13**, 25–106.

Vijande, M., Costales, M., and Fitzsimons, J. T. (1986). Increased sodium appetite and polydipsia in Goldblatt hypertension. *In* "The Physiology of Thirst and Sodium Appetite" (G. deCaro, A. N. Epstein, and M. Massi, eds.), pp. 413–418. Plenum Press, New York.

Vincent, J. D., Poulain, D. A., and Nicolescu-Catargi, A. (1972). Activity of osmosensitive single cells in the hypothalamus of the behaving monkey during drinking. *Brain Res.* **44**, 371–384.

Volicer, L., and Loew, C. (1971). Penetration of angiotensin II into the brain. *Neuropharmacology* **10**, 631–636.

Von Euler, U. S. A. (1953). A preliminary note on slow hypothalamic "osmo-potentials". *Acta Physiol. Scand.* **29**, 133–136.

Wada, M., Kobayashi, H., and Farner, D. S. (1975). Induction of drinking in the white-crowned sparrow, *Zonotrichia leucophrys gambelii*, by intracranial injections of angiotensin II. *Gen. Comp. Endocrinol.* **26**, 192–197.

Waldbillig, R. J., and Bartness, T. J. (1981). Insulin-induced drinking: An analysis of hydrational variables. *Physiol. Behav.* **26**, 787–793.

Walsh, L. L., and Grossman, S. P. (1973). Zona incerta lesions: Disruption of regulatory water intake. *Physiol. Behav.* **11**, 885–887.

Walsh, L. L., and Grossman, S. P. (1975). Loss of feeding to 2-deoxy-D-glucose but not insulin after zona incerta lesions in the rat. *Physiol. Behav.* **15**, 481–486.

Walsh L. L., and Grossman S. P. (1976). Zona incerta lesions impair osmotic but not hypovolemic thirst. *Physiol. Behav.* **16**, 211–215.

Walsh, L. L., and Grossman, S. P. (1977). Electrolytic lesions and knife cuts in the region of the zona incerta impair sodium appetite. *Physiol. Behav.* **18**, 587–596.

Walsh, L. L., and Grossman, S. P. (1978). Dissociation of responses to extracellular thirst stimuli following zona incerta lesions. *Pharmacol. Biochem. Behav.* **8**, 409–416.

Walsh, L. L., Halaris, A. E., Grossman, L., and Grossman, S. P. (1977). Some biochemical effects of zona incerta lesions that interfere with the regulation of water intake. *Pharmacol. Biochem. Behav.* **7**, 351–356.

Wayner, M. J. (1970). Motor control functions of the lateral hypothalamus and adjunctive behavior. *Physiol. Behav.* **5**, 1319–1325.

Wayner, M. J., Kantak, K. M., Barone, F. C., DeHaven, D. L., Wayner, M. J. III, and Cook, R. C. (1981). Effects of LH kainic acid infusions on ingestion and autonomic activity. *Physiol. Behav.* **27**, 369–376.

Weindl., A. (1973). Neuroendocrine aspects of circumventricular organs. *In* "Frontiers of Neuroendocrinology" (W. F. Ganong and L. Martini, eds.), pp. 3–32. Oxford University Press, New York.

Weisinger, R. S., Considine, P., Denton, D. A., Leksell, L., McKinley, M. J., Mouw, D. R., Muller, A. F., and Tarjan, E. (1982). Role of sodium concentration of the cerebrospinal fluid in the salt appetite of the sheep. *Am. J. Physiol.* **242**, R51-R63.

Weisinger, R. S., Considine, P., Denton, D. A., McKinley, M. J., and Mouw, D. (1979). Rapid effect of change in cerebrospinal fluid sodium concentration on salt appetite. *Nature* **280**, 490–491.

Weisinger, R. S., Denton, D. A., McKinley, M. J., Muller, A. F., and Mouw, D. (1985). Cerebrospinal fluid [Na] and salt appetite. *Brain Res.* **326**, 95–105.

Weiss, C. S., and Almli, C. R. (1975a). Polyethylene glycol induced thirst: A dual stimulatory mechanism? *Physiol. Behav.* **14**, 477–482.

Weiss, C. S., and Almli, C. R. (1975b). Lateral preoptic and lateral hypothalamic units: In search of the osmoreceptors for thirst. *Physiol. Behav.* **15**, 713–722.

Weiss, M. L. (1986). Sodium appetite induced by sodium depletion is suppressed by intracerebroventricular captopril. *In* "The Physiology of Thirst and Sodium Appetite" (G. deCaro, A. N. Epstein, and M. Massi, eds.), pp. 405–411. Plenum Press, New York.

Wettendorff, H. (1901). Modifications du sang sous l'influence de la privation d'eau: Contribution à l'étude de la soif. *Trav. Lab. Physiol. Inst. Solvay* **4**, 353–384.

White, S. D., Wayner, M. J., and Cott, A. (1970). Effects of intensity, water deprivation, prior water ingestion and palatability on drinking evoked by lateral hypothalamic electrical stimulation. *Physiol. Behav.* **5**, 611–619.

Williams, D. R., and Teitelbaum, P. (1959). Some observations on the starvation resulting from lateral hypothalamic lesions. *J. Comp. Physiol. Psychol.* **52**, 458–465.

Williams, J. W., Rudy, T. A., Yaksh, T. L., and Viswanathan, C. T. (1977). An extensive exploration of the rat brain for sites mediating prostaglandin-induced hyperthermia. *Brain Res.* **120**, 251–262.

Winquist, R. J. (1986). Possible mechanisms underlying the vasorelaxant response to atrial natriuretic factor. *Fed. Proc.* **45**, 2371–2375.

Winson, J., and Miller, N. E. (1970). Comparison of drinking elicited by eserine or DFP injected into preoptic area of rat brain. *J. Comp. Physiol. Psychol.* **73**, 233–237.

Wirsig, C. R., and Grill, H. J. (1982). Contribution of the rat's neocortex to ingestive control: Latent learning for the taste of sodium chloride. *J. Comp. Physiol. Psychol.* **96**, 615–627.

Wise, R. A. (1968). Hypothalamic motivational systems: Fixed or plastic neural circuits? *Science* **162**, 377–379.

Wise, R. A. (1969). Plasticity of hypothalamic motivational systems. *Science* **165**, 929–930.

Witt, D. M., Keller, A. D., Batsel, H. L., and Lynch, J. R. (1952). Absence of thirst and resultant syndrome associated with anterior hypothalamectomy in the dog. *Am. J. Physiol.* **171**, 780 (Abstr.).

Wishart, T. B., and Mogenson, G. J. (1970). Effects of food deprivation on water intake in rats with septal lesions. *Physiol. Behav.* **5**, 1481–1486.

Wolf, A.V. (1950). Osmometric analysis of thirst in man and dog. *Am. J. Physiol.* **161**, 75–86.

Wolf, A. V. (1958). "Thirst: Physiology of the Urge to Drink and Problems of Water Lack." Charles C. Thomas, Springfield, Ill.

Wolf, G. (1964). Effects of dorsolateral hypothalamic lesions on sodium appetite elicited by DOC and acute hyponatremia. *J. Comp. Physiol. Psychol.* **58**, 396–402.

Wolf, G. (1965). Effect of deoxycorticosterone on sodium appetite of intact and adrenalectomized rats. *Am. J. Physiol.* **208**, 1281–1285.

Wolf, G. (1967). Hypothalamic regulation of sodium intake: Relations to preoptic and tegmental functions. *Am. J. Physiol.* **213**, 1433–1438.

Wolf, G. (1968). Thalamic and tegmental mechanisms for sodium intake: Anatomical and function relations to the lateral hypothalamus *Physiol. Behav.* **3**, 997–1002.

Wolf, G. (1969). Innate mechanisms for regulation of sodium appetite. *In* "Olfaction and Taste (Proceedings of the Third International Symposium)" (C. Pfaffman, ed.), pp. 548–553. Rockefeller University Press, New York.

Wolf, G. (1971). Neural mechanisms for sodium appetite: Hypothalamus positive- hypothalamofugal pathways negative. *Physiol. Behav.* **6**, 381–389.

Wolf, G., and DiCara, L. A. (1971). A third ascending hypothalamic pathway. *J. Exp. Neurol.* **33**, 69–77.

Wolf, G., and Handal, P. J. (1966). Aldosterone-induced sodium appetite: Dose response and specificity. *Endocrinology* **78**, 1120–1124.

Wolf, G., and Miller, N. E. (1964). Lateral hypothalamic lesions: Effects on drinking elicited by carbachol in preoptic area and posterior hypothalamus. *Science* **43**, 585–587.

Wolf, G., and Quartermain, D. (1966). Sodium chloride intake of desoxycorticosterone treated and of sodium deficient rats as a function of saline concentration. *J. Comp. Physiol. Psychol.* **2**, 288–291.

Wolf, G,. and Quartermain, D. (1967). Sodium chloride intake of adrenalectomized rats with lateral hypothalamic lesions. *Am. J. Physiol.* **212**, 113–118.

Wolf, G., and Schulkin, J. (1980). Brain lesions and sodium appetite:an approach to the neurological analysis of homeostatic behavior. *In* "Biological and Behavioral Aspects of Salt Intake" (M. R. Kare, M. J. Fregly, and R. A. Bernard, eds.), pp. 331–339. Academic Press, New York.

Wolf, G., DiCara, L. V., and Braun, J. J. (1970). Sodium appetite in rats after neocortical ablation. *Physiol. Behav.* **5**, 1265–1269.

Wolf, G., Schulkin, J., and Fluharty, S. J. (1983). Recovery of salt appetite after lateral hypothalamic lesions: Effects of preoperative salt drive and salt intake experiences. *J. Comp. Physiol. Psychol.* **97**, 506–511.

Wolf, G., Schulkin, J., and Simon, P. E. (1984).Multiple factors in the satiation of salt appetite. *Behav. Neurosci.* **98**, 661–673.

Wolgin, D. L., Cytawa, J., and Teitelbaum, P. (1976). The role of activation in the regulation of food intake. *In* "Hunger, Basic Mechanisms and Clinical Implications" (D. Novin, W. Wyrwicka, and G. Bray, eds.), pp. 179–192. Raven Press, New York.

Wolny, H. L., Plech, A., and Herman, Z. S. (1974). Diuretic effects of intraventricularly injected noradrenaline and dopamine in rats. *Experientia* **30**, 1062–1063.

Wood, R. J., Rolls, B. J., and Ramsay, D. J. (1977). Drinking following intracarotid infusions of hypertonic solutions in dogs. *Am. J. Physiol.* **232**, 88–92.

Wood, R. J., Maddison, S., Rolls, E. T., Rolls, B. J., and Gibbs, J. (1980). Drinking in the rhesus monkey: Roles of pre-systemic and systemic factors in drinking control. *J. Comp. Physiol. Psychol.* **94**, 1135–1148.

Wood, R. J., Rolls, E. T., and Rolls, B. J. (1982). Physiological mechanisms for thirst in the non-human primate. *Am. J. Physiol.* **242**, 423.

Wright, J. W., Morseth, S. L., and LaCrosse, E. (1984). Angiotensin III-induced dipsogenic and pressor responses in rodents. *Behav. Neurosci.* **98**, 640–651.

Wright, J. W., Morseth, S. L., and Fairley, P. C. (1987).Angiotensin's contribution to dipsogenic additivity in several rodent species. *J. Comp. Physiol. Psychol.* **101**, 361–370.

Zambioni, P., and Siro-Brigiani, G. (1966). Effeto delle catecholamine sulla sete e la diuresi nel ratto. *Boll. Soc. Ital. Biol. Sper.* **42**, 1657–1659.

Zhang, D. M., Stellar, E., and Epstein, A. N. (1984). Together intracranial angiotensin and systemic mineralocorticoid produce avidity for salt in the rat. *Physiol. Behav.* **32**, 677–681.

Zigmond, M. J., and Stricker, E. M. (1973). Recovery of feeding and drinking by rats after intraventricular 6-hydroxydopamine or lateral hypothalamic lesions. *Science* **182**, 717–720.

Zimmer, L. J., Meliza, L., and Hsiao, S. (1976). Effects of cervical and subdiaphragmatic vagotomy on osmotic and volemic thirst. *Physiol. Behav.* **16**, 665–670.

Zolovick, A. J., Avrith, D., and Jalowiec, J. E. (1977). Reversible colchicine-induced disruption of amygdaloid functions in sodium appetite. *Brain Res. Bull.* **5**, 35–39.

Zotterman, Y. (1956). Species differences in the water taste. *Acta Physiol. Scand.* **37**, 60–70.

Index